EXCELLENCE IN PRACTICE Series
Katharine G. Butler, Editor

Perspectives in Applied Phonology

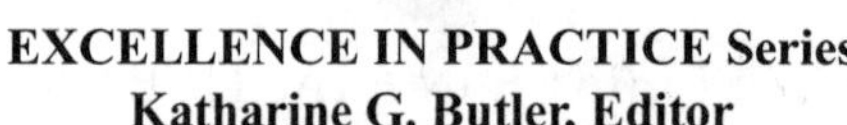

EXCELLENCE IN PRACTICE Series
Katharine G. Butler, Editor

Conversational Management with Language-Impaired Children
Bonnie Brinton and Martin Fujuki

Successful Interactive Skills for Speech-Language Pathologists and Audiologists
Dorothy Molyneaux and Vera W. Lane

Communicating for Learning: Classroom Observation and Collaboration
Elaine R. Silliman and Louise Cherry Wilkinson

Hispanic Children and Adults with Communication Disorders: Assessment and Prevention
Henriette W. Langdon with Li-Rong Lilly Cheng

Family-Centered Early Intervention for Communication Disorders: Prevention and Treatment
Gail Donahue-Kilburg

Building Early Intervention Teams: Working Together for Children and Families
Margaret H. Briggs

Speech, Language, and Hearing Programs in Schools: A Guide for Students and Practitioners
Pamelia O'Connell

Dysphagia: A Continuum of Care
Barbara C. Sonies

Perspectives in Applied Phonology
Barbara Williams Hodson and Mary Louise Edwards

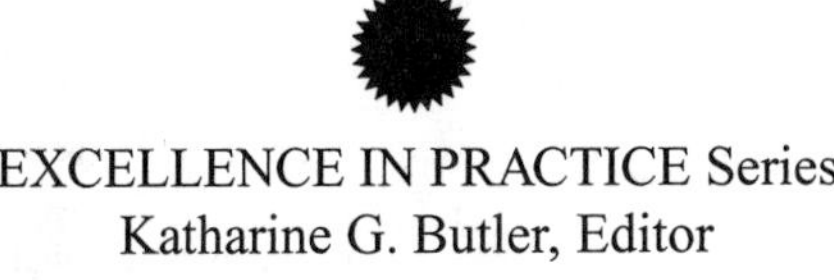

EXCELLENCE IN PRACTICE Series
Katharine G. Butler, Editor

Perspectives in Applied Phonology

Barbara Williams Hodson, PhD, CCC-SLP
Professor
Communication Disorders and Sciences
Wichita State University
Wichita, Kansas

Mary Louise Edwards, PhD
Professor and Chair
Communication Sciences and Disorders
Syracuse University
Syracuse, New York

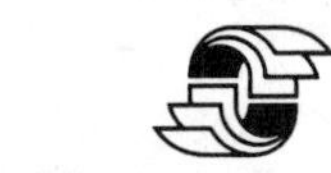

AN ASPEN PUBLICATION®
Aspen Publishers, Inc.
Gaithersburg, Maryland
1997

Library of Congress Cataloging-in-Publication Data

Hodson, Barbara Williams
Perspectives in applied phonology/
Barbara Williams Hodson, Mary Louise Edwards.
p. cm. — (Excellence in practice series)
Includes bibliographical references and index.
ISBN 0-8342-0881-4
1. Articulation disorders. 2. Phonetics.
I. Edwards, Mary Louise. II. Title. III. Series.
RC424.7.H63 1997
616.85'5—dc20
96-43784
CIP

Orders: (800) 638-8437
Customer Service: (800) 234-1660

Editorial Resources: Jane Colilla
Library of Congress Catalog Card Number: 96-43784
ISBN: 0-8342-0881-4

Printed in the United States of America

1 2 3 4 5

Table of Contents

Contributors ix
Forewords xi
Preface xv

Chapter 1—Historical Overview of Clinical Phonology 1
Mary Louise Edwards

A Personal Perspective 1
A Brief History of Clinical Phonology 3
Special Clinical Applications 11
Conclusion 14

Chapter 2—The Categorization of Phonological Impairment 19
David Ingram

A Selective Historical Perspective 20
Current Research on Phonological Impairment 26
The Classification of Phonological Impairment 33
Conclusion 38

Chapter 3—From Articulation to Phonology: The Challenge of Change . . 43
Mary Elbert

A Quick Overview 44
An Experimental (Sentimental) Journey across Three Decades 44
Enduring Concepts 54
Conclusion 55

Chapter 4—Developmental Phonological Disability: Order in Disorder . . 61
Pamela Grunwell

Theoretical Perspectives 62
Clinical Applications 67

Conclusion 81
Appendix 4–A 85
Appendix 4–B. 87
Appendix 4–C. 89
Appendix 4–D 91
Appendix 4–E. 93
Appendix 4–F. 95
Appendix 4–G 97
Appendix 4–H 98
Appendix 4–I 100
Appendix 4–J 102

Chapter 5—Developmental Phonological Disorders: One or Many? 105
Lawrence D. Shriberg

Theoretical Perspectives. 106
Assessment of Childhood Speech Disorders 119
Treatment of Childhood Speech Disorders 126
The Capability-Focus Framework 126
Conclusion 127

Chapter 6—Child Phonology and Infant Vocalizations: Theory and Methodology 133
D. Kimbrough Oller

How Modern Research in Child Phonology Began. 133
A Historical Perspective on How Scientific Progress Can Be Limited by Theory 136
In Search of New Frameworks, or at Least New Protections 141
Suggestions about Methodological Protections in Child Phonology ... 142
Suggestions about Theoretical Growth 148
Conclusion 153

Chapter 7—Phonological Awareness: Connecting Speech and Literacy Problems 157
Joy Stackhouse

What Is Phonological Awareness? 158
The Relationship between Phonological Awareness and Literacy Development. 159
A Stage Model of Literacy Development 162

Why Might Children Fail To Develop Phonological Awareness Skills? 164
Phonological Processing Problems in Children with Reading Impairments 165
Literacy Development in Children with Phonological Impairments 167
Children with Arrested Speech and Literacy Development 170
A Stage Model of Speech Development 176
Zoe: A Longitudinal Case Study of Phonological Awareness Development 179
Conclusion 188
Future Directions 190

Chapter 8—Disordered Phonologies: What Have We Learned about Assessment and Treatment? 197
Barbara Williams Hodson

Clinical Phonology: The Early Years 197
Developments in Evaluation of Children's Phonologies 198
Treatment Practices in the 1990s 202
Cycles Phonological Remediation Approach 206
Client Examples 211
Clinical Phonology: The Next 25 Years 218

Appendix A—Glossary 225
Index 233
About the Contributors 253

Contributors

Mary Louise Edwards, PhD
Professor and Chair
Communication Sciences and Disorders
Syracuse University
Syracuse, New York

Mary Elbert, PhD, CCC-SLP
Professor
Department of Speech and Hearing Sciences
Indiana University
Bloomington, Indiana

Pamela Grunwell, PhD
Head of Department
Department of Human Communication
DeMontfort University
Leicester, United Kingdom

Barbara Williams Hodson, PhD, CCC-SLP
Professor
Communication Disorders and Sciences
Wichita State University
Wichita, Kansas

David Ingram, PhD
Professor
Department of Linguistics
University of British Columbia
Vancouver, British Columbia

D. Kimbrough Oller, PhD
Professor
Psychology and Pediatrics
University of Miami
Miami, Florida

Lawrence D. Shriberg, PhD, CCC-SLP
Professor
Department of Communicative Disorders
University of Wisconsin—Madison
Madison, Wisconsin

Joy Stackhouse, PhD
Senior Lecturer
Department of Human Communication Science
University College London
London, United Kingdom

Forewords

The idea for this book arose in discussion with Dr. Barbara Hodson during the preparation of another manuscript. Dr. Hodson noted that clinical phonology is a young discipline, springing from phonology and from phonologists who became interested in the atypical aspects of phonological acquisition. Their assessment and intervention primarily was in children who were being served in speech and hearing clinics of the 1960s. Also during the 1960s, a panel of linguistists addressed a general session of the American Speech-Language-Hearing Association (ASHA). This panel brought to ASHA information related to the linguistic analyses conducted by specialists in linguistics who had become fascinated with the speech production of adult aphasic clients. Following an exciting and challenging few hours of presentations, a question and answer period brought forth the following question from a graduate student in speech correction: "Well, sirs, it was most enlightening to hear about the brain-behavior characteristics of expressive aphasics. Could you follow up by providing some insights regarding aphasia treatment?" The answer was: "That is neither our discipline nor our purview."

Looking back from the 1960s through to the 1990s, programs in human communication sciences and disorders have done much to draw into their ranks linguists whose primary research interests may be best served by their presence in speech-language-hearing clinics where preschoolers with atypical phonology may be found. Intensive research efforts have been underway for the past three decades, and the authors chosen here to represent clinical phonology have played a central role in its formation, its growth, and its knowledge base. They are among the founders of the discipline, the researcher-clinicians who have reached across the chasm between linguists speech-language pathologists.

Those who have been trained solely in the tradition of normal and disordered articulation processes will encounter a fascinating walk through time, and into the future, as the authors draw upon their own history, experiences, and insights while they construct a carefully drawn path that leads both the naive and the expert to the cutting edge of research. They sketch a cohesive picture of phonological development and disorders from infancy to literacy, each author contributing his or her frame of reference and reflections on the theoretical and the practical. The various points of view demonstrate the agreements and the disagreements to be found in clinical phonology. The discussion of research methodologies leads readers to immersion into a world of scientific inquiry that reveals the rationale for selecting one therapeutic procedure over another. While there is considerable consensus, important distinctions remain across theoretical and real-world measurement of phonological impairments and their treatment.

It is a pleasure to view the future through the eyes of these authors. Readers will find themselves reopening this book time and again as they reflect upon the wisdom of those who have made the study of children's phonological development and disorders their mission.

—Katharine G. Butler, PhD
Editor, Excellence in Practice Series

Hindsight, insight, and foresight. How often we wish we had all three! With this book, we have all three for the subject of applied phonology. Through personal experience and academic legacy, the contributors to this volume understand the roots of applied phonology—its history and its evolution. Their own work shaped the development of this field. Now in retrospect, the authors can retell the progress in applied phonology, not as indifferent historians, but as dedicated scholars and clinicians who sought to make phonological theory work in the proving ground of phonological development and phonological disorders. The authors write insightfully on how applied phonology has come to its current place. Contemporary issues stand in relief to the brave but often uncertain efforts of the past. The story that is traced in these chapters is vibrant with the personal convictions and motives of the authors. It is one thing to know that a theory won adherents, but it is another thing to know how the adherents were won to the theory. The contributors also write prophetically on where applied phonology is likely to go. They lead the reader on an intellectual trajectory, rooted in the past, interpreted in the present, and forecast for tomorrow.

Although science is sometimes portrayed as an "objective" process in which human qualities are muted and repressed, it is unavoidable that science is a human practice. Therefore, science is best understood as a human endeavor, one that is colored and driven by human qualities. Applied phonology has its own history of science, and it is eloquently told by these writers who practiced it, who continue to practice it, and imagine how it will be practiced in the future. Science is not diminished by acknowledging its origins in human efforts and perseverance. To the contrary, science so conceived takes on a greater depth. The charge to the authors of these chapters was essentially to write the story of their own pursuits in applied phonology. The products are scholarly, revealing, and, in the whole, inspiring. The satisfying scholarship in these chapters is replete with good arguments, thoughtful review of the literature, and presentation of data. The revelation is honest and personal. The inspiration takes its spark from the quintessential human inquiry, the desire to know and to change things for the better. A good book lets the reader stand on the author's shoulders for a better view of the subject at hand. With this book, the reader stands on the shoulders of eight authors for an encircling view of applied phonology.

—*Ray Kent*

Preface

A need has existed for a book that pulls together research of individuals who led the way in applied phonology research. Seven of the eight contributors for this book were conducting applied phonology research and publishing their results in the 1970s, and all of these individuals have continued to do so through the 1980s to the present day. The eighth contributor, Stackhouse, who began publishing in the 1980s, has been a frontrunner in terms of investigating phonological awareness abilities of children with expressive phonological impairments. This is an area that increasingly is being recognized as needing attention, and we felt that this book would not be complete without a chapter on this important topic.

We also wanted this book to cross disciplines and to include authors from more than one country. Four of the contributors to this book have backgrounds in linguistics (Edwards, Grunwell, Ingram, Oller), and four hold clinical certification (Elbert, Hodson, Shriberg, Stackhouse). Two reside in the United Kingdom (Grunwell, Stackhouse), one lives in Canada (Ingram), and the other five reside in the United States.

Readers will note some spelling variations (e.g., *realization* and *realisation*; *behavior* and *behaviour*) because of differences in British and American spellings. In light of the fact that both sets of spelling are correct in English-speaking countries, and because this book is likely to be read by individuals in other countries as well as the one in which it is being published, the customary spellings used by the authors in their own countries have been retained.

Moreover, there are certain differences in terms. A glossary includes some specific terminology differences (with the particular phonologist referenced), as well as commonly accepted definitions.

It is our hope that this book will fill a void. Although many of these phonologists have published together before (e.g., book chapters, journal theme issues) and all are referenced in general articulation/phonology textbooks, no previous publication has included original writings by all of these individuals. It is anticipated that the chapter references will provide a springboard for readers to seek out additional research articles by these phonologists.

We especially want to thank Kay Butler for her encouragement to undertake this project and for her excellent Foreword for the Series. We also are delighted to have a Foreword written by one of the world's leading speech scientists, Ray Kent, who has made numerous contributions to applied phonology literature. In addition, we want to acknowledge Aspen staff members who have interacted with us at various stages of this project for their assistance—Loretta Stock, Sandy Cannon, Mary Anne Langdon, and Jane Colilla. We also express our appreciation to Robert Lowe, Linda Louko, Lesley Magnus, and an anonymous reviewer, whose comments contributed immeasurably to the end product. And finally, we thank Wendy Chitwood, Mickie Doran, Dawn Lang, Tera Hamer, and Dana Ingmire for providing preliminary feedback about the chapters from the perspective of graduate students in an applied phonology seminar.

—Mary Louise Edwards
—Barbara Williams Hodson

CHAPTER 1

Historical Overview of Clinical Phonology

Mary Louise Edwards

Phonology, the branch of linguistics that deals with sound systems and sound patterns, has a long history, dating back at least to the time when the alphabetic principle was discovered. However, attempts to apply the principles and concepts of phonology to clinical issues are much more recent, starting only in the late 1960s. Several different theories have been applied clinically in the intervening 25 years, with varying degrees of success. These include distinctive feature theory, generative phonology (in two different versions), natural phonology, and, most recently, various nonlinear models. This introductory chapter, which attempts to provide some historical perspective, includes an overview of these different theories and the major clinical contributions that grew out of them. Natural phonology is highlighted because it gave rise to the phonological process approach, which became the predominant approach to phonological assessment and remediation in the 1980s. This chapter provides the framework for the later chapters of this volume, in which several members of the first generation of clinical phonologists describe their contributions and the evolution of their views over the past two decades.

A PERSONAL PERSPECTIVE

My own involvement in clinical phonology goes back almost to its inception. As a graduate student in linguistics at the Ohio State University in the late 1960s, I was fascinated by the work of one of my young professors, David Stampe. I was particularly interested in his theory of natural phonology, in which he introduced the concept of phonetically motivated natural phonological processes and showed how such processes could account for similarities in the types of sound changes observed in various domains, such as dialect variation and historical language change, as well as phonological acquisition in children (e.g., Stampe, 1969, 1973/1979). My master's thesis (Edwards, 1970/1973), conducted under his direction, was an investigation of children's acquisition of liquids, based on natural phonological processes. In this thesis, I attempted to show that such an analysis would be more revealing and would capture more generalizations than one based on Roman Jakobson's (1941/1968) theory, the predominant theory of phonological acquisition up until that time.

My master's thesis was one of the first serious attempts to apply the theory of natural phonology in the area of language acquisition. Thus it generated a considerable amount of interest among child phonologists and led directly to my being asked to join Carol Stoel, Marcy Macken, and others as a research associate on the Child Phonology Project (CPP) at Stanford University. At that point (1971–1972), the CPP, directed by Professor Charles Ferguson, was attempting to test empirically some of Jakobson's predictions regarding order of acquisition (e.g., Jakobson, 1941/1968, 1971). Specifically, we were investigating the perception and production of several classes of sounds in young children (18 months to 4 years) acquiring American English and Mexican Spanish. My 1974 paper on the perception and production of fricatives, affricates, liquids, and glides by English-learning children reported some of the results from the CPP. A later paper on phonological variation (and the "trade-off phenomenon") in children's speech (Garnica & Edwards, 1977) also grew out of this involvement, as did my doctoral dissertation on fricative acquisition, completed in 1979 under the direction of Charles Ferguson (Edwards, 1979a, 1979b, 1979c).

After funding ended on the English part of the CPP, I replaced David Ingram as research associate in linguistics at the Institute for Childhood Aphasia (ICA), housed at Stanford University and directed by Jon Eisenson. Although I was at the ICA for only one year, my experience there had a profound impact and shaped the direction of my professional career. Many of the severely language-impaired children who were seen at the institute also had severe speech-sound production problems and were very difficult to understand. In the early 1970s, however, *language* was the exciting new frontier, and the focus of the institute was very much on language (i.e., syntax). There was little interest in the children's speech-sound production problems or in "articulation" therapy, which was considered to be boring.

Fortunately, the clinician who was hired as a research assistant, Barbara Bernhardt, from the University of British Columbia, also had a strong linguistics background and shared my interest in phonology. We spent much of that year studying the phonology of the language-impaired children at the institute and devising and carrying out remediation plans for them, based on our analyses of their phonological systems. The research reports that we wrote during that year (e.g., Edwards & Bernhardt, 1973a, 1973b) were never published, in part because we soon moved to different ends of the continent, but the phonological patterns of some of our subjects were discussed at length by Ingram in his seminal book on

Phonological Disability in Children (Ingram, 1976) and have therefore become well known. These reports are some of the earliest attempts to apply Stampe's theory of natural phonology in the clinical realm. (Note that Barbara Bernhardt has recently become known as a major proponent of nonlinear phonology; see, e.g., Bernhardt, 1992; Bernhardt & Gilbert, 1992; Bernhardt & Stoel-Gammon, 1994.)

A BRIEF HISTORY OF CLINICAL PHONOLOGY

As discussed in several places throughout this volume, something that might be described as a revolution took place in the field of speech-language pathology in the 1970s. Specifically, the subdiscipline now known as clinical phonology arose in the 1970s and flourished in the 1980s. In fact, a major purpose of this volume is to bring together and review the contributions of several of the individuals involved in this revolution.

Distinctive Feature Theory

As mentioned earlier, serious attempts to apply theoretical principles and concepts from phonology to clinical populations began in the late 1960s and early 1970s. At that time, a number of researchers began to look to distinctive feature theory (e.g., Chomsky & Halle, 1968; Jakobson, Fant, & Halle, 1952) for insights that would aid in the assessment and treatment of young children with severe speech-sound production difficulties (children who are now typically said to exhibit disordered, delayed, or impaired phonology). In distinctive feature-based analyses, similarities among seemingly separate surface errors (such as [t] for adult /s/ and [p] for adult /f/) are captured in terms of commonalities in the features that are in error, such as stridency or continuancy. Contributions in this vein include those of Menyuk (1968), McReynolds and Huston (1971), Singh and Frank (1972), and Pollack and Rees (1972). (See detailed reviews in Edwards & Shriberg, 1983.)

These early researchers demonstrated that distinctive *features* could indeed provide additional insights into clinical problems, and one assessment procedure grew out of this work (McReynolds & Engmann, 1975). Distinctive feature analysis, however, never really caught on in the field of speech-language pathology, perhaps because of problems inherent in the approach. For example, syllable structure errors such as segment and syllable deletions cannot be dealt with in a satisfactory way using distinctive features. In addition, use of a distinctive feature approach required a more sophisticated knowledge of phonology than was possessed by most clinicians at that time. (The more recent use of features, based on nonlinear theories of phonology, will be mentioned later in this chapter and in Ingram, Chapter 2 of this volume.)

It should be noted here that the use of minimal pairs in phonological remediation, which continues to be a popular approach (see Elbert, Chapter 3 of this volume, and Hodson, Chapter 8 of this volume) owes much, in my view, to distinctive feature theory. For example, to train a feature that is in error a high percentage of the time, McReynolds and Engmann (1975) recommended pairing a phoneme that contains the + aspect of the feature with another phoneme containing the – aspect, with the phoneme pair differing *only* in the feature contrast to be trained; for example, using /p/ vs. /b/ to train the [–voice] feature. Minimal-pair training, as traditionally applied (e.g., Elbert, Rockman, & Saltzman, 1980; Kelman & Edwards, 1994), also typically uses pairs of phonemes that are minimally different in their feature content. Gierut's use of "maximal oppositions" (i.e., *maximally* different minimal pairs, such as /mu/ vs. /gu/) in the late 1980s and 1990s (e.g., Gierut, 1989, 1990) constitutes the most noteworthy exception to this traditional use of minimal pairs. (Note also that incorporating minimal pairs in articulation therapy was advocated by some in the late 1950s and early 1960s; see, e.g., Fairbanks, 1960).

Standard Generative Phonology

There were also several attempts in the early to mid-1970s to apply theoretical concepts from standard generative phonology (e.g., as described by Chomsky & Halle, 1968) in analyzing data from children with severe speech-sound production problems. The specific aspect of generative phonology that was applied at that time was primarily the concept of formal phonological rules, written in distinctive feature notation. (Note the overlap between distinctive feature theory and generative phonology.) Major papers that followed this approach include those by Compton (1970, and to some extent 1975, 1976), Oller (1973), Oller and Kelly (1974), and Lorentz (1974). (See Oller, Chapter 6 of this volume.) These early researchers showed that by using such an approach, they could capture regularities in children's sound errors that would not be evident in a traditional articulation test approach. To illustrate, by combining related "substitution rules," such as p → b/#_ and t → d/#_, into more general rules written in distinctive feature notation (in this case, [–sonorant] → [+voice]/#_), Oller (1973) was able to reduce the total number of rules postulated for his five subjects from 223 to 76, and by doing so he was able to capture many significant generalizations about his subjects' sound changes (e.g., obstruents are voiced in word-initial position). Detailed reviews of these and other papers were presented in Edwards and Shriberg, 1983. This approach, however, using the formal rules of standard generative phonology, also failed to become widespread, perhaps largely because of the technical knowledge of phonology and the many conventions of rule formulation that it required.

Natural Phonology

The other phonological theory to be applied to clinical populations in the early 1970s was Stampe's (1969, 1973/1979) theory of natural phonology, referred to earlier. According to this view, children's sound errors are accounted for by a set of phonetically motivated and innate "natural" phonological processes, such as stopping of fricatives, fronting of velars, and simplification of consonant clusters. The underlying (mental) representations (URs) to which these processes apply are considered to be basically equivalent to the adult surface forms, minus the predictable phonetic detail, such as aspiration on initial voiceless stops in English. So, for example, regardless of how a child might produce the word *soap* (e.g., as [bop], [top], or [do]), the UR would be assumed to be /sop/. (See Edwards, 1995, for a discussion of this as well as other views regarding the nature of children's URs.)

Early attempts to apply Stampe's theory in analyzing the speech of children with multiple misarticulations include Edwards and Bernhardt (1973a, 1973b), mentioned above, Grunwell (1975), Ingram (1976), Oller (1973), and Oller and Kelly (1974). Notice that a few of these articles are also mentioned above under generative phonology. In fact, some of these early papers have to be put in both categories, judging from discussions contained within them. For example, Oller (1973) based his analysis primarily on generative phonological rules, but he also discussed Stampe's theory, pointing out some of the processes common to the children in his study and also in normal phonological development, such as reduction of /s/ plus stop clusters. Similarly, in her analysis procedures, Grunwell (1975) included an analysis that was said to be based on generative phonology (as in Compton, 1970), but she used the term *process* to describe the general rules presented (see Grunwell, Chapter 4 of this volume). So these researchers used formal rules to capture children's general processes or sound changes. (Stampe, 1969, 1973/1979, made a much sharper distinction between processes and rules. For further discussion, see Edwards, 1992.)

Unlike distinctive features and generative-type phonological rules, phonological processes have become more widely accepted and applied in speech-language pathology. Process approaches to the assessment and remediation of speech-sound disorders in children, based more or less closely on Stampe's theory of natural phonology, became commonplace in the 1980s.

Weiner's (1979) *Phonological Process Analysis* was the first published procedure based primarily on phonological processes. Two others appeared a year later (Hodson, 1980, 1986; Shriberg & Kwiatkowski, 1980), followed by Ingram's procedure in 1981. Other process-based analysis procedures continued to be published throughout the 1980s and into the 1990s (e.g., Bankson & Bernthal, 1990; Grunwell, 1985; Khan & Lewis, 1986; Lowe, 1986). In addition, several programs for computer-assisted phonological process analysis also became available (e.g., Hodson, 1985; Long & Fey, 1988; Masterson & Pagan, 1990; Oller & Delgado, 1990; Shriberg, 1986; Weiner, 1983, 1988).

As discussed elsewhere (e.g., Edwards, 1983, 1994), these procedures and programs differ considerably from one another (e.g., in the size and type of sample utilized, the numbers and types of processes assessed, recording and scoring procedures, and so forth). All, however, share the goal of discovering the phonological processes underlying children's sound errors. That is, like distinctive feature analysis and analyses based on phonological rules, phonological process analysis goes beyond simply listing children's sound errors by word position or classifying them as substitutions or omissions. In each case, an attempt is made to account for the child's surface errors in terms of the phonological processes and combinations of processes that would give rise to those errors. (For instance, an error of [d] for initial /s/ would be accounted for by a combination or interaction of stopping and initial voicing.) This type of approach is now well accepted for analyzing the speech of children with many misarticulations and reduced intelligibility (i.e., children with phonological impairments) and for deriving remediation goals, as discussed by Hodson in Chapter 8 this volume. (More detailed reviews of specific procedures and programs are presented in Bernthal & Bankson, 1993, Edwards, 1994, and Kelman & Edwards, 1994. See also Ingram, Grunwell, Shriberg, and Hodson, Chapters 2, 4, 5, and 8 of this volume).

In addition to published procedures and computer programs, guidelines for nonstandardized phonological process analysis have been presented in the literature (e.g., see Edwards, 1994; Kelman & Edwards, 1994). In this type of approach, an analysis is derived without the use of a published "test" or a finite set of processes. In nonstandardized analysis, it is possible to withhold judgment regarding difficult or ambiguous items and to account for them on the basis of how the child deals with similar but more straightforward items (Edwards, 1994). To illustrate, a child's production of [d] for /g/ in the word *goat* (as in [dot]) could be due to either regressive alveolar assimilation (RAA) or velar fronting. If the initial /g/ is produced correctly in words such as *go*, in which alveolar assimilation is not possible, then the [d] for /g/ production in *goat* is probably best attributed to RAA. Most published procedures are not set up in a way that encourages this kind of analytical problem solving.

The reasons for the fairly rapid spread of phonological-process-based assessment and remediation procedures are not entirely clear. The publication of Ingram's book on phonological disability in children in 1976 was certainly a factor. Ingram's was the first book on phonology written expressly for speech-language pathologists, and in it he introduced, defined, and gave examples of many phonological processes exhibited by normally developing and/or phonologically impaired children. As noted elsewhere (e.g., Edwards, 1994), Ingram's book played a major role in promoting the clinical usefulness of phonology in general and phonological processes in particular. Phonological processes are also more transparent and are thus more easily understood than distinctive features and phonological rules (according to personal contact with many working clinicians). Additionally, they involve less formalism and require less academic preparation in phonology. Process-based approaches have continued to predominate into the 1990s, although other phonological approaches have also been developed.

Standard Generative Phonology Revisited

A different application of standard generative phonology from that discussed above was introduced in the late 1970s and early 1980s (Dinnsen, Elbert, & Weismer, 1979, 1980). Instead of focusing on formal phonological rules, written in distinctive features, this approach focuses on the nature of the child's URs on which processes or rules operate. According to Dinnsen et al. (1979, 1980), we should not assume that children's URs are adultlike (Stampe, 1969, 1979). Rather, this has to be established empirically for each individual child.

Dinnsen et al. (1979, 1980) discussed several types of evidence that they believe may be used to determine the nature of the child's URs, such as the existence of optional rules. They focused, however, on "morphophonemic alternations." To illustrate, one of the phonologically impaired children they discuss, Jamie, omitted final stops, producing such forms as [dɔ:] for *dog*. However, when he added the diminutive ending /i/, the final consonant showed up, as in [dɔgi] for *doggie*. Thus he exhibited alternation between Ø and [g] in final position. Dinnsen et al. (1979, 1980) saw this as evidence for an adultlike UR (/dɔg/) and a final-consonant deletion rule. (These researchers did not use the term/concept of *process*.) They contrasted this child with Matthew, who also omitted final stops. When Matthew added the diminutive ending, however, the final stops did not show up, as in [dai] for *doggie*. In the view of these researchers, there was no evidence that Matthew's URs contained final stops and hence no evidence for a final-consonant deletion rule. (According to this approach, if final consonants are not present in the child's URs, they are not available to be deleted.) Dinnsen et al. argued that crucial evidence of this type is needed to justify the existence of rules such as final-consonant deletion. (See Edwards, 1995, for a more detailed discussion of children's URs.)

The view introduced by Dinnsen et al. (1979, 1980) was illustrated by Maxwell (1979) and was more fully articulated by Elbert and Gierut (1986). In these later writings, the concept of underlying representations was replaced by a broader concept referred to as *(productive) phonological knowledge*. This encompasses all the information that is internalized or stored mentally for each morpheme. Elbert and Gierut (1986) recommended using a large sample of single words containing potential minimal pairs and morphonemic alternations to classify the child's productive phonological knowledge according to six predetermined types, from Type 1 (full adultlike knowledge) to Type 6 (least knowledge). Sounds that the child consistently produces correctly (Type 1 knowledge) are not affected by phonological rules in any position or morpheme, whereas sounds that are never produced in an adultlike fashion (Type 6 knowledge) are said to be excluded by "inventory constraints." In essence, if a child's productions are not similar to those of the "ambient" (adult) language, then his or her underlying representations are also considered to be "nonadultlike."

It should be noted that in this approach, determination of the child's URs is based only on production evidence, even though URs are *mental* representations that cannot be directly observed or ascertained. Information about the child's perceptual ability is not considered, nor is information from acoustic analyses. A different approach that does include these additional sources of information is described in Tyler, Edwards, and Saxman (1990).

Elbert and Gierut (1986) were concerned with phonological knowledge in part because they wanted to be able to predict a child's ability to generalize in treatment. Therefore a number of clinical studies (e.g., Gierut, 1989, 1990, 1992) have been based on this view of phonological knowledge since the mid- to late 1980s. These studies have shown that children with phonological difficulties seem to generalize more readily and make more far-reaching changes in their phonological systems if they are first trained on sounds for which they have least phonological knowledge and if these sounds are contrasted (in minimal pairs) with maximally different sounds (i.e., sounds that differ in many features), especially other sounds for which they have limited knowledge. This approach differs considerably from most applications of minimal pairs, in which the pairs differ by just one feature (as in *pat* vs. *bat* or *sea* vs. *tea*) and involve the correct adult sound versus the child's error (e.g., Kelman & Edwards, 1994). (See earlier comments on minimal pairs in this chapter, as well as Elbert and Hodson, Chapters 3 and 8 of this volume.)

Nonlinear Phonology

Several more recent nonlinear theories of phonology (e.g., autosegmental, onset-rime, and feature geometry) have also begun to be applied clinically, particularly since 1990. (See Bernhardt & Stoel-Gammon, 1994, for an excellent introduction. See also Bernhardt & Gilbert, 1992; Chin & Dinnsen, 1991; Schwartz, 1992; and Ingram and Oller, Chapters 2 and 6 of this volume.) Whereas earlier approaches focused on segments (consonants and vowels) and emphasized rules and processes, nonlinear models focus on multitiered representations and incorporate both segmental and prosodic information (Bernhardt & Gilbert, 1992). These approaches include several autonomous levels, or tiers, that are hierarchically organized. For example, the syllable tier (made up of strong and weak syllables) dominates the onset-rime tier. The onset of the syllable consists of all the consonants (up to three in English) preceding the vowel or nucleus, and the rime/rhyme consists of the vowel and any consonants following it in the coda. An example of this type of hierarchical structure for the word *strongly* is shown in Figure 1–1 (based on Bernhardt & Stoel-Gammon, 1994). See Bernhardt (1992) and Bernhardt and Gilbert (1992) for illustrations of nonlinear phonological analysis and examples of how the results of such analyses may be used in planning intervention.

"Feature geometry" (e.g., Bernhardt & Stoel-Gammon, 1994; Chin & Dinnsen, 1991; Sagey, 1986) carries this type of organization below the level of the segment.

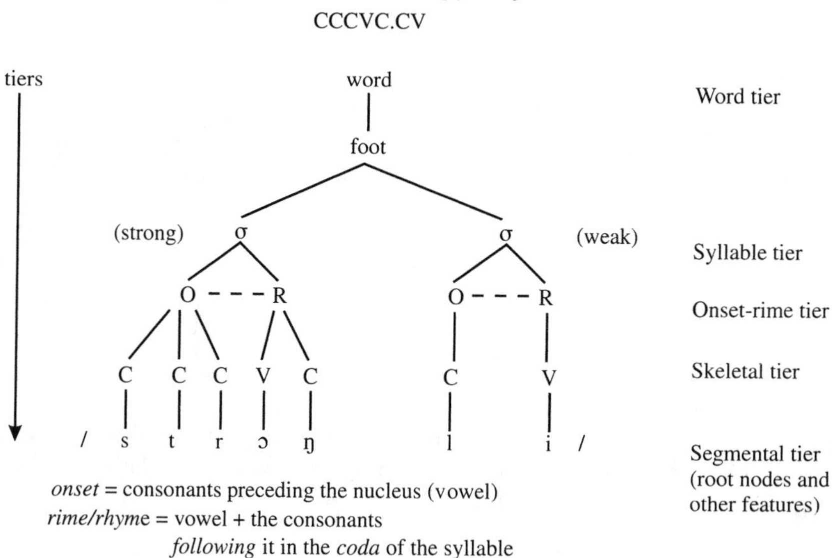

Figure 1–1 Nonlinear Representation of the Word *Strongly. Source*: Adapted from B.H. Bernhardt, and C. Stoel-Gammon, Nonlinear Phonology: Introduction and Clinical Application, *Journal of Speech and Hearing Research*, Vol. 37, pp. 123–143, © 1994, American Speech-Language-Hearing Association.

In earlier feature-based models, each feature was seen as independent. In feature geometry, however, features are organized into hierarchies to capture the fact that some features are dominant over others. The *skeletal tier* contains C and V nodes for nonsyllabic and syllabic elements, respectively. Each C and V dominates a root node that is the structural representation of a phoneme (Chin & Dinnsen, 1991). Each root node in turn dominates four nodes, two binary (+/–) feature nodes ([continuant] and [consonantal]) and two class nodes ([laryngeal] and [supralaryngeal]). The laryngeal node dominates features for voicing, and the supralaryngeal node dominates [soft palate] (for the nasal/non-nasal distinction) and [place] for the articulator nodes ([labial], [coronal], and [dorsal]). Each articulator node dominates binary features such as [round], [anterior], and [back] that indicate how the articulator is used. A feature geometric representation of the labial nasal /m/, based on Chin and Dinnsen (1991) is shown in Figure 1–2. (See Bernhardt & Stoel-Gammon, 1994, for a somewhat different version of feature geometry.)

Chin and Dinnsen (1991) used feature geometry (as presented by Sagey, 1986) to describe and classify consonants in disordered phonological systems, and they

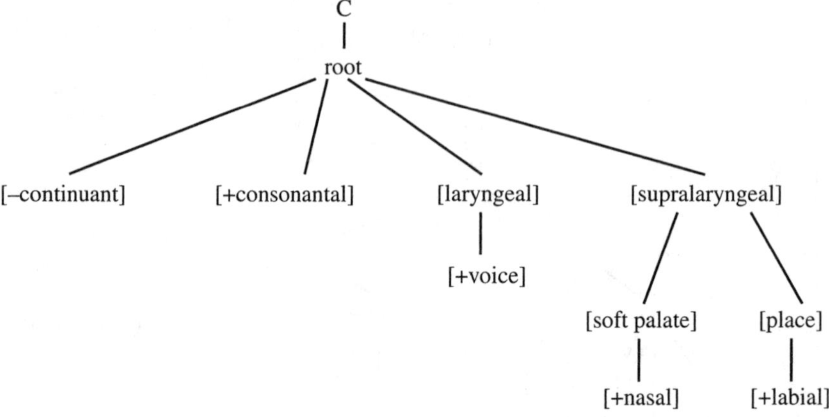

Figure 1–2 Feature Geometric Representation of /m/. *Source:* Adapted with permission from S. Chin, and D. Dinnsen, Feature Geometry in Disorded Phonologies, *Clinical Linguistics and Phonetics,* Vol. 5, pp. 329–337, © 1991, Taylor & Francis, Ltd.

argued that this model provides a better explanation than one based on representations and rules. Specifically, this type of model may be better able to handle phenomena such as assimilation (feature spreading) and coalescence (reassociation of features).

Optimality theory (OT), which is still being developed and refined, is another type of nonlinear model that may hold promise for phonological analysis and intervention. This model focuses on *constraints* rather than rules or processes. For example, Bernhardt and Stemberger (1995) and Stemberger (1995) discussed a number of constraints on phonological output that govern the development of syllable structure in young children. To illustrate, there are constraints on faithfulness that prevent segments from being deleted and require segments that are adjacent in the input to be adjacent in the output. There are also negative constraints that prevent certain types of segments from appearing or that restrict their occurrence to specific positions. Stemberger (1995) discussed many such constraints, including, for instance, Syl>Onset, which requires that syllables must have an onset, and NotComplex(Onset), which prohibits clusters from occurring in syllable onsets. It is too soon to speculate about the possible long-term influence of OT in the field of clinical phonology. Some of us, however, have been struck by the apparent similarities between the constraints of OT and the phonetically motivated processes of natural phonology.

SPECIAL CLINICAL APPLICATIONS

Phonology and Fluency

Research into what is sometimes called "the stuttering-phonology connection" began in earnest at Syracuse University in the late 1980s and continues to the present time (e.g., Louko, Edwards, & Conture, 1990; Wolk, Edwards, & Conture, 1993; Yaruss & Conture, 1996). This research interest was spurred by a number of factors.

For example, on several occasions we noted that young children being seen for their phonological problems sometimes became dysfluent during the course of remediation as their phonology improved. In addition, we frequently observed that the phonological abilities of our young clients who stuttered lagged behind those of their normally fluent peers. In fact, a review of the available literature revealed that approximately 30% to 40% of young children who stutter also have phonological difficulties, as compared to only about 2% to 7% of young children with normal fluency. This led us to begin to seriously think about the relationship between stuttering and phonology (e.g., Wolk, Conture, & Edwards, 1990).

Some of our preliminary research indicated that young children who stutter may exhibit more cluster reduction than their normally fluent peers (Louko et al., 1990). This observation, however, was not borne out in our later, more controlled investigations, in which we compared the phonological systems of children who exhibited disordered phonology only to those of children who exhibited both stuttering and disordered phonology. In this later research, we also sampled many words with clusters, as well as complex syllable shapes (Wolk et al., 1993; Yaruss & Conture, 1996). At this point, we have found no particular phonological patterns that characterize the speech of young children who stutter (see review in Louko, 1995). Moreover, the phonological behavior of young children who stutter *and* exhibit disordered phonology does not appear to differ significantly from that of children who exhibit only disordered phonology. Rather, there is a great deal of variability in the types of phonological patterns exhibited by young children with both stuttering and disordered phonology, just as there is for children with only phonological problems.

One difficulty we have had in pursuing this line of research relates to the lack of a clear theoretical framework. There is no agreed-upon theory of childhood stuttering *or* disordered phonology in children. Hence we have had to look elsewhere for a theoretical model that might account for the relationship between the two disorders. At this point, the covert repair hypothesis, or CRH (e.g., Postma & Kolk, 1993), seems to hold the most promise.

According to the CRH, individuals who stutter may demonstrate an impairment in their phonological encoding such that the activation of target phonemes is somewhat delayed (Kolk, Conture, Postma, & Louko, 1991). During this delay, target phonemes are in competition with other phonemes. This increases the likelihood that phonological encoding errors will become part of the speaker's phonetic plan. During the internal monitoring process, it is assumed that speakers can detect such errors in their phonetic plan (Levelt, 1993). They may then interrupt their ongoing speech to repair these errors *before* they are produced. Speech dysfluencies are thought to arise as a byproduct of this detection and repair process when a speaker disrupts ongoing speech in an attempt to repair such errors *covertly*. According to this view (e.g., Yaruss & Conture, 1996), it is hypothesized that children's speech dysfluencies are related to their speech errors because such errors provide an opportunity for error detection and self-repair, and hence for the occurrence of dysfluencies. Yaruss and Conture (1996), however, found that the CRH was better able to account for *nonsystematic* (e.g., slip-of-the-tongue) errors than for systematic errors. This is a problem because, by definition, errors that characterize the speech of children with disordered phonology are largely systematic. Further empirical research on the relationship between stuttering and disordered phonology is clearly needed—for example, research on how the CRH might explain this relationship. In addition, the connection between stuttering and disordered phonology has clinical implications. It is not known, for instance, if the long-term prognosis is worse for children who exhibit both disorders.

Intervention

Many of our young clients who were being seen for fluency concerns also had phonological skills that were not age appropriate. Therefore we developed a unique remediation group at Syracuse University in the late 1980s based on the principles of the existing stuttering groups, such as using a reduced rate of speech and increased pause time (e.g., Conture, 1990), but also incorporating phonological goals and building on some of the earlier remediation procedures described, for example, in Tyler, Edwards, and Saxman (1987), such as modified cycles. (See Chapter 8.) The specific techniques used in the stuttering-phonology (S-P) group are described in more detail in Conture, Louko, and Edwards (1993), along with preliminary findings from several children who participated in the group over a period of time.

The approach used in the S-P group was basically an *indirect* one in which we did not call attention to or overtly correct the children's sound errors. Our goal was to improve their phonology without exacerbating their stuttering. Extensive modeling of correct productions was infused throughout the session in age-appropriate games and activities. In spite of the indirect nature of the remediation, the phonological skills of the children in the S-P group improved, and they became more intelligible. Just as important, this was done without a detrimental effect on their fluency.

The success of the S-P group led to the formation of a preschool phonology group based on many of the same principles. It is very difficult (if not impossible) to predict which children with phonological problems may be at risk for becoming dysfluent in the course of remediation. In part for that reason, we decided to use an indirect and naturalistic approach in our preschool phonology group. As with the S-P group, we adopted what we have called a "modified cycles" framework (Kelman & Edwards, 1994; Tyler et al., 1987), with several phonological processes being targeted sequentially in one cycle and with each session focusing on just one particular phoneme or cluster (Hodson & Paden, 1991; see also Chapter 8). In our phonology group, the auditory "bombardment" takes place through extensive and repeated modeling of the target sound in meaningful words used in games and activities throughout the session. In addition, the intervention is indirect, with no overt correcting of sound errors. Children are reinforced for their participation in the activities, which are as naturalistic as possible. That is, words and sounds are produced as a natural part or consequence of the activity. (See Kelman & Edwards, 1994, for details of this preschool phonology group.)

Phonological Awareness

Although not based on a specific theory of adult phonology, a considerable amount of emphasis has been placed in recent years on the area of phonological awareness or metaphonology. This has for some time been of concern to reading specialists and individuals interested in learning disabilities (e.g., see Blachman, 1984; Vellutino & Scanlon, 1987), and more recently it has also become an area of interest for researchers and clinicians in the area of speech-language pathology (e.g., Catts, 1991, 1993; Kamhi, Lee, & Nelson, 1985). Much of this research has concerned the phonological awareness skills and later reading and/or spelling abilities of children with language disorders. However, some research has focused specifically on the metaphonological skills and/or later reading and spelling abilities of children with developmental phonological disorders. Examples include the work of Bird and Bishop (1992), Bird, Bishop, and Freeman (1995), Clarke-Klein (1994), Green and Edwards (1992), and Webster and Plante (1992).

To give one example, Green and Edwards (1992) presented seven phonological awareness tasks modified from the reading literature to 10 preschool-aged (preliterate) children with impaired phonology and 10 with age-appropriate phonology. In this research, the children with phonological impairments performed significantly worse on several of the tasks, all of which involved production (e.g., rhyme knowledge, rhyme production, sentence division, and bisyllabic word division). There were no significant differences on the receptive tasks, including rhyme detection and phoneme detection. Results of this study suggest that children with phonological impairments (but without other language problems) may be at some risk for later reading difficulties, given that they exhibit poorer phonological awareness skills than their phonologically normal peers.

Metaphonologically based treatment programs have been devised for children with phonological impairments (e.g., Chabon & Prelock, 1991). In addition, it has been proposed that speech-language pathologists should play an active role in promoting phonological awareness in all the children they serve (e.g., Catts, 1991). See Stackhouse, Chapter 7 of this volume.

CONCLUSION

In this chapter, I have attempted to provide some historical perspective on the area of clinical phonology as it has developed over the course of the past 25 years. This overview, of course, reflects my own particular biases, although I have tried to be as even-handed as possible. I hope that the reader will benefit from my introduction to the work of the other authors, as well as my mention of issues that are dealt with in more depth in later chapters.

It will be interesting to see what developments arise in the field of clinical phonology in the next 25 years. To what extent will our assessment and remediation techniques be influenced by new phonological theories, new understandings from other disciplines, and new technologies? Is there another revolution in the offing? Whatever happens, we can anticipate more challenges and discoveries as we look forward to a new century and embark on the next 25 years of clinical phonology.

The author thanks Barbara Hodson, Linda J. Louko, and Robert Lowe for helpful suggestions on an earlier draft of this chapter.

REFERENCES

Bankson, N., & Bernthal, J. (1990). *Bankson-Bernthal Test of Phonology*. Chicago: Riverside.

Bernhardt, B.H. (1992). The application of nonlinear phonological theory to intervention with one phonologically disordered child. *Clinical Linguistics and Phonetics, 6,* 283–316.

Bernhardt, B.H., & Gilbert, J.G. (1992). Applying linguistic theory to speech-language pathology: The case for non-linear phonology. *Clinical Linguistics and Phonetics*, *6,* 123–145.

Bernhardt, B.H., & Stemberger, J.P. (1995). *Nonlinear phonology and child phonological development: A constraint-based approach*. Manuscript in preparation.

Bernhardt, B.H., & Stoel-Gammon, C. (1994). Nonlinear phonology: Introduction and clinical application. *Journal of Speech and Hearing Research, 37,* 123–143.

Bernthal, J.E., & Bankson, N.W. (1993). *Articulation and phonological disorders* (3rd ed.). Englewood Cliffs, NJ: Prentice Hall.

Bird, J., & Bishop, D.V.M. (1992). Perception and awareness of phonemes in phonologically impaired children. *European Journal of Disorders of Communication, 27,* 289–311.

Bird, J., Bishop, D.V.M., & Freeman, N.H. (1995). Phonological awareness and literacy development in children with expressive phonological impairments. *Journal of Speech and Hearing Research, 38*, 446–462.

Blachman, B. (1984). Language analysis skills and early reading acquisition. In G. Wallach & K. Butler (Eds.), *Language learning disabilities in school age children* (pp. 271–287). Baltimore: Williams & Wilkins.

Catts, H. (1991). Facilitating phonological awareness: Role of speech-language pathologists. *Language, Speech, and Hearing Services in Schools, 22,* 196–203.

Catts, H. (1993). The relationship between speech-language impairments and reading disabilities. *Journal of Speech and Hearing Research, 36,* 948–958.

Chabon, S., & Prelock, P. (1991). *Meta magic: A metalinguistic approach to the training of closed syllables*. Tucson, AZ: Communication Skill Builders.

Chin, S., & Dinnsen, D. (1991). Feature geometry in disordered phonologies. *Clinical Linguistics and Phonetics*, *5*, 329–337.

Chomsky, N., & Halle, M. (1968). *The sound pattern of English*. New York: Harper & Row.

Clarke-Klein, S.M. (1994). Expressive phonological deficiencies: Impact on spelling development. *Topics in Language Disorders*, *14*, 40–55.

Compton, A.J. (1970). Generative studies of children's phonological disorders. *Journal of Speech and Hearing Disorders, 35*, 315–339.

Compton, A.J. (1975). Generative studies of children's phonological disorders: A strategy of therapy. In S. Singh (Ed.), *Measurements in hearing, speech, and language* (pp. 55–90). Baltimore: University Park.

Compton, A.J. (1976). Generative studies of children's phonological disorders: Clinical ramifications. In D.M. Moorhead & A.E. Moorhead (Eds.), *Normal and deficient child language: Selected readings* (pp. 61–96). Baltimore: University Park.

Conture, E.G. (1990). *Stuttering* (2nd ed.). Englewood Cliffs, NJ: Prentice Hall.

Conture, E.G., Louko, L.J., & Edwards, M.L. (1993). Simultaneously treating stuttering and disordered phonology in children: Experimental treatment, preliminary findings. *American Journal of Speech-Language Pathology, 2,* 72–81.

Dinnsen, D.A., Elbert, M., & Weismer, G. (1979, November). *On the characterization of functional misarticulations*. Paper presented at the annual meeting of the American Speech-Language-Hearing Association, Atlanta, GA.

Dinnsen, D.A., Elbert, M., & Weismer, G. (1980). Some typological properties of functional misarticulation systems. In W.O. Dressler (Ed.), *Phonologica* (pp. 83–88). Innsbruck: Innsbrucker Beitrage zur Sprachwissenschaft.

Edwards, M.L. (1973). The acquisition of liquids. *Working Papers in Linguistics*, *15*, 1–54. (Original master's thesis completed 1970)

Edwards, M.L. (1979a). *Patterns and processes in fricative acquisition: Longitudinal evidence from six English-learning children*. Unpublished doctoral dissertation, Stanford University.

Edwards, M.L. (1979b). Phonological processes in fricative acquisition. *Papers and Reports on Child Language Development*, *17*, 98–105.

Edwards, M.L. (1979c). Word-position in fricative acquisition. *Papers and Reports on Child Language Development*, *16*, 67–76.

Edwards, M.L. (1983). Issues in phonological assessment. *Seminars in Speech and Language, 4*, 351–374.

Edwards, M.L. (1992). In support of phonological processes. *Language, Speech, and Hearing Services in Schools, 23*, 233–240.

Edwards, M.L. (1994). Phonological process analysis. In E.J. Williams & J. Langsam (Eds.), *Children's phonology disorders: Pathways and patterns* (2nd ed., pp. 43–65). Rockville, MD: American Speech-Language-Hearing Association.

Edwards, M.L. (1995). Developmental phonology. In H. Winitz (Ed.), *Human communication disorders: A review* (Vol. 4, pp. 31–79). Timonium, MD: York.

Edwards, M.L., & Bernhardt, B.H. (1973a). *Phonological analyses of the speech of four children with language disorders.* Unpublished manuscript, Institute for Childhood Aphasia, Stanford University.

Edwards, M.L., & Bernhardt, B.H. (1973b). *Twin speech as the sharing of a phonological system.* Unpublished manuscript, Institute for Childhood Aphasia, Stanford University.

Edwards, M.L., & Shriberg, L.D. (1983). *Phonology: Applications in communicative disorders.* San Diego: College Hill.

Elbert, M., & Gierut, J. (1986). *Handbook of clinical phonology: Approaches to assessment and treatment.* San Diego: College Hill.

Elbert, M., Rockman, B., & Saltzman, D. (1980). *Contrasts: The use of minimal pairs in articulation training.* Austin, TX: Exceptional Resources.

Fairbanks, G. (1960). *Voice and articulation drill book* (2nd ed.). New York: Harper Brothers.

Garnica, O.K., & Edwards, M.L. (1977). Phonological variation in children's speech: The trade-off phenomenon. *Working Papers in Linguistics, 22*, 81–87.

Gierut, J. (1989). Maximal opposition approach to phonological treatment. *Journal of Speech and Hearing Disorders, 54*, 9–19.

Gierut, J. (1990). Differential learning of phonological oppositions. *Journal of Speech and Hearing Research, 33*, 540–549.

Gierut, J. (1992). The conditions and course of clinically induced phonological change. *Journal of Speech and Hearing Research, 35*, 1049–1063.

Green, M.K., & Edwards, M.L. (1992, November). *Phonological awareness skills of phonologically disordered preschoolers.* Poster session presented at the annual convention of the American Speech-Language-Hearing Association, San Antonio, TX.

Grunwell, P. (1975). The phonological analysis of articulation disorders. *British Journal of Disorders of Communication, 10*, 31–42.

Grunwell, P. (1985). *Phonological Assessment of Child Speech (PACS).* Windsor, UK: NFER-Nelson.

Hodson, B.W. (1980). *Assessment of phonological processes.* Danville, IL: Interstate.

Hodson, B.W. (1985). *Computer Analysis of Phonological Processes* [Computer program]. Stonington, IL: PhonoComp.

Hodson, B.W. (1986). *Assessment of Phonological Processes-Revised (APP-R).* Austin, TX: Pro-Ed.

Hodson, B.W., & Paden, E.P. (1991). *Targeting intelligible speech* (2nd ed.). Austin, TX: Pro-Ed.

Ingram, D. (1976). *Phonological disability in children.* New York: American Elsevier.

Ingram, D. (1981). *Procedures for the phonological analysis of children's language.* Baltimore: University Park.

Jakobson, R. (1968). *Child language, aphasia, and phonological universals* (A.R. Keiler, Trans.). The Hague: Mouton. (Original work published 1941)

Jakobson, R. (1971). The sound laws of child language and their place in general phonology. In A. Bar-Adon & W.F. Leopold (Eds.), *Child language: A book of readings* (pp. 75–82). Englewood Cliffs, NJ: Prentice Hall.

Jakobson, R., Fant, G., & Halle, M. (1952). *Preliminaries to speech analysis: The distinctive features and their correlates* (Tech. Rep. 13, MIT Acoustics Laboratory). Cambridge, MA: MIT Press.

Kamhi, A.G., Lee, R., & Nelson, L.K. (1985). Word, syllable, and sound awareness in language disordered children. *Journal of Speech and Hearing Disorders, 50*, 207–212.

Kelman, M.E., & Edwards, M.L. (1994). *Phonogroup: A practical guide for enhancing phonological remediation.* Eau Claire, WI: Thinking Publications.

Khan, L.M.L., & Lewis, N.P. (1986). *Khan-Lewis Phonological Analysis (KLPA).* Circle Pines, MN: American Guidance Service.

Kolk, H., Conture, E.G., Postma, A., & Louko, L.J. (1991, November). *The covert-repair hypothesis and childhood stuttering.* Presented at the annual meeting of the American Speech-Language-Hearing Association, Atlanta.

Levelt, W. (1993). Monitoring and self-repair in speech. *Cognition, 14*, 41–104.

Long, S., & Fey, M. (1988). *Computerized Profiling* [Computer program]. Ithaca, NY: Ithaca College, Department of Speech Pathology and Audiology.

Lorentz, J. (1974). A deviant phonological system of English. *Papers and Reports on Child Language Development, 8*, 55–64.

Louko, L.J. (1995). Phonological characteristics of young children who stutter. *Topics in Language Disorders, 15*, 8–59.

Louko, L.J., Edwards, M.L., & Conture, E.G. (1990). Phonological characteristics of young stutterers and their normally fluent peers: Preliminary observations. *Journal of Fluency Disorders, 15*, 191–210.

Lowe, R.J. (1986). *The ALPHA (Assessment Link Between Phonology and Articulation) Test of Phonology.* East Moline, IL: LinguiSystems.

Masterson, J.J., & Pagan, F.G. (1990). *Macintosh Interactive System for Phonological Analysis (Mac-ISPA).* University: University of Mississippi, Department of Communicative Disorders.

Maxwell, E.M. (1979). Competing analyses of a deviant phonology. *Glossa, 13*, 181–214.

McReynolds, L.V., & Engmann, D. (1975). *Distinctive feature analysis of misarticulations.* Baltimore: University Park.

McReynolds, L.V., & Huston, K. (1971). A distinctive feature analysis of children's misarticulations. *Journal of Speech and Hearing Disorders, 36*, 156–166.

Menyuk, P. (1968). The role of distinctive features in children's acquisition of phonology. *Journal of Speech and Hearing Research, 11*, 138–146.

Oller, D.K. (1973). Regularities in abnormal child phonology. *Journal of Speech and Hearing Disorders, 38*, 36–47.

Oller, D.K., & Delgado, R. (1990). *Logical International Phonetic Programs (LIPP)* [Computer program]. Miami, FL: Intelligent Hearing Systems.

Oller, D.K., & Kelly, C.A. (1974). Phonological substitution processes of a hard-of-hearing child. *Journal of Speech and Hearing Disorders, 39*, 65–74.

Pollack, E., & Rees, N. (1972). Disorders of articulation: Some clinical applications of distinctive feature theory. *Journal of Speech and Hearing Disorders, 37*, 451–461.

Postma, A., & Kolk, H. (1993). The covert-repair hypothesis: Prearticulatory repair processes in normal and stuttered dysfluencies. *Journal of Speech and Hearing Research, 36*, 472–487.

Sagey, E. (1986). *The representation of features and relations in non-linear phonology.* Unpublished doctoral dissertation, Massachusetts Institute of Technology.

Schwartz, R. (1992). Clinical applications of recent advances in phonological theory. *Language, Speech, and Hearing Services in Schools, 23*, 269–276.

Shriberg, L.D. (1986). *PEPPER: Programs to Examine Phonetic and Phonologic Evaluation Records* [Computer program]. Hillsdale, NJ: Lawrence Erlbaum.

Shriberg, L.D., & Kwiatkowski, J. (1980). *Natural process analysis (NPA): A procedure for phonological analysis of continuous speech samples*. New York: John Wiley.

Singh, S., & Frank, D.C. (1972). A distinctive feature analysis of the consonantal substitution pattern. *Language and Speech, 15*, 209–218.

Stampe, D. (1969). The acquisition of phonetic representation. In R.T. Binnick, A. Davison, G.M. Green, & J.L. Morgan (Eds.), *Papers from the fifth regional meeting, Chicago Linguistic Society* (pp. 433–444). Chicago: Chicago Linguistic Society.

Stampe, D. (1979). *A dissertation on natural phonology*. New York: Garland. (Original dissertation completed 1973)

Stemberger, J.P. (1995, June). *The development of syllable structure in English, with emphasis on codas*. Paper presented at the UBC International Conference on Phonological Acquisition, Vancouver, BC.

Tyler, A.A., Edwards, M.L., & Saxman, J.H. (1987). Clinical application of two phonologically based treatment procedures. *Journal of Speech and Hearing Disorders, 52*, 393–409.

Tyler, A.A., Edwards, M.L., & Saxman, J. (1990). Acoustic validation of phonological knowledge and its relationship to treatment. *Journal of Speech and Hearing Disorders, 55*, 251–261.

Vellutino, F., & Scanlon, D. (1987). Phonological coding, phonological awareness, and reading ability: Evidence from a longitudinal and experimental study. *Merrill-Palmer Quarterly, 33*, 321–363.

Webster, P.E., & Plante, A.S. (1992). Effects of phonological impairment on word, syllable, and phoneme segmentation and reading. *Language, Speech, and Hearing Services in Schools, 23*, 176–182.

Weiner, F. (1979). *Phonological Process Analysis* [Test]. Baltimore: University Park.

Weiner, F. (1983). *Process Analysis by Computer (PAC)* [Computer program]. State College, PA: Parrot Software.

Weiner, F. (1988). *Process Analysis: Version 2.0* [Computer program]. State College, PA: Parrot Software.

Wolk, L., Conture, E.G., & Edwards, M.L. (1990). Comorbidity of stuttering and disordered phonology in young children. *South African Journal of Communication Disorders, 37*, 15–20.

Wolk, L., Edwards, M.L., & Conture, E.G. (1993). Co-existence of stuttering and disordered phonology in young children. *Journal of Speech and Hearing Research, 36*, 906–917.

Yaruss, J.S., & Conture, E.G. (1996). Stuttering and phonological disorders in children: Examination of the covert repair hypothesis. *Journal of Speech and Hearing Research, 39*, 349–364.

CHAPTER 2

The Categorization of Phonological Impairment

David Ingram

The study of phonological development in the late 1960s was a period of great excitement and anticipation, driven by two major forces. One was the advent of powerful theoretical proposals, such as generative phonology (Chomsky & Halle, 1968) and natural phonology (Stampe, 1969), which invited their application to both normal children and children with phonological impairments (Ingram, 1976). The other was the collection of data itself. Little was known at the time about development in either group of children. Data-based study of the language of these children was undertaken with full expectations that we would determine significant developmental milestones, based on linguistic generalizations, on both populations. As well, it was anticipated that research would identify the uniqueness of phonological impairment and establish effective procedures for assessment and intervention based upon our findings.

In retrospect, an accurate assessment is that our eyes were bigger than our stomachs; that is, the expectations were greater than the means to achieve them. Today, we are still groping with many of the basic questions that were raised 25 years ago: What methods do we use to assess children? What are the developmental milestones? What linguistic characteristics distinguish normal children from children with impairments? What are the most effective principles for intervention?

In light of the above assessment, this chapter has two goals. First, it takes a brief look at the past and discusses examples of both the mistakes and the gains that have been made. Such examples provide an important background for some of the beliefs I hold today about phonological acquisition in both normal children and children with phonological impairments. The second goal is to present some of these beliefs, including a preliminary linguistic typology of children with phonological impairments.

A SELECTIVE HISTORICAL PERSPECTIVE

This brief historical retrospective begins by discussing two mistakes that have been made in the study of phonological impairment. The word *mistake* is used loosely here to refer to influences that have not positively affected the course of research.

Mistake 1: The Medical Model

The first of these forces is what I refer to as the influence of the medical model (see Ingram, 1987). By *medical model*, I mean the approach to health problems that has been developed by the medical profession. The general model works something like this. Someone comes to the doctor because he or she does not feel well. The following sequence of events then occurs (in many but by no means all instances): first, there is a blood test; next, the blood test is analyzed for some abnormality; next, once the abnormality is determined, the patient's problem is classified as some disease; last, this categorization is used to place the patient into a predetermined program of treatment.

It is argued here that this model has been applied to the field of speech-language pathology without much in the way of discussion or justification. The traditional steps for phonological remediation are as follows:

1. Elicit the child's speech through a test instrument that is relatively quick to administer; our articulation tests are the equivalent to a blood test.
2. Assess the results through a scoring system that likewise is relatively quick to do, often yielding a numerical result and possibly the identification of specific speech errors.
3. Use the results to place the child into some superficial category of phonological impairment based on the results of Step 2 (e.g., open-syllable syndrome, tetism).
4. Use the child's newly found categorization to place the child into a predetermined program of treatment that is needed for this type of child.

This model has an initial appeal to it, particularly with children who have just one or two dominant phonological difficulties. Its general problem, however, is that in many instances it is too simplistic when applied to language, which is a complex, abstract, rule-based cognitive system. Take, for example, Step 1, which has led to the development of articulation tests. Such tests can be of normative value, determining where a child is in relation to his or her peers. Articulation tests per se, however, are not often of much value for fully understanding the nature of a child's linguistic system, whether for theoretical purposes or for purposes of planning intervention. Concerning Step 3, we have not been particularly successful in determining an effective typology of impairment. This is not surprising in that there is also no established typology for the ways that normal children differ from one another. This is a worthy goal, but the elicitation of phonological data through articulation tests is not the means to obtain substantive data sufficient to develop such a typology (see also Shriberg, 1993). Without an effective Step 3, the success of Step 4 will always be restricted, though some success has been achieved, as will be discussed below.

What we need instead of the medical model is a developmental model, one that attempts to study the child's underlying phonological system and the course of acquisition for both normal children and those with phonological impairments. Such a model should have all of the following properties: (a) assessment proceeds until enough data are obtained to characterize the complete range of the child's patterns; (b) intervention strategies are developed that are based on the unique patterns of each child's system, not a predetermined categorization except perhaps of the most general kind (see below); and (c) intervention will need to be based on linguistic principles on how the mind is equipped to acquire language.

Mistake 2: The Linguistic Model

The second mistake is what I will call the influence of the linguistic model. By *linguistic model*, I mean the application of linguistic theories to the understanding of language acquisition in both normal children and children with impairment. At first glance, this might appear to be contrary to the developmental model just outlined, which assumes that research into phonological acquisition requires the use of linguistic theory. The problem being identified, however, is the premature application of linguistic models to developmental issues; that is, the application of new theories before their explanatory power has been completely tested.

It is on this point that our colleagues in the medical profession would probably be quite surprised. In medicine, researchers are quite cautious about testing new theories or treatments before allowing them to be used widely. In medicine, there are testing agencies that watchdog such activities. In speech-language pathology, however, we have no such agencies. Instead, the reverse takes place: The instant a new theory appears on the horizon, it is followed by proposals about how it better describes normal acquisition and, much worse, how it can be used in intervention.

An example of this problem can be seen in the following hypothetical case of a child who is referred to a speech-language pathologist (SLP) for a phonological problem. An analysis of the child's system yields the following description. The child has just four word-initial consonants—[b], [p], [d], and [t]—but no other stops. Sample forms are *pot* [pat], *ball* [ba], *dog* [da], *cake* [tet], and *goat* [dot]. Let us assume that the SLP concludes that working to establish the complete stop inventory is of primary importance for treatment. Here are four phonological analyses on these data, based on distinct phonological theories:

1. *Traditional phonemic theory*: The child has four word-initial phonemes—/p/, /b/, /t/, and /d/.
2. *Phonological process analysis*, based on natural phonology: The child has applied the phonological process of fronting, changing [k] to [t] and [g] to [d].
3. *Jakobson distinctive feature theory*: The child has acquired the distinctive features [labial] and [voice]; /p/ is [+labial] [–voice], /b/ is [+labial] [+voice], /t/ is [–labial][–voice], /d/ is [–labial][+voice].
4. *Nonlinear phonology*: radical underspecification: The child has acquired the distinctive features [coronal] and [voice]; /b/ is [–coronal] [+voice], /p/ is [–coronal], [d] is [+voice], and [t] is not specified for any features. [coronal] is underspecified because it is higher in the feature hierarchy than [labial]; [–voice] is not specified because it is a default feature. Markedness is t > p, d > b.

These are four very distinct phonological analyses of the small set of data in question. What then, are the implications for treatment? They are as follows: regardless of analysis, teach [g] and [k], which are the missing stops. The alternative theories in this instance do not lead to different treatment proposals. I refer to this situation as "theory as description." Although theoretical work is of fundamental importance, we need to exert caution in its extension to practice.

The identification of the two problems above does not mean that progress in the understanding of phonological acquisition has not been made. Next, I will identify two general results over recent years that are more positive, one in the area of descriptive results on phonological acquisition, the other in the area of intervention.

Gain 1: Patterns of Phonological Development

We now have a much better understanding of the patterns of phonological acquisition that children follow. Controversy does exist, and it is likely that each of the findings about to be presented would be challenged by one researcher or another. Yet there are findings today that I feel are fundamental for our understanding phonological acquisition and that will need to be accounted for by any theory of phonological acquisition. These are given as 10 basic assumptions, with the word *assumption* rather than *finding* used to capture their controversial nature (a more detailed discussion of these is in Ingram, 1991):

1. In the first year of life, infants show the ability to perceive a broad range (and possibly all) of the acoustic characteristics of speech sounds in at least simple syllables.
2. Children begin receptive vocabulary development around age 1:0 and have a receptive vocabulary on the order of 250 words around 1:6.

3. Productive vocabulary acquisition at first proceeds very slowly, beginning at approximately 1:0 to 1:6:

Age	0:8	0:10	1:0	1:3	1:6	1:9
Number of Words	0	1	3	19	22	118

4. Around 1:6, a marked increase appears to take place in productive vocabulary acquisition. This increase is often referred to as the *word spurt* (see above).
5. Phonological analysis of the child's first words indicates that there is phonological organization from the onset of acquisition. The organization, however, is restricted to a few basic syllable shapes and phonological features.
6. The child's first distinctive features are not applied across the board but are usually restricted to specific sounds.
7. Children do not begin acquisition by attempting to express all the phonemes of the language. Instead, they attempt a restricted set.
8. The child's patterns of matching and substitution for the target language phonemes show the same restrictions as mentioned in Assumption 6 above.
9. Phonologically organized speech sounds show three patterns of development over the first 6 months of acquisition: (a) lexical (i.e., restricted to single words), (b) gradual (i.e., spreading slowly from one word to several), and (c) abrupt (i.e., suddenly occurring in several words).
10. Despite some individual variation, children within a specific linguistic community will develop a *basic set* of phonologically organized speech sounds. Importantly, these basic sets will differ from language to language.

Here are a few examples of how phonological acquisition looks, based on these assumptions. Below is an example of one English child's acquisition of word-initial stop consonants across six stages (or time periods):

Time	*Consonants in Phonetic Inventory*					
1				d		
2		b		d		
3		b		d		s
4	p	b		d		s
5	p	b	t	d		s
6	p	b	t	d	k	s

The child's gradual development of contrasts supports Assumption 6 above. For example, [voice] first appears as a contrast for labials, then alveolars, and has yet to be acquired for velars.

The example below demonstrates Assumptions 8 and 9. Here we see one child's acquisition of the English stops /b/, /p/, /d/, and /t/ across four stages. This example differs from the previous one, which referred only to the appearance of consonants in the phonetic inventory. Here we are considering how the child's consonants are used in relation to the phonemes in the adult language (which are shown within slashes). Parentheses indicate a sound that is used only once, and the asterisk marks highly frequent sounds. Other sounds that are unmarked are used more than once but not as frequently as those with asterisks.

Stage	*/b/*	*/p/*	*/d/*	*/t/*
1			(d)	
2	*b		d	
3	*b		*d	d
4	*b	(b)	*d	d,t

The acquisition of /d/ shows a gradual emergence of [d], which is infrequent at Stage 1, used at Stage 2, and highly frequent in Stages 3 and 4. This is a very common pattern in the emergence of a speech sound. /b/, however, shows an abrupt emergence at Stage 2. /p/ shows the lexical pattern, with only one word with a [b] for /p/ at Stage 4.

Assumption 10 is based on very recent and mostly unpublished research findings (see Ingram, 1992). It requires the extensive study of languages and the determination of the initial inventories that children use. Below are some preliminary results of mine for four languages concerning what appears to be their basic set of word-initial consonants. By *basic set*, I mean the set of consonants that mark a point at which individual differences between children begin to be lost:

French		*English*				*Italian*				*Quiché*				
m		m	n			m	n			m	n			
b	d	b	d	g		b	d		g	p	t	ʧ	k	ʔ
p	t	p	t	k		p	t	ʧ	k				x	
f	s	f	s		h	f	s							
	l					v								
		w					l			w	l			

We see numerous differences across these inventories. French, for example, has velar consonants, but they are acquired relatively later in French than in the other languages. Meanwhile, French, Italian, and Quiché show the early acquisition of [l], which is acquired relatively later by English-speaking children. Such results are solid evidence that phonological acquisition is more than just overcoming articulatory limitations. Note, for example, the early use of [v] in Italian, which is notoriously late for English children. Pye, Ingram, and List (1987) have shown that the functional load of a sound is of great importance. The more words a child acquires that contain a particular sound, the more likely it is that the sound will be acquired early.

Preliminary results indicate these same differences when children with phonological impairment are compared. For example, Bortolini, Ingram, and Dykstra (1993) examined a group of normal Italian children matched to a group of Italian children with phonological impairment. The results showed virtually identical inventories (i.e., Italian children with an impairment will nonetheless show an early [v], just like Italian normal children). These results provide strong support for the claim that the phonological impairment is indeed a linguistic, not just an articulatory, deficit.

Gain 2: Phonological Intervention

A second gain in our knowledge that can be identified is in the area of phonological intervention. It is by no means the case that everyone agrees on how to do phonological intervention. In fact, there was probably more agreement 25 years ago than there is today. The difference, however, is that today proposals are based upon principles of acquisition; they are not ad hoc suggestions based on intuition or just trial and error. (I say "just trial and error" because trial and error will always be a part of treatment, but treatment should be also theory driven whenever possible.)

Here are four claims about phonological acquisition that have important clinical implications. Each is described briefly, then followed by its implication for phonological intervention:

1. Children's receptive development is in advance of their production. Phonologically, children show perception of phonemic oppositions that may not show up in their production until months later. *Implication:* Initiate intervention with a concentration on developing receptive knowledge. Do not expect correct production to occur simultaneously with receptive development.
2. Children acquire a linguistic system, not specific rules. Phonologically, children are developing a system of phonological oppositions, not specific sounds. *Implication*: Present the child with linguistic material that demonstrates a sound's role in the linguistic system. For example, if a child does not have /s–/, present the child with words with /s–/ that are similar to other words in his system with other sounds (e.g., *six* vs. *fix* vs. *mix*). Second, systematically present a range of speech sounds, not just one.
3. Language acquisition is gradual. The internalization of the linguistic system takes time. It involves the representation of the phonological form of words in the mind and the ability to retrieve that information and translate it into speech production. Therefore, not surprisingly, this process takes several

months, and neither receptive nor productive development is instantaneous. *Implication*: Allow time for children to develop a phonological unit into their receptive knowledge. Do not expect receptive knowledge, or later production, to be established instantaneously.

4. Language acquisition is sensitive to linguistic input. Recent research on cross-linguistic phonological acquisition indicates that the first sounds of children are more influenced by their linguistic prominence in the language than by their assumed articulatory difficulty (see Pye et al., 1987). *Implication*: The phonological information presented to the child should be robust enough to establish its importance in the system. For example, teaching the child a series of words with /s–/ will require the number of words to be sufficiently large as to demonstrate its linguistic value.

Any approach to phonological intervention needs to take these findings into consideration. One approach to phonological intervention is very much founded on these four claims (among others). This is the cyclical model of Hodson and Paden (Hodson & Paden, 1991; Hodson, 1994; and Hodson, Chapter 8 of this volume). This approach demonstrates the effectiveness of intervention procedures when they are founded on basic assumptions on the nature of phonological acquisition.

CURRENT RESEARCH ON PHONOLOGICAL IMPAIRMENT

The previous section has provided a brief assessment of both errors and gains that have been made over the last 25 years of research into the nature of phonological acquisition. Here we turn our attention to current research in this area. This will be done by first discussing the theoretical approach of nonlinear phonology that underlies most of the current research. A basic knowledge of nonlinear phonology is needed to understand and assess the importance of this research as it becomes more and more available. This section is followed by a summary of my own recent research on phonological impairment, including a tentative descriptive classification.

Nonlinear Phonology

The caution expressed above about the premature application of linguistics theories is distinct from the need for researchers to work within a linguistic theory. Eventually, theories will result in useful applications. One excellent example of this has been the application of natural phonology to the description and remediation of children with phonological impairments. The identification of phonological processes has provided a descriptive means for grouping children's error patterns into general terms such as *stopping and fronting* (see Edwards and Hodson, Chapters 1 and 8 of this volume).

At this point, natural phonology within linguistics is an old theory. After being developed by Stampe (1969) and worked on in the 1970s, it was adapted quickly by those working in phonological acquisition and was developed even more by the latter researchers than by theoretical linguists. In more recent years, phonological theory has evolved into an approach known as nonlinear phonology. This approach is the dominant one in linguistics and is becoming the most widely used approach in phonological acquisition. It has also been applied to work with children with phonological impairments (see Bernhardt, 1992; Bernhardt & Stoel-Gammon, 1994).

It is premature in my view to claim that nonlinear phonology will revolutionize our approach to phonological assessment and remediation. The advisement above concerning premature application is just as relevant for work in this new theory as it is for earlier ones. Note that two of the theories proposed in my hypothetical accounts on the analysis of the stop consonants were nonlinear accounts of the data. At the same time, nonlinear phonology holds promise, and anyone interested in phonological remediation should have some basic knowledge of it. The references above provide a starting point.

It is not my purpose here to provide a tutorial on nonlinear phonology. What I would like to do, however, is give an assessment of the major aspects of the theory in relation to their potential application to the field of phonological impairment. This assessment will focus on the topics of feature hierarchy, phonological representations, and prosodic structure.

Feature Hierarchy

The notion of phonological feature is basic and is used in a range of theories. In earlier theories, features were seen as comprising bundles or groupings that corresponded to what have been called phonemes. A phoneme such as English /b/, for example, would be an abbreviation for a set of features such as [+consonantal] [–vocalic] [–continuant] [+anterior] [–coronal] [+voice]. Those features that lead to differences in meanings between words are called *distinctive features*.

Nonlinear phonology keeps much of this approach to features. It differs, however, in at least two fundamental ways. One is that features are seen as part of a greater structure or *hierarchy* such that some features are ranked higher than others. Figure 2–1 provides a summary of the feature hierarchy given in Bernhardt and Gilbert (1992) for English. Within the hierarchy, some features are more basic than others and can therefore be predicted. For example, the hierarchy begins at the root node, where four features attach, and two lower nodes, the laryngeal node and the place node. The laryngeal node contains two features, whereas the place node contains three lower nodes (i.e., the labial, coronal, and dorsal). (See Bernhardt & Gilbert, 1992, for details; the use of this particular hierarchy here is purely demonstrative.)

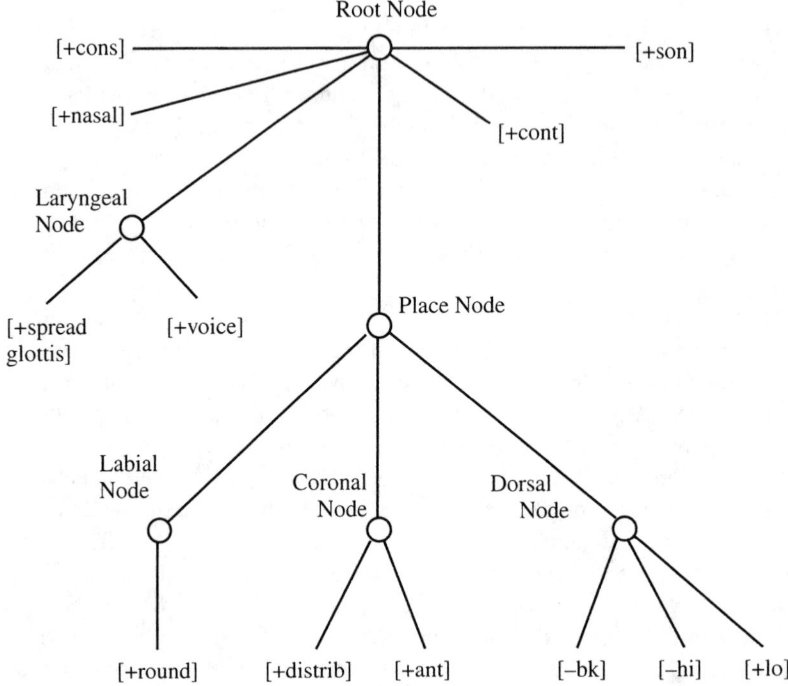

Figure 2–1 Feature Geometry for English. *Source:* Reprinted with permission from B.H. Bernhardt, and J.G. Gilbert, Applying Linguistic Theory to Speech-Language Pathology: The Case for Non-Linear Phonology, *Clinical Linguistics and Phonetics*. Vol. 6, p. 128, © 1992, Taylor & Francis, Ltd.

A second aspect of nonlinear phonology is that the theory has altered the features that are being used within the hierarchy from the more traditional terms. The change has been toward developing a theory of features that is based on the articulators of speech (e.g., the lips, tongue blade, tongue body, and larynx). Features that are not articulator based—for example, [velar]—have been replaced by [dorsal], the feature for the tongue body. Understanding current feature theory requires an understanding of these new features and how they participate in the feature hierarchy.

The potential appeal of the feature hierarchy to those working within phonological acquisition is that it can account for how children's features are acquired. We could propose that the features at the top of the hierarchy are acquired first, followed by those below. This is a proposal that is essentially Jakobsonian in nature, except that the feature system is much more developed than at the time of Jakobson

(1941/1968). In remediation, we could establish where the child is in his or her feature acquisition and then determine which features to add on the basis of the feature hierarchy (see Bernhardt & Gilbert, 1992).

Much research will be needed before we can say with confidence that these proposals are valid. One difficulty resides in the feature hierarchy itself. There are many proposals in the phonological literature, and there is much debate about its actual nature. It is difficult to apply a feature hierarchy when its details are still in such a state of uncertainty. Second, we know from numerous studies that children show varied developmental paths in their feature acquisition (e.g., Ferguson & Farwell, 1975). Toward this end, Rice and Avery (1995) have established a feature hierarchy for acquisition that allows children much choice regarding which features they will begin to acquire. Last, my own work on feature acquisition suggests that children can follow virtually any course of feature acquisition in the early stages and that they only begin to look alike when they reach some set of shared or *core* features (i.e., those that underlie the basic set of sounds in the inventories given above). If these preliminary results on normal acquisition are borne out in future work, it is not obvious what contribution the notion of a feature hierarchy will make to phonological remediation.

Representations

A fundamental aspect of phonological theory for years has been the notion of a phonological representation (i.e., the distinction of an underlying representation that is more abstract than the surface phonetic representation). The examination of the nature of the more abstract representation has been a central issue within nonlinear phonology, particularly the question of which features are present and absent.

To examine this issue, let us consider a consonantal system with the phonemes /b/, /p/, /t/, /d/, and /f/. Such a system would involve the representation of the features [labial], [coronal], [voice], and [continuant]. In general terms, two ways have been suggested to represent these features. One is known as radical underspecification (RU). RU proposes that only marked features are shown underlyingly; other features are supplied by redundancy rules. Possible redundancy rules might be the following: obstruents are unmarked for [–labial], [–voice], [+coronal], and [–continuant]. Our system above would then have the following underlying representation:

	/	*b*	*p*	*t*	*d*	*f*	/
labial		+	+			+	
coronal		–	–			–	
voice		+			+		
continuant						+	

All the features not specified would be filled in by the redundancy rules above. An advantage of this approach is that the number of specifications indicates how marked the system is. In this case, we see that /t/ is the least marked segment and that /b/ and /f/ are the most marked.

An alternative to RU is contrastive specification (CU), which proposes that all and only distinctive features are marked underlyingly. In our example above, we have the following contrasts (i.e., minimal pairs that differ only by a single feature): +/–voice: /b/ /p/, /t/ /d/; +/–continuant /f/ /p/; +/–labial /b/ /d/, /p/ /t/. This would result in the following underlying representation:

	/	*b*	*p*	*t*	*d*	*f*	/
labial		+	+	–	–		
coronal							
voice		+	–	–	+		
continuant			–			+	

Blank spaces would be filled in with redundancy rules as well, but these would be more specific to the individual system. For example, we would need to claim that if [+continuant], then [+labial]; if [+labial], then [–coronal]; otherwise [+coronal]; and so forth.

The discussion of these alternatives is currently underway concerning their application to normal phonological acquisition. The limited literature to date suggests that RU is a better model for the study of acquisition (Dinnsen, 1996; Ingram, 1995; Stemberger & Stoel-Gammon, 1991). One reason for this preference is that the specifications and redundancy rules make predictions about the child's order of acquisition of speech sounds and the kinds of errors that he or she makes. For example, in the RU representation above, the predictions about acquisition order are t > d, p > b, f, based on the number of marked features. Further, the redundancy rules look a lot like the phonological processes of natural phonology. For example, if obstruents are marked for [+continuant], a phoneme without the feature [continuant] should be redundantly [–continuant]. Thus the child who is acquiring /s/ but has not acquired the feature [continuant] will redundantly produce /s/ as [t] (e.g., stopping).

The proponents of nonlinear phonology argue that it captures both the underlying knowledge of the child and the error patterns, whereas natural phonology is more restricted to error patterns. In this sense, nonlinear phonology is an improvement, and it is of value for speech-language pathologists to consider what children know as well as their errors. It is less obvious, however, how to translate this theory at this point into any changes in practice. The field for a long time has discussed assessment and remediation in relation to minimal pairs (e.g., Ingram, 1976).

One possible application that I have pursued in recent work is in the area of assessment. In Ingram (1981) and (1976), I suggested that assessment include the determination of children's phonetic inventories as well as their phonological processes. Such suggestions, however, lead only to inventories of phonemes. The application of nonlinear phonology to these inventories can provide better insight into which features a child has acquired and which ones need to be acquired. This can be shown by examining the word-initial consonantal phonological inventories of a child with a phonological impairment, based on data in Shriberg and Kwiatkowski (1979). (The sounds that the child produced are within [ ], and the target English phonemes are within / /):

[m] /m/	[n] /n/	
[b] /b/	[d] /d, g, ð/	
	[t] /p, t, k, s/	
[w] /w, l, r/		[h] /f, h/

This child has the phonological processes of fronting and stopping. What may be less apparent from just examining these inventories is the pervasive use of the [voice] feature. In Ingram (1990), a detailed CU analysis of these data indicated that [voice] is the most used feature in the child's system, allowing the child to distinguish the [d] /d, g, ð/ from [t] /p, t, k, s/ and the continuants [w] /w, l, r/ from [h] /f, h/. This finding coupled with others results in a characterization of one kind of phonological impairment in which [voice] is used despite problems with supralaryngeal features.

Prosodic Structure

The third aspect of nonlinear phonology of primary importance is its emphasis on distinct levels of prosodic structure. Although mention of the syllable in phonology is common, nonlinear phonology has focused much more directly on developing our knowledge of distinct prosodic levels above the segment. Again, as with the aspects above, there are a variety of proposals in the phonological literature. One widely cited view is that there is a hierarchy of prosodic structure, called appropriately the *prosodic hierarchy* (Nespor & Vogel, 1986). One common set of prosodic categories that make up the prosodic hierarchy is as follows (where > means "consists of"; e.g., a phonological word consists of feet): phonological word > foot > syllable > mora.

The prosodic structure below the foot deserves further elaboration. In an adaptation of the approach in Demuth and Fee (1995), a syllable consists of an onset consonant and a rhyme. The rhyme contains a nuclear vowel, optionally followed by a coda. The coda can be either a consonant or vowel. The elements that fill the rhyme are moras, or timing units. This results in the following structure:

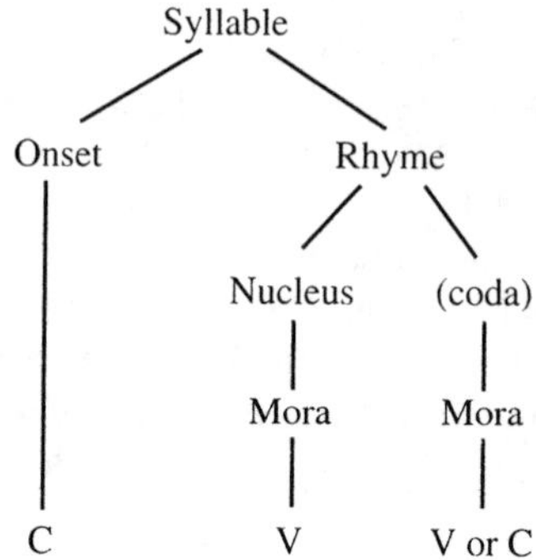

This structure is proposed to be universal (i.e., it underlies the phonological structure of languages).

Demuth and Fee (1995) attempted to account for how children might acquire a syllable structure of this kind. They proposed on the basis of the analysis of acquisition data, that the stages below are the first three stages that children follow. In Stage 1, the *core syllable stage*, children begin acquisition with a core syllable that is a CV (i.e., a syllable consisting of a single-consonant onset and a nucleus and therefore a single mora, e.g., [dɑ]). In Stage 2, the *minimal word stage*, words consist of minimal words (i.e., binary feet). There are two possible binary foot structures:

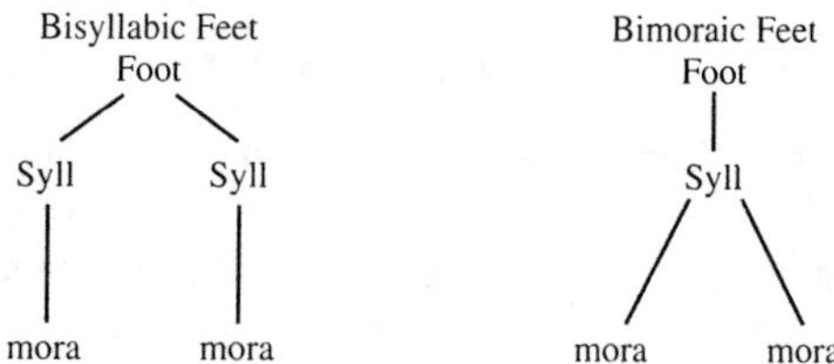

These two structures yield three possible syllable structures: CVCV, CVC, and CVV (e.g., [badi], [kit], and [ki:]). In Stage 3, the *stress feet stage*, children use multiple-foot structures that also carry stress.

The Demuth and Fee paper is one of the first attempts to account for prosodic acquisition within the nonlinear model (see Fikkert, 1994). It also accounts for some unexplained patterns that have been described in the literature. Stemberger (1992), for example, observed that his daughter at one stage showed variable pronunciations of words of the following kind: *bite* [bɑj] and [bɑt], and *grape* [dɑj] and [dɑp]. Note that all these forms comply with the minimal word stage (i.e., they all have two moras).

If further research supports these stages, they have obvious clinical potential. The remediation of a child's speech at the onset of phonological acquisition can take the child through these stages. One child, for example, might use CVCV minimal words, whereas another might use CVV ones. The recognition of moraic structure in the latter case would be another example of children with phonological impairment showing compensatory development. They may delete final consonants, but they are using another means to construct minimal words.

THE CLASSIFICATION OF PHONOLOGICAL IMPAIRMENT

The study of normal and nonnormal development has at its core the question of whether the latter is simply a delayed version of the former or has its own distinct properties. This is the case regardless of the linguistic domain. For example, researchers who study grammatical acquisition in children with specific language impairment have spent a great deal of time trying to determine whether these children have a specific linguistic or processing deficit (see Rice, 1994).

The same question exists for those who study children with phonological impairment. In this case, the processing accounts can be claims that these children have either auditory processing deficits and/or articulatory deficits. A specific phonological deficit can be proposed as well (e.g., that these children cannot form appropriate phonological representations).

Research to answer this question has a logical sequence to it. First, we need to select a phonological theory within which to work. As discussed in the previous section, many current researchers have selected nonlinear phonology for this purpose. Second, we need to determine the course of normal acquisition and the extent to which normal children vary among each other. This is an ongoing and incomplete process at this time. Third, we need to determine the patterns used by children with phonological impairment and compare them to those of normal children.

Our progress in this third area, the study of phonological impairment, is restricted in several ways. One inherent way is that it is tied to progress in normal acquisition, the findings on which are still far from completed. Further, our database at this time must be recognized as relatively limited. Even exceptions to this such as the Wisconsin database (see Shriberg, Chapter 5 of this volume), in which 64 children have been studied, are situations in which the data are still being analyzed. These data are restricted primarily to English-speaking children, with data from other languages just beginning to appear. Although theoretical proposals can be offered, we have a great deal of description ahead before we can offer, with confidence, a theoretical account of phonological impairment.

Toward this end, my own research has been directed to establishing a better descriptive understanding of the patterns of phonological impairment, both for

English-speaking children and for children from other linguistic communities. This research will be summarized in the next three sections, looking first at the cross-linguistic data, next at some recent results on English-speaking children, and last at a tentative descriptive typology based on these findings.

Cross-Linguistic Research

The cross-linguistic research is of particular importance because it is the richest means to isolate the influence of articulatory versus linguistic factors in phonological impairment. For example, if phonological development in all children is constrained by articulatory maturation, then all children, regardless of linguistic community, should follow similar developmental patterns. Let us call this the biological theory of phonological acquisition. We have seen that data from normal children disprove this theory. This is not to deny that there are articulatory constraints, but children at a very early stage of word acquisition are capable of adapting their articulations to the language that they are acquiring.

The influence of articulation becomes more interesting when children with phonological impairments are brought into the question. Here we can identify two distinct theories on how such children should look:

1. *The linguistic theory*: All speech development is determined by articulatory and linguistic factors. *The prediction*: Children with phonological impairments will look like younger normal children within their linguistic communities.
2. *The linguistic/articulatory theory*: Normal speech development is determined by articulatory and linguistic factors, but phonological delay is determined only by articulatory factors. *The prediction*: Children with phonological impairments will look similar to one another, regardless of linguistic community.

Although it is too early to decide between these two theories, preliminary results thus far support the linguistic theory. We have known for some time from group studies that English-speaking children with phonological impairments look similar to normal children (e.g., Ingram, 1981; Shriberg, 1993; Stoel-Gammon, 1985). Data from other language communities, however, have been slower in coming. One early exception is the work on Swedish by Magnusson (1983) and Nettelbladt (1983), who studied children with phonological impairments. These studies did not concentrate on a direct comparison of their results, but such a comparison can be done. Below are my analyses of the word-initial consonantal inventories of a normal Swedish child at age 2:2 and those of Nettelbladt's 10 children with phonological delay:

Swedish:

Normal

m	n	
p	t	
b	d	
f	θ	h

Phonological Impairment

m	n		
p	t		
b	d		
f	s		h
v			
		j	

We can see that the two inventories are very similar. For example, the normal child is still lacking the velar stops and the voiced fricative /v/. The phonological delay group also lack velar stops, yet they show the early use of /v/, a pattern also found with Italian children.

Bortolini, Ingram, and Dykstra (1993) directly compared word initial consonants in nine normal children and nine Italian children with phonological impairments. Frequency criteria were used to indicate whether sounds were infrequent (parentheses), used, or frequent (asterisks). Results are as follows:

Italian:

Normal

*p	*t	*ʧ	*k
*b	*d		g
*f	*s		
*v	(z)		

Phonological Impairment

*p	*t	(ʧ)	*k
*b	d		(g)
*f	s		
v			

Here we see the early use of an affricate and the striking use of /v/, both later acquisitions for English-speaking children. The /v/, in fact, is one of the latest acquisitions by English-speaking normal children, yet it is one of the earlier acquisitions by the Italian children with phonological delay. We find, however, that it is a much more frequent sound in the input to Italian children than it is in the input to English-speaking ones.

Other more recent studies include work by Topbas (1992) on Turkish. Below is a comparison of the initial consonants of normal Turkish children at 1:9 with those of a child with a phonological impairment at 6:0.

Turkish:

Normal

m	n		
b	d		
p	t	ʧ	k
		j	

Phonological Impairment

m	n	
b	d	
p	t	ʧ
		j

The Turkish inventory is striking due to the lack of early fricatives despite a system of eight fricatives, both voiced and voiceless. We often think of a lack of fricatives in English-speaking children as a sign of delay, yet this is normal for Turkish children. We see the same lack of fricatives, yet we see the early affricate just as in the normal data. Findings similar to those above can be found for Brazilian Portuguese in Yavas and Lamprecht (1988) and for Dutch in an extensive recent study by Beers (1995).

In summary, preliminary data from a small range of languages support the phonological rather than the articulatory account of phonological delay. This results in two preliminary conclusions: (a) normal children show early phonological inventories unique to their linguistic environment, and (b) children with phonological delay show systems like normal children in their own linguistic environment rather than like phonologically delayed children from other environments.

Data on English-Speaking Children

General comparisons such as those above are important to show the influence of the linguistic environment on phonological development. Such studies obscure, however, the differences that may exist between individual children. Although children with phonological impairments may generally look like their same-language peers, they may show more subtle linguistic differences. Results such as those just cited therefore do not rule out the possibility that there may be distinct types of phonological impairment. The determination of a typology of phonological impairment will require many detailed analyses of individual children.

My own single-subject phonological analyses have led me to a descriptive linguistic typology of phonological impairment. This typology is descriptive in the sense that it has evolved from the analysis of individual children. It is linguistic in that it concentrates on the phonological patterns that the children display. Such a linguistic typology can be contrasted with those developed from a medical model (see Shriberg, Chapter 5 of this volume). It is also not an explanatory typology in that the underlying mechanisms that lead to each type are not established but are only speculative at this time (see Ingram, 1989, for a discussion of description vs. explanation in first-language acquisition).

Two forms of information are at the center of the typology. One is the examination of the phonological systems of the children; the other is the comparison of the system in relation to the child's vocabulary size. The latter issue has been relatively unexplored in the study of children with phonological impairments. The typology is proposed with full recognition of its highly tentative nature:

- *Type 1: Children with Phonological Delays*. These are children who show an age delay in development but who have relatively intact relations holding between developmental stage and vocabulary and between laryngeal and supralaryngeal development. That is, they show the phonological patterns of younger normal children, and they have vocabularies that are commensurate with their phonological level. To explain this type of child, we need to establish the factor that causes the delay.

- *Type 2: Children with Developmentally Distinct Phonologies.* These are children who have acquired relatively large vocabularies but who express them with a severely impaired phonological system. Case studies on such children have been discussed in several places, including Leonard (1985). They are cited as evidence that some children with phonological impairments do not look like younger normal children. I have argued elsewhere, however (Ingram, 1987), that these children are using patterns typical of younger children, but only patterns used in the very earliest stages of development. This observation led me to propose the following hypothesis about when a young child's system does not look like those of younger normal children: *The extent to which the phonology of a child with a phonological impairment differs from that of a younger normal child is the consequence of an inverse relation between the child's stage of phonological acquisition and the size of the child's vocabulary.*
- *Type 3: Children with Socially Influenced Phonological Patterns.* The above type can eliminate some of the published cases of unusual phonological patterns, but not all of them. For those cases that remain, it is possible to speculate that an additional social pressure has been at work that forces the child to use a particularly uncommon speech pattern. One possibility is that the child may be aware of his or her speech difficulties and try extreme measures to improve. Another possibility for school-age children is that the social environment may involve teasing or other undue pressure to force the child to correct an error. Unusual patterns may even be introduced during intervention. One such case can be found in Compton (1970). Compton reported on a child who was saying *sock* as [kak]. To alter this, the clinician had him practice an extended [sss] before *sock*. The result of this effort was that the child changed the production to [skak]. Such a change could well be the goal of the clinician, who may have the establishment of consonant clusters in mind. The point here, however, is that the intermediate production is not common in normally developing children. The establishment of this type will require detailed examinations of the child's entire linguistic environment.
- *Type 4: Children with Supralaryngeal Developmental Delays.* These are children with advanced development of the feature [voice] relative to place distinctions made in the supralaryngeal region. We have already seen a case study showing this pattern. Data suggesting that this type exists have come from the study of larger samples of English-speaking normal children compared to samples from children with phonological impairments (Ingram, 1990) and also from results from Italian children (Bortolini et al., 1993). Ingram (1990) observed that normal children tend to acquire the stop series [b, d, g] before any voice distinctions emerge. The children with phonological impair-

ment, however, had a greater tendency to show incomplete stop series with at least one voice contrast (e.g., systems such as [b], [d], [t], or [b], [d], [p], [t]). There was even one case of a child with only a voice contrast but no place (i.e., [t], [d]). In the study on Italian children, it was found that the normal children showed twice as many voice errors as place errors, whereas the children with phonological impairments showed twice as many place errors as voice errors. The proposed account would be the delayed maturation of the supralaryngeal musculature in relation to that of the larynx. At the same time, the child's ability to organize a linguistic system is intact and compensates to the best of its ability in light of the specific maturational delay.

CONCLUSION

The research over the last 25 years has made great gains in our understanding of phonological acquisition in both normal children and children with phonological impairments. Here I have tried to provide a historical overview on this research and give an assessment of the current state of affairs. In both cases, this has been a highly selective and personal point of view, with other chapters in this volume providing other views and interpretations.

Regarding the historical perspective, I have identified both positive and negative influences in both research and application. Regarding research, a strong positive contribution has been the range of descriptive findings that have come forth. Although our data collection is far from complete, we understand a great deal more now than we did 25 years ago. We also have been able to make use of some of these findings to develop research-based applications in remediation, such as allowing time for children to internalize new linguistic knowledge before they express it and presenting children with a range of phonological material, not just one sound at a time.

At the same time, I have identified what I feel are less positive contributions to our development of effective remediation. One of these contributions is the persistence of the medical model approach, which assumes that language can be treated in the same mechanical fashion as medical problems. Articulation tests in more complex cases of phonological impairment are not comprehensive analytic procedures, and remedial decisions based on them are questionable in a number of ways. At the same time, I have warned against the premature application of new theoretical proposals, which require much more clinical testing than usually practiced before they are presented to SLPs. Such suggestions may not be of direct service to the children they are expected to benefit and may turn off SLPs to future proposals as well.

The discussion of this historical perspective was followed by an assessment of current research in the field. The first part of this assessment presented the current theoretical approach of nonlinear phonology. The caution against premature application does not mean that theoretical models should not be explored to better our understanding of phonological acquisition. This model provides interesting proposals about feature hierarchies, the nature of children's representations, and prosodic patterns. I expressed some reservations on the applicability of feature hierarchies but also stated that the nonlinear approach to representations and prosodic structure is likely to yield useful results both in theory and application.

The last section presented my own research on cross-linguistic acquisition and the development of a descriptive taxonomy of phonological impairment. The cross-linguistic data are very limited at this time, but they show that overall, children with phonological impairments look more like the normal children in their linguistic community than like children with phonological impairments in other linguistic environments. If this finding is maintained, it is strong evidence for the linguistic interpretation of impairment over one of just articulatory constraints. These children are capable of phonological acquisition and use their phonological abilities to compensate for those factors that are causing their delay.

The descriptive typology is presented to provide a preliminary understanding of how individual children may vary from each other. There appear to be maturational and social factors that may contribute to the individual patterns that we see. The preliminary typology suggests that we need to pay more attention to (a) vocabulary size in relation to the child's phonological system, (b) the social and clinical environment, and (c) the distinct articulators involved in phonology, such as the larynx as opposed to the tongue. The typology is not at a stage such that it yields established clinical implications, but the hope is that more research on it may lead to that point.

REFERENCES

Beers, M. (1995). *The phonology of normally developing and language-impaired children*. Unpublished PhD dissertation, University of Amsterdam.

Bernhardt, B. (1992). Developmental implications of nonlinear phonological theory. *Clinical Linguistics and Phonetics, 6*, 259–281.

Bernhardt, B., & Gilbert, J. (1992). Applying linguistic theory to speech-language pathology: The case for non-linear phonology. *Clinical Linguistics and Phonetics, 6*, 123–145.

Bernhardt, B., & Stoel-Gammon, C. (1994). Nonlinear phonology: Introduction and clinical application. *Journal of Speech and Hearing Research, 37*, 123–143.

Bortolini, U., Ingram, D., & Dykstra, K. (1993, June). *The acquisition of the feature [voice] in normal and phonologically delayed Italian children*. Paper presented at the Symposium on Research in Child Language Disorders, University of Wisconsin, Madison.

Chomsky, N., & Halle, M. (1968). *The sound pattern of English*. New York: Harper & Row.

Compton, A. (1970). Generative studies of children's phonological disorders. *Journal of Speech and Hearing Disorders, 35*, 315–339.

Demuth, K., & Fee, J. (1995). *Minimal words in early phonological development.* Unpublished manuscript, Brown University and Dalhousie University.

Dinnsen, D. (1996). Context-sensitive underspecification and the acquisition of phonemic contrasts. *Journal of Child Language, 23*, 57–79.

Ferguson, C., & Farwell, C. (1975). Words and sounds in early language acquisition. *Language, 51*, 419–439.

Fikkert, P. (1994). *On the acquisition of prosodic structure.* Unpublished PhD dissertation, University of Leiden.

Hodson, B. (1994). Determining phonological intervention priorities: Expediting intelligibility gains. In E. Williams & J. Langsam (Eds.), *Children's phonology disorders: Pathways and patterns* (pp. 67–87). Rockville, MD: American Speech-Language-Hearing Association.

Hodson, B., & Paden, E. (1991). *Targeting intelligible speech: A phonological approach to remediation* (2nd ed.). Austin, TX: Pro-Ed.

Ingram, D. (1976). *Phonological disability in children.* London: Edward Arnold.

Ingram, D. (1981). *Procedures for the phonological analysis of children's language.* Baltimore: University Park.

Ingram, D. (1987). Categories of phonological disorder. In *First international symposium on specific language disorders in children* (pp. 88–99). Middlesex, UK: Association for All Speech Impaired Children.

Ingram, D. (1989). *First language acquisition: Method, description, and explanation.* Cambridge, UK: Cambridge University Press.

Ingram, D. (1990, November). *The acquisition of the feature [voice] in normal and phonologically delayed English children.* Paper presented at the annual meeting of the American-Speech-Language-Hearing Association, Seattle, WA.

Ingram, D. (1991). Toward a theory of phonological acquisition. In J. Miller (Ed.), *Research perspectives on language disorders* (pp. 55–72). Boston: College Hill.

Ingram, D. (1992). Early phonological acquisition: A crosslinguistic perspective. In C. Ferguson, L. Menn, & C. Stoel-Gammon (Eds.), *Phonological development* (pp. 147–158). Parkton, MD: York.

Ingram, D. (1995). The acquisition of negative constraints, the OCP, and underspecified representations. In J. Archibald (Ed.), *Phonological acquisition and phonological theory* (pp. 63–79). Hillsdale, NJ: Lawrence Erlbaum.

Jakobson, R. (1968). *Child language, aphasia, and phonological universals* (A. Keiler, Trans.). The Hague: Mouton. (Original work published 1941)

Leonard, L. (1985). Unusual and subtle phonological behavior in the speech of phonologically disordered children. *Journal of Speech and Hearing Research, 24*, 389–405.

Magnusson, E. (1983). *The phonology of language disordered children* (Travaux de l'Institut de Linguistique de Lund, No. 17). Lund: CWK Gleerup.

Nespor, M., & Vogel, I. (1986). *Prosodic phonology.* Dordrecht, the Netherlands: Foris.

Nettelbladt, U. (1983). *Developmental studies of dysphonology in children.* Lund: CWK Gleerup.

Pye, C., Ingram, D., & List, H. (1987). A comparison of initial consonant acquisition in English and Quiché. In K.E. Nelson & A. van Kleeck (Eds.), *Children's language* (Vol. 6, pp. 175–190). Hillsdale, NJ: Lawrence Erlbaum.

Rice, K., & Avery, P. (1995). Variability in a deterministic model of language acquisition: A theory of segmental elaboration. In J. Archibald (Ed.), *Phonological acquisition and phonological theory* (pp. 23–42). Hillsdale, NJ: Lawrence Erlbaum.

Rice, M. (1994). Grammatical categories of children with specific language impairment. In R. Watkins & M. Rice (Eds.), *Specific language impairment in children* (pp. 69–89). Baltimore: Paul H. Brookes.

Shriberg, L. (1993). Four new speech and prosody-voice measures for genetics research and other studies in developmental phonological disorders. *Journal of Speech and Hearing Research, 36*, 105–140.

Shriberg, L., & Kwiatkowski, J. (1979). *Natural process analysis.* Madison: University of Wisconsin, Department of Communicative Disorders.

Stampe, D. (1969). The acquisition of phonetic representation. In R.T. Binnick, A. Davison, G.M. Green, & J. Morgan (Eds.), *Papers from the fifth regional meeting of the Chicago Linguistic Society* (pp. 443–454). Chicago: Chicago Linguistic Society.

Stemberger, J. (1992). A performance constraint on compensatory lengthening in child phonology. *Language and Speech, 35*, 207–218.

Stemberger, J., & Stoel-Gammon, C. (1991). The underspecification of coronals: Evidence from language acquisition and performance errors. In C. Paradis & J.F. Prunet (Eds.), *The special status of coronals: Internal and external evidence* (pp. 181–199). New York: Academic Press.

Stoel-Gammon, C. (1985). Phonetic inventories, 15–24 months: A longitudinal study. *Journal of Speech and Hearing Research, 28*, 505–512.

Topbas, C. (1992, August). *A pilot study of phonological acquisition for Turkish children and its implications for phonological disorders.* Paper presented to the Sixth International Conference on Turkish Linguistics, Anadolu University, Eskisehir, Turkey.

Yavas, M., & Lamprecht, R. (1988). Processes and intelligibility in disordered phonology. *Clinical Linguistics and Phonetics, 2*, 329–345.

Chapter 3

From Articulation to Phonology: The Challenge of Change

Mary Elbert

The slogan "Lifelong learning is the key to success" has become a catchphrase of the 1990s for everything from early childhood education to elder hostels, but throughout the years, not just the 1990s, it certainly has been more than a slogan for speech-language pathologists. In a profession that is constantly developing and changing in the midst of research and practice, it is a way of life.

Undergraduates in the discipline of speech-language pathology often express frustration when there are no clear-cut, unequivocal answers to clinical questions. This can be either terribly frustrating or extremely challenging. There is a certain excitement in becoming aware that there is still much to be discovered and that each person in the profession has the potential to contribute to the body of knowledge that constitutes the basis of our work. Obviously, those of us who have been committed to research in the area of child phonology have considered it a challenge.

In thinking about this chapter, I have recalled the way in which the area of child phonology has changed since the late 1960s when I was a graduate student. At that time, my research exhibited a strong behaviorist perspective on the issue of generalization. My experimental procedures still owe a debt to behaviorism, but my view of generalization has become more cognitively based. This change in perspective on my part and on the part of many colleagues reflects an area of study undergoing dynamic growth. My focus in this chapter will be on some of the changes that have occurred and how the research of many people has contributed to these changes and to the substantial increase in our knowledge base.

A QUICK OVERVIEW

To begin with, in the late 1960s and early 1970s, we talked about "articulation," not "phonology." Van Riper had just published his fourth edition of *Speech Correction: Principles and Methods* (1963), and McDonald's (1964) work focused on the influence of context on articulation. This emphasis soon changed. On the horizon was the *Fisher-Logemann Test of Articulation Competence* (Fisher & Logemann, 1971), which introduced a place-voice-manner pattern analysis, and results of studies by Compton (1975) and Weber (1970) suggested that there was a linguistic component to speech-sound problems.

The landmark work of McReynolds and her colleagues (McReynolds & Bennett, 1972; McReynolds & Engmann, 1975; McReynolds & Huston, 1971) introduced distinctive feature analysis as a basis for discovering patterns of speech errors described in terms of distinctive features. It was the publication of Ingram's *Phonological Disability in Children (*1976) that introduced speech-language pathologists to the linguistic concepts of phonological processes. From that point on, our work turned in a direction that was to change our thinking about assessment and treatment of disordered speech. Numerous researchers, many of whom are contributors to this book, explored the possibilities of describing children's speech-sound problems as phonological processes.

AN EXPERIMENTAL (SENTIMENTAL) JOURNEY ACROSS THREE DECADES

Decade 1: Late 1960s and Early 1970s

My own research journey began during my early graduate education and my master's thesis under the direction of Ralph Shelton. The thesis, published in the *Journal of Speech and Hearing Research* in 1967, was entitled "A Task for Evaluation of Articulation Change: I. Development of Methodology" (Elbert, Shelton, & Arndt, 1967). As far as I know, this was the first use of what is now known as a probe measure—that is, an ongoing measure of change. Previously, all measures of change had been based on pre-post articulation tests or other global measures. This early research demonstrated the use of a method for measuring change and also a fact that had been recognized by clinicians but never before demonstrated experimentally: Cognate sounds of treated sounds changed without direct treatment. This change was attributed to the similarity in features. The fact that other unrelated sounds did not change provided further support for this finding. Specifically, my study demonstrated that if you teach /s/, the cognate sound /z/ will also change even if it is not treated; however, /r/ will not change. This early work solidified my interest in clinical research and began my career-long interest in trying to understand the process of generalization.

There were a number of investigations of articulation generalization during the late 1960s and early 1970s and continuing into the 1980s. One type of generalization demonstrated in a number of studies was that in which a target sound taught in a few exemplar words was extended to untaught words containing the same sound (Arndt, Elbert, & Shelton, 1971; Elbert & McReynolds, 1975, 1978, 1985; Elbert et al., 1967; Hoffman, 1983; McReynolds, 1972; McReynolds & Elbert, 1981; Mowrer, 1971; Powell & Elbert, 1984; Shelton, Elbert, & Arndt, 1967). This basic finding has been replicated many times; thus it seems clear that children extend their correct use of a sound taught in only a few exemplars to a larger set of untrained items containing the same sound.

Other types of generalization have been observed to occur *across word positions* (Elbert & McReynolds, 1975, 1978; McReynolds, 1972; Powell & McReynolds, 1969; Rockman, 1983) and across more complex linguistic units (Gierut, 1985; McLean, 1970; McReynolds, 1972; Wright, Shelton, & Arndt, 1969). A gradient of correct production has been demonstrated from imitative tasks, to reading, to spontaneous speech.

A more complex type of generalization has been observed in *across-sound* generalization. The earlier, more behaviorally based work showing generalization to cognate sounds was greatly extended by the work of McReynolds and her colleagues (McReynolds & Bennett, 1972; McReynolds & Engmann, 1975; McReynolds & Huston, 1971) using a linguistic approach.

McReynolds and Huston (1971) studied a group of 10 children who had multiple articulation errors and analyzed these errors using a *distinctive feature* analysis based on the Chomsky and Halle (1968) distinctive feature system. They discovered that the children's errors could be described according to specific features. There were two different patterns of feature errors, however. For some children, most of the sound errors could be attributed to errors on a few features, such as stridency, continuancy, or voicing. This proved to be a very economical way of characterizing the errors. Other children displayed a different pattern: they had many features in error, but all at low percentages. The first pattern was described as a *phonetic* problem. The children did not produce the sounds; instead, they omitted the sounds or used a few sounds as substitutions for most other sounds. The second pattern was described as a *phonemic* pattern. The children did produce the sounds but used them inappropriately. Thus McReynolds and Huston concluded that

> according to our results, articulation problems cannot be regarded solely as problems in motor productions; they also consist of inappropriate phonemic rules. Consider that children lacking features in their repertoires also evidence inappropriate rule behavior. Inappropriate use of features contributes considerably to the articulation problems of these children. To a large extent, therefore, we would agree with

> individuals who contend that articulation problems should be considered within the framework of a phonological system, as systems at variance with adult phonemic systems. (p. 165)

Some of the children in Pattern 1 (errors described by a few features) were studied further by McReynolds and Bennett (1972). These participants were provided treatment on sounds containing the feature most in error. The results of this experimental study indicated that training a feature in one sound resulted in increased correct production of other sounds that also contained that feature.

Children with Pattern 1 errors have been the children most often studied in other experimental treatment investigations (e.g., Elbert & McReynolds, 1975, 1978). They are the children with very low baseline scores who simply do not produce a sound correctly. When they are trained to produce the sound correctly in a few contexts, they generalize across many untrained items containing the sound and across some other phonetically similar sounds. These types of generalization patterns support the conclusion that the problem is primarily phonetic—that is, once the children learn the motor skill required to produce the sound, they are able to use that sound appropriately.

McReynolds and her colleagues suggested that the children with errors that fit in Pattern 2—producing the sounds but using them inappropriately—constituted an entirely different subgroup that would require a different form of treatment. This suggestion was largely ignored for many years; however, more recent developments may have inadvertently filled the gap and provided such treatment. And that leads us into a new era.

Decade 2: Late 1970s and 1980s

Assessment

As mentioned in the overview, Ingram (1976) described children's speech-sound errors as phonological processes. This description was based on Stampe's (1973) theory of natural phonology. The assumption underlying this theory was that children possessed adultlike mental representations of sounds and that the sounds were changed through phonological processes into simplified productions. This assumption has been challenged (Dinnsen & Elbert, 1984); however, Edwards (1992) has defended Stampe's theory. Edwards has cautioned that even if we disagree with the assumption about adultlike underlying representations, we should not disregard the whole theory because the concept of phonological processes has contributed a great deal to the study of child phonology.

It is true that the notion of describing children's errors as phonological processes has had great appeal and has been adopted widely. On the whole, this description of speech-sound errors has seemed less complicated and less abstract than the procedures for distinctive feature analysis. Initially, there were a number of texts and manuals describing procedures for analysis of children's speech according to phonological processes (Bernthal & Bankson, 1981; Grunwell, 1987; Hodson, 1980; Ingram, 1981; Khan & Lewis, 1986; Shriberg & Kwiatkowski, 1980; Weiner, 1979). A point of agreement across authors was that speech-sound errors should be considered as "patterns of error," not just individual errors on a number of single sounds. This agreement marks an important landmark in the assessment and treatment of children with phonological disorders. Although the notion of patterns of error had been considered related to distinctive features, it had never been demonstrated as clearly. Grouping errors into categories such as errors of final-consonant deletion or of stopping (using stops as a substitute for fricatives) was a user-friendly way of utilizing a complex theory.

Another linguistic approach applied to children with speech-sound problems was based on standard generative phonological analysis. This approach differed from the previous approaches based on other linguistic theories. For instance, the distinctive feature approach made claims about the relationship among error sounds, and the phonological process approach described the relationship of error sounds to the ambient system; however, the *standard generative phonological approach* made claims about the child's *internalized representations* of *lexical items* (underlying representations; Dinnsen & Elbert, 1984; Elbert, Dinnsen, & Powell, 1984; Elbert, Dinnsen, & Weismer, 1984).

By determining whether a child's *underlying representations* were adultlike, it became possible to describe individual differences. Using generative phonological analyses, researchers have been able to profile information about an individual's phonological system on a continuum that describes a particular child's *productive phonological knowledge* from least to most knowledge (Elbert, 1989; Elbert & Gierut, 1986; Gierut, Elbert, & Dinnsen, 1987). These categories are based on an analysis of the child's productions on single-word tests and spontaneous speech. Thus the term *productive phonological knowledge* is based solely on speech productions, not on perception. The child may perceive sounds in an adult fashion but not produce sounds in an adult way. On this continuum, the category of "most productive phonological knowledge" includes all the sounds that a child uses entirely appropriately (adultlike usage). At the other end of the continuum, the category of "least productive phonological knowledge" contains a list of sounds that the child never produces (phonetic inventory constraints). Other categories between these two end points contain sounds that are produced but are used inappropriately, either due to phonological rules or because the sounds are produced only in certain specific positions in words (positional constraints). I have described one child in terms of these categories (Elbert, 1992) as an illustration of how a child's system could include some sounds that are adultlike, but produce other sounds only in one position and never produce some sounds. Further, the error patterns are described in terms of error types. A child may have an error pattern of final-consonant deletions, but this pattern may be divided into subsets in which some final-consonant sounds never occur in the system in any position, not just final position, and other sounds occur in initial position but not final. For example, a child may have a pattern of final-consonant deletion in which fricatives and velar stops are not produced in word final position; however, the velars are produced in initial position in words, and the fricatives are not produced in any position. In this case, the velars would be considered as positional constraints because the child shows some productive phonological knowledge of the sounds. The fricatives would be considered phonetic inventory constraints because they never occur in any position and thus would fall into the category of least phonological knowledge.

This type of analysis and characterization of sounds has implications for treatment. Teaching sounds from the category of least phonological knowledge has been shown to influence other sounds in error within the system. Sounds for which the child already possesses some knowledge may show change without direct treatment (Gierut et al., 1987; Powell, Elbert, & Dinnsen, 1991). Therefore our suggestion has been to teach sounds from within the category of least phonological knowledge to bring about the greatest change in the system. Powell (1991) presented an expanded illustration of how this approach could be applied to treatment target selection with one client.

Elbert et al. (1984) combined information about a child's unique productive phonological knowledge with information about treatment targets and the linguistic relationships that exist among sounds and proposed a set of predictions about generalization patterns. It seems clear that children's knowledge about the sound system of the language as they enter treatment, combined with other factors, exerts a strong influence over subsequent learning.

Treatment

Thus, during the 1980s, the term *articulation disorders* was replaced by the term *phonological disorders* to describe problems with speech-sound production. This change in theory and terminology has influenced both assessment and treatment practices. On the whole, the influence has been greater in assessment procedures.

The impact of adopting the new term *phonological disorders* on treatment procedures is by no means insignificant. The specific activities used during treatment sessions to improve speech-sound production need careful consideration. How does one implement new theory as treatment procedures or activities? Exactly what constitutes phonological remediation, as distinct from articulation remediation?

Several authors offer opinions on what constitutes phonological treatment as opposed to articulation treatment. For instance, Stoel-Gammon and Dunn (1985) described phonological remediation as (a) based on the systematic nature of phonology; (b) characterized by *conceptual*, rather than motoric, activities; and (c) ultimately aimed at *generalization*. Bernthal and Bankson (1993) stated that phonological treatment procedures that have been proposed in the literature consist primarily of suggestions regarding goals for remediation that are likely to facilitate generalization to an entire class of sounds. Conceptually oriented teaching tasks such as *contrast training* have been suggested to facilitate the reorganization of the phonological system.

The one treatment procedure generally considered to be conceptual, minimal contrasts (Elbert, Rockman, & Saltzman, 1980; Weiner, 1981; Winitz, 1975), has been in our clinical literature for many years. In this procedure, pairs of words that differ on only one sound are presented to the child (e.g., *bow* and *boat*), and the child is asked to say both words. For the child who omits final consonants, the two words are produced identically and lead to miscommunication. This procedure is intended to illustrate to the child that sound usage is important to communication and thus contributes to more adultlike conceptualization of the sound system. This, in turn, contributes to adultlike usage of final sounds. In this instance, stops are produced correctly in word-initial position but deleted in word-final position. The clinician assumes that the final-consonant deletion is not a motor problem but reflects a conceptual problem related to syllable structure (open vs. closed syllables). Treatment focuses on cognitive awareness of final-consonant contrasts (Bernthal & Bankson, 1993). Stoel-Gammon and Dunn (1985) pointed out that communication breaks down if the child fails to produce the sound that distinguishes the words. Although this situation supposedly forces the child to become aware of the error and change an underlying concept, it is not clear whether the child's improvement in production is due to a cognitive restructuring of a concept or the production practice and feedback. Cognitive and productive factors have been combined.

Weiner (1981) investigated the use of minimal contrasts in treatment with two preschool children with phonological disorders. He described his treatment procedures as conceptual rather than motoric and provided data to support the effectiveness of the treatment. His claims for the effectiveness of the conceptual treatment were challenged by Shelton (1982), who pointed out that Weiner's study was confounded due to the use of other procedures used in combination with the minimal contrasts. The children also were given instruction on how to say the words, an auditory model, and verbal and token reinforcement for correct responses. These additional procedures, which are characteristic of motoric treatment, may have influenced the results and obscured the effect of a purely conceptual treatment.

Other authors have also investigated minimal pairs (Dodd & Iacano, 1989; Hoffman, Norris, & Monjure, 1990; Monahan, 1986; Tyler, Edwards, & Saxman, 1987). Lowe (1994) has presented and discussed in detail a number of variations on the basic minimal-pair paradigm that have appeared in the literature.

In a recent investigation, Saben and Costello-Ingham (1991) completed a descriptive study with two children and asked if the use of minimal-word-pair treatment, unaccompanied by direct motoric treatment, would be successful in modifying speech-sound productions. The answer was no. The sounds selected for treatment were not present in the phonetic inventories of the two subjects at the initiation of treatment, and this may have been the crucial aspect. Although the treatment was intended to be conceptual, production responses were required from the subjects, and the subjects were unable to produce acceptable responses until imitation procedures were used. Thus the conceptual and motor components needed to be mixed in treatment. In their discussion, the authors suggested that minimal-pair treatment may be appropriate for phonemes for which a child has some degree of productive knowledge and may not be appropriate for errors for which productive knowledge is absent.

It appears that phonological treatment tasks can be described on a continuum from purely motoric treatment to purely conceptual treatment, with most procedures mixing the two elements to some degree. The traditional production approach, which teaches the sound first in isolation and moves toward more complex productions, would be an example of a motoric treatment. The minimal-contrast procedure, although claimed to be a conceptual treatment, is an example of a mixed treatment because it incorporates production into the contrast training. A purely conceptual treatment with no production component has not yet been reported in the literature on children with phonological disorders.

One treatment approach generally identified as phonological is the cyclical approach (Hodson & Paden, 1991). This is probably the best known phonological treatment approach. In this approach, several sounds involved in a particular pattern are targeted for treatment for a limited time and then recycled later. This treatment approach is focused on encouraging gradual changes across the phonological system rather than on motor practice of a single sound at a time.

Decade 3: The 1990s and on to 2001

Assessment

The results from a number of studies published during the 1990s have contributed to both assessment and treatment issues. Several large-*N* studies helped to give us an overview of normally developing populations as well as children with phonological disorders. Specifically, Smit (1993a, 1993b) provided information on phonological error distributions in singleton consonants and in consonant clusters from the Iowa-Nebraska Articulation Norm Project (Smit, Hand, Freilinger, Bernthal, & Bird, 1990). Shriberg and his colleagues (Shriberg, Gruber, & Kwiatkowski, 1994; Shriberg & Kwiatkowski, 1994; Shriberg, Kwiatkowski, & Gruber, 1994) provided descriptive profiles of children with developmental phonological disorders and both short-term and long-term normalization information on these children. The search for a consistent sequence of phonological acquisition across children is of continuing high interest to speech-language pathologists. Dinnsen, Chin, Elbert, and Powell (1990) proposed that the acquisition of features rather than individual sounds described the pattern of growth in phonetic inventories. Using features as the basis for change in phonetic inventories accounts for the variability that exists among children in the acquisition of specific speech sounds.

Treatment

In the area of treatment, there has been continued interest in the use of minimal pairs; however, this interest has focused on the number of feature differences between the two members of a minimal pair.

In earlier work, minimal pairs were often chosen on the basis of creating a contrast between a target sound and an error sound substitution without particular attention to the feature differences represented. These minimal pairs might differ on only one feature or several. For instance, a clinician might select minimal pairs contrasting /t/ and /k/ ("tea," "key") for the common error pattern involving a dental stop replacing a velar stop. In this case, the two sounds differ only on one feature (place) and can be described as minimal pairs having a minimal feature opposition. An example of a minimal pair with maximal opposition would be to contrast "me" and "key" (place, voice, manner).

Gierut (1992) and Williams (1993) used the idea of minimal pairs that were maximally contrastive and described qualitative and quantitative changes in the phonological systems of children with phonological disorders as a result of treatment on this type of minimal pairs. These studies extended the use of minimal-pair contrasts from earlier work and raised theoretical issues regarding the type of learning that might occur with the different types of contrasts.

Powell (1991) presented a plan for selecting treatment targets with a view toward maximizing the effects of generalization. His plan was based on results from treatment efficacy research and emphasized the importance of determining intervention priorities. Powell et al. (1991) presented data on the contribution of stimulability to generalization in preschool children during treatment. Their results indicated that treatment may be most efficient when priority is given to linguistically significant sounds that are nonstimulable. That is, stimulable sounds can be expected to change without direct treatment.

A series of award-winning articles was published in 1992 in *Language, Speech, and Hearing Services in Schools* as a clinical forum. As editor of the journal, Kamhi organized the forum in response to an earlier article written by Fey (1985/1992). Several authors (Edwards, 1992; Elbert, 1992; Hodson, 1992; Hoffman, 1992; Kamhi, 1992; Schwartz, 1992) responded to Fey, and these articles, taken together, presented a coherent summary of the state of the art in the early 1990s.

Throughout these articles, there was a general acceptance of the term *phonological disorder* or *disordered phonology* to describe problems involving the speech-sound system. Although there were some differences of opinion on the use of terms such as *rules* versus *processes* (Edwards, 1992), there was more agreement than disagreement. All of the authors within the forum generally agreed that the goal of phonologically oriented treatment was to facilitate phonological reorganization so that correct production would develop. Another important point stressed throughout the articles was that when new terms grow out of a new theory, new clinical treatment practices are warranted. Kamhi (1992) and Schwartz (1992) argued for the need to establish a consistency between theory and practice.

An innovative way of viewing treatment with a child with a phonological disorder was presented in a 1993 issue of *Seminars in Speech and Language* entitled "Persistent Sound System Disorder: Nature and Treatment." Shelton (1993b) organized the issue around the speech-sound problems of one child and invited a number of clinical investigators to analyze this child and his treatment plan from a variety of different perspectives (Elbert, 1993; Hodge, 1993; Hoffman, 1993; McCauley, 1993; Ruscello, 1993; Shelton, 1993a; Tessier, 1993; Vance, 1993). From these various perspectives, Shelton concluded that "both articulatory and phonological concepts contribute to the understanding of children's speech-sound system and related language disorders, but neither is sufficient by itself as a framework for clinical work" (p. 175).

Another line of research that has emerged stresses phonological awareness. Howell and Dean (1991) proposed metalinguistic awareness as the basis of new treatment procedures designed to accelerate change in phonological development. *Metalinguistic awareness* has been defined by Cazden (1972) as "the ability to reflect upon language as well as to comprehend and produce it" (p. 303) and by Tunmer and Herriman (1984) as "the ability to reflect upon and manipulate the structural features of spoken language itself as an object of thought, as opposed to simply using the language system to comprehend and produce sentences" (p. 12). In Howell and Dean's view, children with phonological disorders have problems in learning pronunciation patterns rather than in articulating speech sounds. They suggested that the majority of children with phonological disorders can imitate or use sounds contrastively in some positions and thus do not need to learn to produce the sound. They are in agreement with Grunwell (1987) that phonological disorders arise more in the mind than in the mouth of the child. Discussion of this type of treatment was presented in a 1995 clinical forum in *Clinical Linguistics and Phonetics* (Bleile & Hand, 1995; Grundy, 1995; Klimacka, 1995; Miccio, 1995; Nettelbladt, 1995).

The notion that a conceptual component needs to be included in treatment has been a part of our literature for many decades. Bernthal and Bankson (1993) stated that perceptual training includes conceptualization or phonological contrast training as well as traditional discrimination tasks. Van Riper (1963) proposed that children need to know the characteristic features of sounds and to learn to define perceptually the standard pattern of a sound through ear training (e.g., discrimination of [s] from [t]) in the first step of treatment. The aim of this practice was to help the child internalize a model of the sound without interference from production attempts. Winitz (1984) also strongly endorsed clinical procedures that emphasize intensive auditory discrimination training. LaRiviere, Winitz, Reeds, and Herriman (1974) introduced a sorting procedure as a conceptualization task to be used for the treatment of certain types of phonological problems. Hodson and Paden (1983, 1991) included an auditory bombardment component (listening at a low level of amplification to numerous repetitions of words containing the target sound or sequence) in their treatment plan as an aid to increase awareness of sounds.

Activities such as ear training and auditory bombardment could be classified as speech-sound discrimination procedures; however, these types of activities can be, to a great extent, conceptual or metalinguistic (e.g., sorting word pairs into two categories that reflect the presence of a phoneme and the absence of a phoneme; Bernthal & Bankson, 1993; Klein, Lederer, & Cortese, 1991; Locke, 1980a, 1980b). It appears that several terms being introduced into the literature are somewhat overlapping. *Conceptualization, metalinguistic awareness*, and *discrimination* all seem to refer to procedures that deal with recognition, listening, and heightened auditory awareness rather than production of speech sounds. Although different authors may have more specific definitions, the distinctions among the terms, if they exist, are unclear. The only clear distinction seems to be between the broader categories of conceptual versus motoric procedures.

It appears that at least two different types of errors, phonetic and phonemic, occur for children with speech-sound problems and that different treatments or different treatment components might be needed for the two (Elbert, 1992). To have consistency between theory and treatment, we need to be sure that our theory is broad enough to include different types of errors. Some errors may be due to articulatory constraints, others to conceptual difficulties, and still others to a combination. We may be able to avoid unnecessary confrontation and confusion by acknowledging that as researchers we are dealing with and talking about different types of problems.

My interest in considering different error types and subgroups of children with speech-sound problems began with the literature of the 1970s, particularly from the McReynolds and Huston (1971) and McReynolds and Bennett (1972) studies, which described two subgroups of children with speech-sound disorders. Subsequent data have added to my conviction.

ENDURING CONCEPTS

Several concepts have withstood the effects of time and continue to contribute to our knowledge of assessment and treatment of phonological disorders. Two that come to mind readily are distinctive features and stimulability.

Distinctive Features

Early on, feature distinctions were discussed by Jakobson and Halle (1956) as a basis for learning the sound system of the language. Many researchers have pursued this notion, and I have referred to several within this chapter. The fact that children seem to learn feature distinctions in their development of phonetic inventories (Dinnsen et al., 1990) and that features may be the basis for a great deal of generalized learning is well documented (e.g., Gierut, 1989; McReynolds & Bennett, 1972). Some facts about the generalization of sounds as a result of treatment are so well established as to serve as predictions (Elbert & Gierut, 1986).

Stimulability

The second concept concerns *stimulability*. The ability of children to imitate speech sounds that are absent from the phonetic inventory has been a topic of interest since the beginning of our profession. Stimulability has been studied and defined in a number of ways. It has been found to be a powerful variable in prediction of change with or without treatment (for review, see Bernthal & Bankson, 1993). More recently, Powell et al. (1991) provided experimental data suggesting that nonstimulable sounds are likely to require direct treatment, whereas stimulable sounds may change without any direct treatment. This finding has implications for planning treatment. Stimulability seems to emerge as a power variable throughout the literature. Although it is not always considered in every treatment approach or research investigation, it should be considered as part of the explanation of change that occurs in developing phonological systems.

A natural follow-up to the data on stimulability has been explored by Miccio and Elbert (1996). In this pilot work, a treatment program designed to increase the size of the phonetic inventory by "teaching" stimulability was implemented. The rationale for this treatment is that sounds that become stimulable will not need direct treatment later. This type of research is an example of attempting to build new information on the basis of strong findings from past research.

Certainly there has been a substantial increase in our knowledge base on phonological assessment and treatment over the last three decades. I would urge the next generation of clinical researchers to maintain a historical perspective so that research information obtained in earlier decades can serve as a basis for current investigations. Information should be additive. Replication of effects provides a solid base for our clinical work.

CONCLUSION

In my own clinical work, I have tried to derive principles from the research literature and apply these principles to individual clients. The key word is *individual.* The population of children with phonological disorders is not a homogeneous population.

So a first principle is to try to understand the unique phonological system of the individual and the unique personal characteristics and environment of the individual. For a child with a relatively mild problem, the analysis of the phonological system can be relatively quick. For the child who presents a moderate to severe phonological problem, the data gathering should include sufficient information on the individual so that we can describe the phonetic inventory, the phonemic inventory, the phonotactic usage (e.g., syllable structure), and stimulability. From this data set, we must organize the information in such a way as to be able to describe error patterns that emerge. These error patterns could be described in terms of place, voice, manner or distinctive features, phonological processes, or a generative phonological analysis. The important issue is to study the individual phonological system in sufficient depth to understand the dimensions of the problem.

Once the analysis is completed, treatment decisions must be made. The goal is to select the targets and procedures that will cause the greatest change in the system in the shortest amount of time. Earlier, I reviewed some of the research literature pertinent to this point, but the final choice will depend on a careful consideration of all of the factors.

A third principle involves a careful examination of the changes in the individual's system during treatment. In our profession, all of us need to be clinical researchers. After collecting information, analyzing the system, and devising a treatment plan, we must monitor the changes that occur and try to understand the factors that may have influenced the change. Ultimately, this is how we build a scientific basis for our work.

As we approach the 21st century, we look forward to the advances in knowledge that will come with the "second generation" of clinical researchers. A number of these talented people are already making their mark in the literature. Let's hear it for the Baby Boomers.

I thank Adele Miccio for helpful comments and suggestions; and Shani Goldberg, Kelly Hamsley, and Debi Giddens for editorial assistance. This work was supported in part by a grant from the National Institutes of Health (DC00260).

REFERENCES

Arndt, W.B., Elbert, M., & Shelton, R.L. (1971). Prediction of articulation improvement with therapy from early lesson sound production task scores. *Journal of Speech and Hearing Research, 14,* 149–153.

Bernthal, J.E., & Bankson, N.W. (1981). *Articulation disorders.* Englewood Cliffs, NJ: Prentice Hall.

Bernthal, J.E., & Bankson, N.W. (1993). *Articulation and phonological disorders* (3rd ed.). Englewood Cliffs, NJ: Prentice Hall.

Bleile, K.M., & Hand, L. (1995). Metalinguistics. *Clinical Linguistics and Phonetics, 9*, 25–28.

Cazden, C. (1972). *Child language and education.* New York: Holt, Rinehart & Winston.

Chomsky, N., & Halle, M. (1968). *The sound pattern of English.* New York: Harper & Row.

Compton, A.J. (1975). Generative studies of children's phonological disorders: A strategy of therapy. In S. Singh (Ed.), *Measurement procedures in speech, hearing and language* (pp. 55–92). Baltimore: University Park.

Dinnsen, D.A., Chin, S.B., Elbert, M., & Powell, T.W. (1990). Some constraints on functionally disordered phonologies: Phonetic inventories and phonotactics. *Journal of Speech and Hearing Research, 33*, 28–37.

Dinnsen, D.A., & Elbert, M. (1984). On the relationship between phonology and learning. In M. Elbert, D.A. Dinnsen, & G. Weismer (Eds.), *Phonological theory and the misarticulationg child* (ASHA Monograph No. 22, pp. 59–68). Rockville, MD: American Speech-Language-Hearing Association.

Dodd, B., & Iacano, T. (1989). Phonological disorders in children: Changes in phonological process use during treatment. *British Journal of Disorders of Communication, 24*, 333–351.

Edwards, M.L. (1992). In support of phonological processes. *Language, Speech, and Hearing in Schools, 23*, 233–240.

Elbert, M. (1989). Generalization in treatment of articulation disorders. In L. McReynolds & J. Spradlin (Eds.), *Generalization strategies in the treatment of communication disorders* (pp. 31–43). Toronto: B.C. Decker.

Elbert, M. (1992). Consideration of error types: A response to Fey's "Articulation and phonology: Inextricable constructs in speech pathology." *Language, Speech, and Hearing Services in Schools, 23*, 241–246.

Elbert, M. (1993). Analysis and treatment from a phonologically oriented perspective. *Seminars in Speech and Language, 14*, 119–127.

Elbert, M., Dinnsen, D.A., & Powell, T.W. (1984). On the prediction of phonological generalization learning pattern. *Journal of Speech and Hearing Disorders, 49*, 309–317.

Elbert, M., Dinnsen, D.A., & Weismer, G. (1984). *Phonological theory and the misarticulating child.* (ASHA Monograph No. 22). Rockville, MD: American Speech-Language-Hearing Association.

Elbert, M., & Gierut, J.A. (1986). *Handbook of clinical phonology: Approaches to assessment and treatment.* San Diego: College Hill.

Elbert, M., & McReynolds, L.V. (1975). Transfer of /r/ across contexts. *Journal of Speech and Hearing Disorders, 40*, 380–387.

Elbert, M., & McReynolds, L.V. (1978). An experimental analysis of misarticulating children's generalization. *Journal of Speech and Hearing Research, 21*, 136–150.

Elbert, M., & McReynolds, L.V. (1985). The generalization hypothesis: Final consonant deletion. *Language and Speech, 28*, 281–290.

Elbert, M., Rockman, B., & Saltzman, D. (1980). *Contrasts: The use of minimal pairs in articulation training*. Austin, TX: Exceptional Resources.

Elbert, M., Shelton, R.L., & Arndt, W.B. (1967). A task for evaluation of articulation change: I. Development of methodology. *Journal of Speech and Hearing Disorders, 44*, 459–471.

Fey, M.E. (1992). Articulation and phonology: Inextricable constructs in speech pathology. *Language, Speech, and Hearing Services in Schools, 23*, 225–232. (Original work published 1985)

Fisher, H., & Logemann, J. (1971). *Fisher-Logemann Test of Articulation Competence*. Boston: Houghton Mifflin.

Gierut, J.A. (1985). *On the relationship between phonological knowledge and generalization learning in misarticulation children*. Unpublished doctoral dissertation, Indiana University.

Gierut, J. (1989). Maximal opposition approach to phonological treatment. *Journal of Speech and Hearing Disorders, 54*, 9–19.

Gierut, J. (1992). The conditions and course of clinically induced phonological change. *Journal of Speech and Hearing Research, 35*, 1049–1063.

Gierut, J.A., Elbert, M., & Dinnsen, D.A. (1987). A functional analysis of phonological knowledge and generalization learning in misarticulating children. *Journal of Speech and Hearing Research, 30*, 462–479.

Grundy, K. (1995). Metaphon: Unique and effective? *Clinical Linguistics and Phonetics, 9*, 20–36.

Grunwell, P. (1987). *Clinical phonology* (2nd ed.). Baltimore: Williams & Wilkins.

Hodge, M. (1993). Assessment and treatment of a child with a developmental speech disorder: A biological-behavioral perspective. *Seminars in Speech and Language, 14*, 128–141.

Hodson, B. (1980). *The assessment of phonological processes*. Danville, IL: Interstate.

Hodson, B. (1992). Applied phonology: Constructs, contributions, and issues. *Language, Speech, and Hearing Services in the Schools, 23*, 247–253.

Hodson, B., & Paden, E. (1983). *Targeting intelligible speech: A phonological approach to remediation*. San Diego: College Hill.

Hodson, B., & Paden, E. (1991). *Targeting intelligible speech: A phonological approach to remediation* (2nd ed.). Austin, TX: Pro-Ed.

Hoffman, P.R. (1983). Interallophonic generalization of /r/ training. *Journal of Speech and Hearing Disorders, 48*, 215–221.

Hoffman, P.R. (1992). Synergistic development of phonetic skill. *Language, Speech, and Hearing Services in the Schools, 23*, 254–260.

Hoffman, P.R. (1993). A whole-language treatment perspective for phonological disorder. *Seminars in Speech and Language, 14*, 142–152.

Hoffman, P.R., Norris, J.A., & Monjure, J. (1990). Comparison of process targeting and whole language treatments for phonologically delayed preschool children. *Language, Speech, and Hearing Services in the Schools, 21*, 102–109.

Howell, J., & Dean, E. (1991). *Treating phonological disorders in children: Metaphon—theory to practice*. San Diego: Singular.

Ingram, D. (1976). *Phonological disability in children*. New York: Elsevier.

Ingram, D. (1981). *Procedures for the phonological analysis of children's language*. Baltimore: University Park.

Jakobson, R., & Halle, M. (1956). *Fundamentals of language*. The Hague: Mouton.

Kamhi, A.G. (1992). The need for a broad-based model of phonological disorders. *Language, Speech, and Hearing Services in Schools, 23*, 261–268.

Khan, L., & Lewis, N. (1986). *Khan-Lewis Phonological Analysis*. Circle Pines, MN: American Guidance Service.

Klein, H., Lederer, S., & Cortese, E. (1991). Children's knowledge of auditory/articulatory correspondences: Phonologic and metaphonologic. *Journal of Speech and Hearing Research, 34*, 559–564.

Klimacka, L. (1995). Managing disordered phonological development with the Metaphon approach. *Clinical Linguistics and Phonetics, 9*, 36–42.

LaRiviere, C.H., Winitz, H., Reeds, J., & Herriman, E. (1974). The conceptual reality of selected distinctive features. *Journal of Speech and Hearing Research, 17*, 122–133.

Locke, J.L. (1980a). The interference of speech perception on the phonologically disordered child. Part I: A rationale, some criteria, the conventional tests. *Journal of Speech and Hearing Disorders, 45*, 431–444.

Locke, J.L. (1980b). The interference of speech perception on the phonologically disordered child. Part II: Some clinically novel procedures, their use, some findings. *Journal of Speech and Hearing Disorders, 45*, 444–468.

Lowe, R.T. (1994). *Phonology assessment and intervention applications in speech pathology*. Baltimore: Williams & Wilkins.

McCauley, R. (1993). A comprehensive phonological approach to the assessment and treatment of sound system disorders. *Seminars in Speech and Language, 14*, 153–165.

McDonald, E.T. (1964). *Articulation testing and treatment: A sensory motor approach*. Pittsburgh: Stanwix House.

McLean, J.E. (1970). Extending stimulus control of phoneme articulation by operant techniques. In F.L. Girardeau & J.E. Spradlin (Eds.), *A functional approach to speech and language* (ASHA Monograph No. 14, pp. 24–47). Rockville, MD: American Speech-Language-Hearing Association.

McReynolds, L.V. (1972). Articulation generalization during articulation training. *Language and Speech, 15*, 149–155.

McReynolds, L.V., & Bennett, S. (1972). Distinctive feature generalization in articulation training. *Journal of Speech and Hearing Disorders, 37*, 462–470.

McReynolds, L.V., & Elbert, M. (1981). Generalization of correct articulation in clusters. *Applied Psycholinguistics, 2*, 119–132.

McReynolds, L.V., & Engmann, D. (1975). *Distinctive feature analysis of misarticulations*. Baltimore: University Park.

McReynolds, L.V., & Huston, K. (1971). A distinctive feature analysis of children's misarticulations. *Journal of Speech and Hearing Disorders, 36*, 155–166.

Miccio, A.W. (1995). Metaphon: Factors contributing to treatment outcomes. *Clinical Linguistics and Phonetics, 9*, 28–35.

Miccio, A.W., & Elbert, M. (1996). Enhancing stimulability: A treatment program. *Journal of Communication Disorders, 29*, 335–352.

Monahan, D. (1986). Remediation of common phonological processes: Four case studies. *Language, Speech, and Hearing Services in the Schools, 17*, 199–206.

Mowrer, D.E. (1971). Transfer of training in articulation therapy. *Journal of Speech and Hearing Disorders, 36*, 427–445.

Nettelbladt, U. (1995). The Metaphon approach to phonological therapy from a Swedish perspective. *Clinical Linguistics and Phonetics, 9*, 42–49.

Powell, T.W. (1991). Planning for phonological generalization: An approach to treatment target selection. *American Journal of Speech-Language Pathology, 1*, 21–27.

Powell, T.W., & Elbert, M. (1984). Generalization following the remediation of early- and late-developing consonant clusters. *Journal of Speech and Hearing Disorders, 49*, 211–218.

Powell, T.W., Elbert, M., & Dinnsen, D.A. (1991). Stimulability as a factor in the phonological generalization of misarticulating preschool children. *Journal of Speech and Hearing Research, 34*, 1318–1328.

Powell, J., & McReynolds, L.V. (1969). A procedure for testing position generalization from articulation training. *Journal of Speech and Hearing Research, 12*, 629–645.

Rockman, B.K. (1983). *An experimental investigation of generalization and individual differences in phonological training*. Unpublished doctoral dissertation, Indiana University.

Ruscello, D.M. (1993). A motor skill learning treatment program for sound system disorders. *Seminars in Speech and Language, 14*, 106–118.

Saben, C.B., & Costello-Ingham, J. (1991). The effects of minimal pairs treatment on the speech-sound production of two children with phonologic disorders. *Journal of Speech and Hearing Research, 34*, 1023–1040.

Schwartz, R.G. (1992). Clinical applications of recent advances in phonological theory. *Language, Speech, and Hearing Services in Schools, 23*, 269–276.

Shelton, R. (1982). Response to Weiner. *Journal of Speech and Hearing Disorders, 47*, 336.

Shelton, R.L. (1993a). Grand rounds for sound system disorder. Conclusion: What was learned. *Seminars in Speech and Language, 14*, 166–178.

Shelton, R.L. (Ed.). (1993b). Persistent sound system disorder: Nature and treatment [special issue]. *Seminars in Speech and Language, 14*.

Shelton, R.L., Elbert, M., & Arndt, W.B. (1967). A task for evaluation of articulation change: II. Comparison of task scores during baseline and lesson series testing. *Journal of Speech and Hearing Research, 10*, 578–585.

Shriberg, L.D., Gruber, F.A., & Kwiatkowski, J. (1994). Developmental phonological disorders III: Long-term speech-sound normalization. *Journal of Speech and Hearing Research, 37*, 1151–1177.

Shriberg, L., & Kwiatkowski, J. (1980). *Natural process analysis (NPA): A procedure for phonological analysis of continuous speech samples*. New York: John Wiley.

Shriberg, L.D., & Kwiatkowski, J. (1994). Developmental phonological disorders I: A clinical profile. *Journal of Speech and Hearing Research, 37*, 1100–1126.

Shriberg, L.D., Kwiatkowski, J., & Gruber, F.A. (1994). Developmental phonological disorders II: Short-term speech-sound normalization. *Journal of Speech and Hearing Research, 37*, 1127–1150.

Smit, A.B. (1993a). Phonologic error distribution in the Iowa-Nebraska Articulation Norms Project: Consonant singletons. *Journal of Speech and Hearing Research, 36*, 533–547.

Smit, A.B. (1993b). Phonologic error distribution in the Iowa-Nebraska Articulation Norms Project: Word-initial consonant clusters. *Journal of Speech and Hearing Research, 36*, 931–947.

Smit, A.B., Hand, L., Freilinger, J.J., Bernthal, J.E., & Bird, A. (1990). The Iowa Articulation Norms Project and its Nebraska replication. *Journal of Speech and Hearing Disorders, 55*, 779–798.

Stampe, D. (1973). *A dissertation on natural phonology*. Unpublished doctoral dissertation, University of Chicago.

Stoel-Gammon, C., & Dunn, C. (1985). *Normal and disordered phonology in children.* Austin, TX: Pro-Ed.

Tessier, D.S. (1993). A description of Matthew's therapy. *Seminars in Speech and Language, 14*, 100–105.

Tunmer, W.E., & Herriman, M.L. (1984). The development of metalinguistic awareness: A conceptual overview. In W.E. Tunmer, C. Pratt, & M.L. Herriman (Eds.), *Metalinguistic awareness in children* (pp. 12–35). New York: Springer-Verlag.

Tyler, A.A., Edwards, M.L., & Saxman, J.H. (1987). Clinical application of two phonologically based treatment procedures. *Journal of Speech and Hearing Disorders, 52*, 393–409.

Van Riper, C. (1963). *Speech correction: Principles and methods* (4th ed.). Englewood Cliffs, NJ: Prentice Hall.

Vance, R. (1993). Assessment of Matthew's language skills. *Seminars in Speech and Language, 14*, 91–99.

Weber, J.L. (1970). Patterning of deviant articulation behavior. *Journal of Speech and Hearing Disorders, 35*, 135–141.

Weiner, F. (1979). *Phonological process analysis.* Baltimore: University Park.

Weiner, F. (1981). Treatment of phonological disability using the method of meaningful minimal contrast: Two case studies. *Journal of Speech and Hearing Disorders, 46*, 97–103.

Williams, A.L. (1993). Phonological reorganization: A qualitative measure of phonological improvement. *American Journal of Speech-Language Pathology, 2*(2), 44–51.

Winitz, H. (1975). *From syllable to conversation*. Baltimore: University Park.

Winitz, H. (1984). Auditory consideration in articulation training. In H. Winitz (Ed.), *Treating articulation disorders: For clinicians by clinicians* (pp. 21–49). Baltimore: University Park Press.

Wright, V., Shelton, R., & Arndt, W. (1969). A task for evaluation of articulation change: III. Imitative task scores compared with scores for more spontaneous tasks. *Journal of Speech and Hearing Research, 12*, 875–884.

CHAPTER 4

Developmental Phonological Disability: Order in Disorder

Pamela Grunwell

In the early 1970s, I began teaching phonetics and linguistics to student speech-language therapists. (Joy Stackhouse was one of my first students.) To ensure that my teaching had clinical relevance, I was encouraged to observe the treatment of children and adults with a wide range of communication disorders. I was fascinated and perplexed. I had just completed a degree in phonetics and linguistics, and during my work for that degree, I had, from personal choice, immersed myself in different theories of phonology. Yet here in speech therapy clinics, no one had heard of distinctive features, minimal pairs, or phonological rules! I became involved in the treatment of one little boy who had a severe speech disorder of nonorganic origin, a "functional articulation disorder." Given my linguistic training, it was inevitable that I should expect to be able to analyze this child's speech patterns, and I did so, using various techniques of phonological analysis (Grunwell, 1975). My colleagues were astounded when I showed them that this child had his own phonological system (i.e., that there was order in disorder). Thus it was that I found myself in the vanguard of a revolution—the linguistic revolution that transformed the theoretical framework for the assessment, diagnosis, and treatment of speech and language disorders in the 1970s and 1980s (Crystal, 1981, 1982; Grunwell, 1982; Ingram, 1976).

The impact of linguistics upon our characterization and treatment of *children's speech disorders* has been fundamental. It has made us redefine the nature of developmental speech disorders by identifying the phonological dimension. Phonological methods of analysis and assessment enable us to discern patterns, or *order in disorder,* and thereby provide systematic intervention programs. The phonological framework for assessment, diagnosis, and treatment proposed in this chapter is based on three theoretical parameters: (a) system, (b) structure, and (c) stability. The first part of this chapter defines and illustrates these concepts with reference to normal mature phonologies and disordered child phonologies. The second part describes the applications of these concepts in the assessment and treatment of disordered child phonologies. The third and final part of the chapter discusses the implications of these approaches to applied clinical phonology. All examples in this chapter are based on the speech of children learning to pronounce various accents of British English; the target pronunciations of some words are therefore different from American English pronunciations.

THEORETICAL PERSPECTIVES

When phonological concepts first began to be applied in the clinical context, much emphasis was placed on the distinction between phonetics and phonology (Crystal, 1981; Grunwell, 1982). In *phonetic* descriptions, one is concerned with the range of sounds a speaker is, or is capable of, producing. A phonetic description can be expressed in articulatory, auditory, or acoustic terminology or a combination of two or more of these. Auditory-articulatory descriptions are the most common and familiar and will be used in this chapter. In *phonological* descriptions, one is concerned with identifying the sounds that function in languages, or in a particular language, to signal meaning differences and with stating the regularities in the occurrence of just these sounds.

The reason for the emphasis on distinguishing phonetics and phonology in the early stages of the development of clinical phonology is historical and is in part pinpointed by Crystal (1981):

> Phonetics has been a routine part of a speech pathologist's training for decades; linguistics, by contrast is of recent origin. Skills in ear-training and phonetic transcription, and associated descriptive and analytical abilities, can thus be taken for granted in a way that linguistic knowledge cannot—and this affects in a direct way the types of assessment and remediation it proves possible to do. (p. 2)

Crystal, in the passage from which this quotation is drawn, is seeking to draw attention to the fact that the concepts and techniques used in phonological analysis are crucially different from those used in phonetic analysis and that they are part of linguistics. The early emphasis on the distinction between phonetics and phonology also resulted from traditional clinical descriptions of speech disorders, especially in children. Up until the mid-1970s, it was customary to label all speech disorders as articulation disorders, thus implying some motoric or anatomical basis for the disorder. There thus existed the curious diagnosis, mentioned above, of "functional articulation disorder" for which no such organic basis could be identified (Powers, 1959, 1971). With the introduction of linguistic, specifically phonological, concepts and techniques, it became evident that the puzzling phenomenon of a "functional articulation disorder" was more appropriately characterized as a *phonological disorder*: "a linguistic disorder manifested by the use of abnormal patterns in the spoken medium of language" (Grunwell, 1981b, p. 9). Hence there was a strong and understandable clinical motivation to disassociate phonetics, aligned with traditional motorically based articulation disorders, from phonology, aligned with the newly discovered linguistically based phonological disorders.

Theoretically, however, most phoneticians do not draw such a sharp distinction. From their viewpoint, there is a close relationship between phonetics and phonology. Here are two definitions of the "domain of phonetics" provided by eminent phoneticians and phonologists:

> All human beings have substantially the same speech apparatus, so that the total repertory of human sounds is effectively the same for the whole species, but the selection made from this total repertory varies quite considerably from community to community. The study of speech as a universal phenomenon is *phonetics*. The study of the systematic organisation of selected speech sounds in the spoken forms of individual languages has variously been called *functional phonetics, phonemics* or more commonly nowadays, *phonology*. The business of *phonology* is to abstract, describe and classify as neatly as we can the recurrent sound units used to build up the spoken forms of a given language and to state the rules for their use. (Henderson, 1971, pp. 38–39)

> Phonetics is the study of the sensible manifestation of language. It is, therefore, concerned with the acoustical properties of speech, with the motor behaviour of the vocal organs that produce the acoustical signal, and with the way the signal is processed in the human auditory system. In studying these topics sight must never be lost of the fact that we are dealing with *manifestations of language* [italics added], and not just with arbitrary acoustical signals produced by the human vocal tract and perceptible to our auditory system. Linguistic considerations and, in particular, facts concerning the limitations that different languages impose on the phonetic shape of words and utterances must therefore be taken into account on a par with articulatory and acoustic data. (Halle & Stevens, 1979, p. 335)

These definitions suggest that rather than adopting the viewpoint of "phonetics versus phonology," it is more appropriate to think in terms of "phonetics *and* phonology." Clearly one cannot employ phonological concepts and techniques without phonetic knowledge, and that knowledge informs clinical assessment and treatment. Further clinical assessment, diagnosis, and treatment need to take into account the interaction between phonetics and phonology (see Grundy & Harding, 1995; Grunwell, 1990). Grunwell's (1990) short definition of *phonology* embodies this viewpoint: "Phonology is concerned both with the signalling of meanings and with the physical phonetic substance whereby meanings are transmitted" (p. 4).

The primary and most well-developed application of phonology in the clinical context is in the assessment of developmental speech disorders, especially developmental phonological disorders. Phonological assessment procedures use the techniques of phonological analysis. The aim of phonological analysis is to provide a description and classification of the sound differences in speech on the basis of their communicative functions and systematic organization as the spoken medium of language. We now therefore consider the key concepts for phonological analysis (i.e., system, structure, and stability).

System

As has already been stated, phonological analysis is primarily concerned with identifying, describing, and classifying the sound differences in a language, or in an individual's speech, that signal meaning differences. Therefore the concept of a system of sounds that fulfills this function is basic to phonological analysis. A system is a set or inventory of different sound units that are in a relationship of replacement or substitutability.

Twelve different consonant sounds of English may replace each other in the context [–ɪn] and by so doing create 12 different words or linguistic meanings. Each of these sound units is therefore said to have *contrastive function*: it is in contrast to, and different from, all other units in this system. The relationship of replacement or contrastivity is termed a *paradigmatic* relationship. A paradigm is basically a list. *Minimal pairs* (i.e., two words that differ in one sound segment) or *minimal sets* (i.e., several words that differ in one sound segment) exemplify the function of phonological contrasts, the operation of a system. There are 24 contrastive consonants in English: that is, 24 consonant phonemes.

We now need to consider what makes the sound units or elements in the phonological system contrastive. It is because they are different in their phonetic (or what is theoretically described as their phonemic) content. At this point, phonological analysis interacts with phonetic description to identify the phonetic properties or *features* that are the basis for each segment's contrastivity. For example:

> /tɪn/ vs, /dɪn/ involves a *voicing* difference between *voiceless* and *voiced* apico-alveolar plosives

/tɪn/ vs. /sɪn/ involves a *manner of articulation* difference between voiceless apicoalveolar *plosive* and *fricative*

/tɪn/ vs. /kɪn/ involves a *place of articulation* difference between voiceless *apicoalveolar* and *velar* plosives.

Every unit in a phonological system is contrastive and therefore phonetically distinct from the other units as a consequence of its phonetic content or properties. It is, however, characteristic for contrastive units in phonological systems to be related to each other in terms of shared properties or constituents, as can be seen from the examples above. This phenomenon results in symmetrical patterning in phonological systems. Part of the English consonant system provides an interesting example:

	m		n		ŋ
p	b	t	d	k	g

This is a subsystem of contrasts that is totally symmetrical in that all three types of contrasts are functioning: manner (oral vs. nasal stop), voice (voiced vs. voiceless), and place of articulation (labial vs. alveolar vs. velar).

Symmetry is therefore another concept in phonological analysis that needs to be considered in the clinical context as a basis for identifying unusual phonological systems. From this consideration of the concept of system in phonology, it is evident that an adequate phonological system must function to signal, through sound differences, the meaning differences required by the language or the speaker. Second, the sound differences that perform this phonological function operate in a phonetically systematic set of combinations that result in economical combinations of phonetic features, or what otherwise might be called symmetrical systems, in the phonologies of natural languages.

Structure

Another dimension of phonological analysis is also concerned with describing the organization of sound systems in languages. This dimension, or parameter, is based on the concept of structure. In this dimension, phonological analysis is concerned with describing the organization of sound units into larger units involving patterns of combination and distribution and therefore relationships of co-occurrence and sequence. The descriptions of the possible combinations of units and, by implication, the restrictions on these possibilities must make reference to a basic structural unit of organization, the *syllable*. The structure of the syllable is as follows:

C	V	C
consonant	vowel	consonant
initial position	essential element	final position

The distribution and co-occurrence of consonant sounds in English are two of the most important aspects of English phonology. For example, there is a structural restriction on the range of consonants that can occur in syllable-initial position such that /ŋʒ/ are excluded and a similar restriction in syllable-final position such that /hwj/ are excluded. There are restrictions on the distribution of consonants and also on the combinations of consonants. For example, in English, the maximum number of consonants that may occur in initial position in a syllable is three; there are, however, restrictions on the combinations and order of the three consonants that may occur in this sequence. They are as follows:

C1 is /s/
C2 is /p t k/
C3 is /w r l j/
but /w/ cannot follow /sp/ or /st/, and /l/ cannot follow /st/.

Thus [spwɪŋ], [stwɪŋ], and [stlɪŋ] are impermissible forms of English. These clusters do not conform to the *phonotactic possibilities* of English phonology. *Phonotactics* describes the possible distributions and combinations of sounds that occur in the phonological system of a language.

The description of these structural patterns in a phonology states the *syntagmatic* relationships between phonological units: the relationships of co-occurrence and sequence and of structural contrast. A *syntagma* is basically a structure. In most phonologies, there are different systems of contrasts at different positions in syllable structure. This presents another concept, the presence or absence of structural symmetry. This needs to be considered in the clinical assessment of phonological systems.

Stability

Mature phonological systems are internally stable: that is, the number of terms in the system is finite and mutually exclusive. Thus phonological systems can be definitively described and the terms in the system do not overlap with each other. The technical term for this condition is *homeostasis*. The stable nature of phonological systems ensures that the systemic and structural patterns of organization are predictable. We shall see in the next section that this is in marked contrast to the nature of developing and disordered child phonologies.

CLINICAL APPLICATIONS

Assessment

As has already been indicated, the primary clinical application of phonology has been in assessment. Clinical phonological assessments evaluate the system, structure, and stability of disordered phonologies. Clearly, an assessment needs to evaluate an individual's performance against a normative reference point or a standard. In phonological assessments, this norm is generally taken to be the characteristics of the adult mature phonological system.

Procedures and Tools

Appendixes 4–A through 4–D provide frameworks for such an assessment. Their use is exemplified employing a data sample collected using a screening assessment procedure known as PACS TOYS (see further below). The data sample is given in Appendix 4–A.

The Phoneme Realization Chart (Appendix 4–B) is from Phonological Assessment of Child Speech (PACS; Grunwell, 1985). This procedure is not in fact a phonological assessment. Although it facilitates an organized presentation of the child's realizations of the adult phonemic systems in four word and syllable positions, it does not compare the child's systems with the adult systems. A similar procedure is available for the examination of the child's realizations of the adult systems of initial clusters and final clusters (Appendix 4–C). These two charts are efficient techniques for organizing a data sample into categories that subsequently can be analyzed phonologically. As such, they are preliminary procedures in a clinical phonological assessment. The categories they employ reflect the three theoretical parameters defined in the preceding section. The child's realizations of the contrasts in the adult *system* are recorded for four positions in *structure* for both singleton targets and clusters. These charts include a simple version of the traditional technique of error analysis that classifies the child's realizations as correct, zero (i.e., omission), or incorrect. There is no subclassification of the incorrect realizations (cf. the traditional categories of "substitution" and "distortion"; Grunwell, 1987). By examining these charts, it is possible to gain an impression of the extent to which the child's pronunciations match the adult targets and of the amount of stability or variability in the child's realizations. In this way, they provide a preliminary indication of the stability or instability of the child's realizations. They do not, however, enable us to analyze the phonological implications of the child's "errors": that is, to identify whether, and to what extent, they involve loss(es) of phonological contrasts.

Recently, a new version of the Phoneme Realization Chart has been published as part of a phonological screening assessment (PACS TOYS; Grunwell & Harding,

1995). The Extended Phoneme Realization Chart (Appendix 4–D) subclassifies the incorrect realizations into the following developmental categories:

- *Almost Mature*. The realizations in this category are "nearly correct" because they differ from a correct, accurate match in minor subphonemic features or properties (e.g., dental realizations of target alveolars: /s/ → [s̪]). These realizations are therefore recognizable as the target but have phonetic characteristics that are different from the typically correct realizations.
- *Developmentally Immature*. These realizations can be classified as evidencing well-established developmental simplifying patterns (or processes; see Edwards, Chapter 1 of this volume); they may involve early patterns such as stopping (/ʃ/ → [t]) or later patterns such as fronting (/ʃ/ → [s]).
- *Atypical*. These are realizations that are not known to be an attested typical immaturity and may have the characteristics of a phonologically unusual type of realization (see Leonard, 1985). There are some easily identified examples of atypical realizations, such as /t/ → [s] and /f/ → [d]. Others are more unusual and may even be deemed idiosyncratic, such as the use of click realizations (e.g., Bedore, Leonard, & Gandour, 1994; Grundy, 1995a, p. 336; Grunwell, 1992a, p. 469, 1992b).
- *Other*. This category includes all incorrect realizations that cannot be confidently classified in the preceding categories. A "not sure" classification has been recognized in other clinical analytical assessment procedures as a useful category (see Crystal, 1982; 1992; Duckworth, Allen, Hardcastle, & Ball, 1990).

It will be observed that zero realizations are not identified as a separate category in this extended developmental classification. Certain instances of zero realizations will be classified as *developmentally immature* (e.g., the omission of word-final consonants). Other instances of zero realizations will be classified as *atypical* (e.g., the omission of word-initial consonants).

Like the original Phoneme Realization Chart, the extended version provides preliminary information about the extent to which the child's pronunciations match the adult's and about the amount of variability. In the context of a screening assessment, the extended chart is also designed to contribute to a developmental differential diagnosis by enabling an examination of the frequency of occurrence of the different types of developmental errors. As indicated by Grunwell and Harding (1995), if the errors are exclusively developmentally immature, further detailed investigation may not be required immediately, and the child's pronunciation abilities can be reviewed a few months later. When there are developmentally immature and atypical patterns or exclusively atypical patterns (a rare occurrence, but see Grunwell, 1992a, 1992b), further investigations are clearly indicated.

Notwithstanding this additional information, the extended chart does not provide a phonological analysis and assessment of the child's consonant realizations. The PACS analytical assessment procedure that is designed to carry out a comparison of the child and adult consonant systems is the Contrastive Assessment Chart (or Contrastive Phones Chart in PACS TOYS; see Appendix 4–E). This chart analyzes the matches and mismatches between the child and adult consonant systems in the three frequently occurring positions in structure, using a simple graphic display. Examination of a completed chart provides direct information about the target contrasts that are present and those that are lost in the child's system.

The chart also details the variability in the child's matches and mismatches with the adult targets. This aspect of the assessment can be refined further if the number of occurrences of each child realization is recorded, thus documenting the relative stability of variable realizations of the targets (Appendix 4–F). The contrastive assessment thus directly assesses the child's pronunciation patterns on all three theoretical parameters identified in the preceding section.

This analytical assessment procedure has a further clinical advantage in that it provides a simple method of reassessment. Comparisons between earlier and later assessments using this procedure are straightforward (see Grunwell, 1992b).

Examination of the charts enables identification of positive changes, such as an increase in the number of contrasts correctly signaled or the number of targets accurately realized. Other changes, such as different distribution patterns and increases or decreases in the amount of variability, can also be detected. This method of reassessment can be further refined by using numerical indicators.

Grunwell (1992c) proposed that the following phonological performance indicators be used when comparing contrastive assessments at two (or more) points in time:

1. *Number of targets attempted against number possible*—in case of sampling bias or avoidance of targets by child
2. *Number of consonants used*—typically should increase over time
3. *Number of stable correct matches*—should clearly increase over time
4. *Number of stable incorrect mismatches*—should decrease over time
5. *Number of variable matches/mismatches*—variability may be an indicator of potential and/or ongoing change
6. *Number of variable matches/mismatches involving correct matches*—a subindicator of No. 5 and a particularly positive type of variability, indicating potential and/or ongoing stabilization of a correct match

These calculations are made separately for each position in word and syllable structure. In addition, in word-final position, three indices measure the occurrence of zero realizations:

7. *Number of stable zero realizations*—should decrease over time
8. *Number of variable zero realizations*—an indicator of the gradual emergence of final consonants
9. *Number of variable zero realizations involving correct matches*—a subindicator of No. 8, which like No. 6 is particularly positive, indicating potential and/or ongoing stabilization of a correct match

These indicators provide detailed measures of changes in a child's pronunciation patterns that can be used to discover whether positive changes have taken place when this is not easily apparent from our examination of the contrastive assessments. They can also be used to inform treatment planning so that it is sensitive to the child's pattern of development (Appendix 4–G).

Another aspect of contrastive assessment and reassessment is the developmental dimension. The PACS Developmental Assessment (Grunwell, 1985) is based on a meta-analysis of studies of the development of consonants in English-speaking children (Grunwell, 1981a). Exhibit 4–1 profiles the phonological development of the system of English consonant contrasts. Complementary to this profile is the Chronology of Phonological Processes (Figure 4–1), which charts the gradual disappearance of developmental simplifying processes from children's speech patterns (Grunwell, 1981a). Using the PACS Developmental Assessment with a Contrastive Assessment, one can identify the developmental stage a child has achieved and, on reassessment, gauge what degree of developmental progress a child has made (Appendix 4–H). It must be acknowledged that this profile has one shortcoming: it does not contain any structural information; indeed it conflates all positions in structure. This may be misleading if a child has different systems in different positions that when conflated suggest a more developed system than is the case. Reference back to the Contrastive Assessment Chart would ensure that the profile would not be misinterpreted. It is sometimes thought that this profile has another shortcoming in that it is usually difficult to map a clinical contrastive assessment precisely onto a developmental stage. In fact, this is by no means a shortcoming because it is a diagnostic indicator. This confirms that the pronunciation patterns and development of the child being assessed do not conform to those of normal development (i.e., the child has a developmental phonological disorder).

Characterization of Developmental Phonological Disorders

Using the theoretical concepts and assessment procedures described above, one can define the characteristics of developmental phonological disorders from either of two different perspectives: the phonological or the developmental.

From a phonological perspective, the characteristics are defined by reference to the concepts of system, structure, and stability. In regard to system, the following characteristics have been identified:

Exhibit 4–1 Profile of Phonological Development: Phonological System

				Labial		Lingual
Stage I (0:9–1:6)	Nasal Plosive Fricative Approximant					
Stage II (1:6–2:0)	m p b w			n t d		
Stage III (2:0–2:6)	m p b w			n t d		(ŋ) (k g) h
Stage IV (2:6–3:0) Stage V (3:0–3:6)	m p b f w			n t d s (l)	j	ŋ k g h
Stage VI (3:6–4:0) (4:0–4:6)	m p b f v w			n t d s z l (r)	ʧ ʤ ʃ j	ŋ k g h
Stage VII (4:6+)	m p b f v w	θ	ð	n t d s z l r	ʧ ʤ ʃ ʒ j	ŋ k g h

Source: Copyright © 1981, Pamela Grunwell.

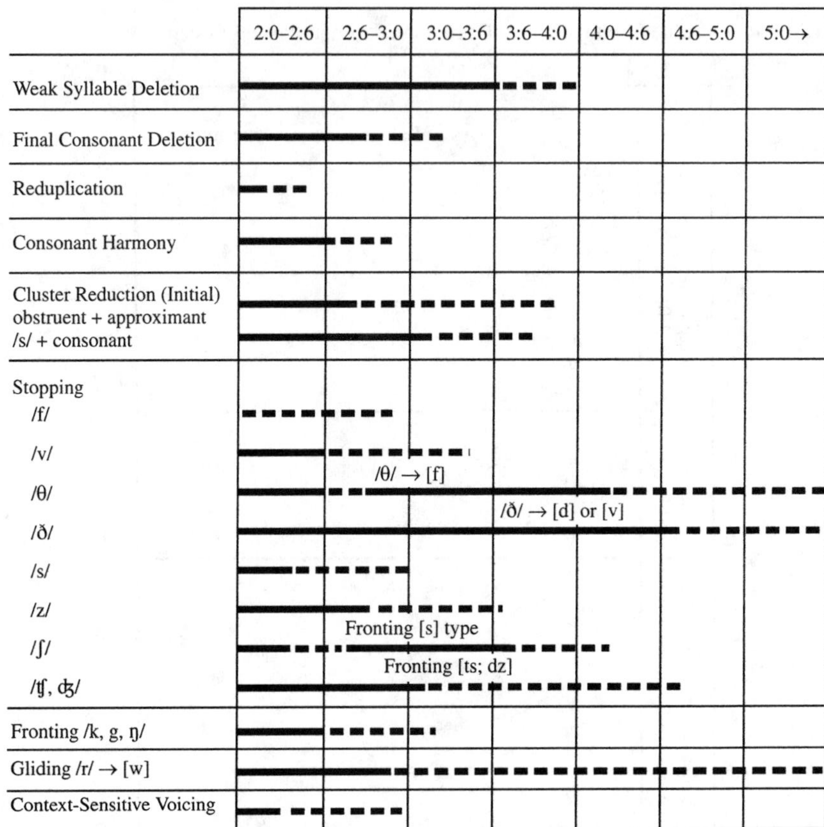

Figure 4–1 Chronology of Phonological Processes. *Source*: Copyright © 1981, Pamela Grunwell.

---

1. There are in large part systematic correspondences between the adult system and the child's realizations of the targets in that system.
2. The child's system is smaller than the adult system, and therefore the child's realizations of adult targets involve loss(es) of phonological contrasts (e.g., /t/ and /s/ → [t]) as in *tin* and *sin* becoming [tɪn]).
3. There is a tendency for one child phone to realize several adult targets, thus entailing multiple loss of phonological contrasts (e.g., /t s ʃ θ ʧ/ → [t], as in *tin, sin, shin, thin,* and *chin* becoming [tɪn]).
4. There tends to be a relationship between the phonetic properties of the adult target and the phonetic properties of the child realization (e.g., target /s/:

voiceless apicoalveolar fricative; realization [t]: voiceless apicoalveolar plosive).

5. There is a tendency for child systems to be asymmetrical and uneconomical in regard to the occurrence of potential combinations of phonetic features, as in the example below:

m	n	
p b	t	g

In regard to structure, the following characteristics have been identified:

1. The child's phonotactic patterns tend to be less complex than those in the adult pronunciations.
2. The child's realizations tend to involve systematic simplifications of complex adult structures (e.g., /st/ → [t]).
3. The simplifications of complex adult structures tend to involve loss(es) of phonological contrasts, which together with other realizations may entail multiple losses of phonological contrasts (e.g., /st/ → [t], as in *stick* and *tick* becoming [tɪk] also possibly *sick* and *thick* becoming [tɪk]).
4. There tends to be a relationship between the phonetic properties of the adult target and the phonetic properties of the child realization, as is evident from the examples above.
5. There is a tendency for structural asymmetry: that is, the use of different—sometimes very different—consonant systems at different positions in structure (for an example, see Appendix 4–I).

With regard to stability, the tendency for systematic correspondences between the adult and child systems has to be qualified as follows:

1. There is a tendency for some variability in the child's realizations of adult targets (e.g., /s/ → [t; s]).
2. In some instances, variability is potentially progressive, as in the example for No. 1.
3. In other instances, variability is not progressive (e.g., /s/ → [t; d]).
4. Extreme variability occurs where there are several different realizations of one target; this can be the situation for several targets (e.g., see Appendix 4–F).
5. There is a tendency for disordered child phonological systems to be variable but static.

Variability in a system or in a child's realizations of target consonants tends to be indicative of change and potential development. It would appear that this is not so in the pronunciation patterns of children with developmental phonological disorders. These children, therefore, have disordered phonologies and disordered development.

A number of characterizations of developmental phonological disorders have been proposed using a developmental perspective. A general classification logically requires three categories:

1. *Delayed Development.* A child appears to be developing pronunciation patterns in a normal way but at a slower rate than normal.
2. *Uneven Development.* A child is using patterns from two (or more) different stages of pronunciation development. Some of the patterns may be age appropriate; others may be delayed or advanced (i.e., chronological mismatch).
3. *Different Development.* A child is using patterns that do not normally occur in pronunciation development; thus these patterns are unusual and atypical and may be deemed idiosyncratic.

It is often found that children with phonological disorders evidence delayed, uneven, and different development.

A more specific and perhaps better known developmental classification is that based on phonological process analysis (see Edwards, Chapter 1 of this volume; also Grunwell, 1985; Stoel-Gammon & Dunn, 1985). There are five categories in this classification:

1. *Persisting Normal Processes.* Normal patterns remain in the child's pronunciation patterns long after the age at which they would normally have disappeared (i.e., *delayed development*, such as the presence of final-consonant deletion in a child aged 3:6).
2. *Chronological Mismatch.* Earlier patterns co-occur with some patterns characteristic of later stages of development (i.e., *uneven development*, such as the presence of final-consonant deletion with the co-occurrence of initial clusters in a child aged 3:6).
3. *Unusual Processes.* Patterns occur that are rarely attested in normal development (i.e., *atypical development*, such as the occurrence of click substitutions; Bedore et al., 1994).
4. *Systematic Sound Preference.* One type of consonant is used for a large range of target consonants (with multiple loss of phonological contrasts; e.g., /t d k g s z ʃ ʧ ʤ tr/ → [d]).
5. *Variable Use of Processes.* More than one realization is used for the same target consonant (cf. variability discussed above; e.g., /k/ → [t d k g]).

As is evident from the above definitions, one can use this classification without having carried out a full phonological process analysis. All that is required is a knowledge of normal and unusual patterns of pronunciation development and a developmental profile. Both these classifications of developmental characteristics are therefore compatible with the assessment procedures described in the preceding section.

Treatment

From the outset, phonology influenced treatment planning and delivery simply in that treatment was based on a phonological assessment. Therapy goals and activities were thus expressed in the terminology of the particular assessment procedure used: features were trained, rules were attacked, processes were eliminated, contrasts were introduced. In relatively few instances, however, were explicit principles specified to guide the decision-making process of treatment planning—what to treat, when, and how (see Edwards, 1983; Hodson & Paden, 1983, 1991; Lancaster & Pope 1989). Over a period of more than 20 years, such a set of principles has been developed empirically by stating the rationale behind every treatment decision in the planning of therapy for children with developmental phonological disorders (Grunwell, 1975, 1983, 1988a, 1988b, 1992b, 1994; Grunwell & Dive, 1988; Grunwell, March, & Russell, 1990; Grunwell & Russell, 1990; Grunwell, Yavas, Russell, & Le Maistre, 1988). Gradually, through this long-term process, the phonological factors that are employed in treatment planning and delivery have been identified, refined, and defined. This section, therefore, discusses the concepts and principles of phonological therapy that have been developed to complement the approach to assessment described in the preceding section. A case study follows to demonstrate how the two interact.

At a general level, the philosophy of phonological therapy needs to be established. This can be expressed as *the premises of phonological therapy*:

1. The child has a developmental phonological disorder (i.e., a disorder in learning to pronounce the phonological system); therapy must be aimed at remediating this disorder.
2. In learning to pronounce this phonological system, children are developing a system of sound contrasts that function to signal meaning contrasts.
3. In learning their phonology, children are organizing their phonological system (i.e., not just learning the correct pronunciation of individual words).
4. The cognitive organization of the phonological system is based on similarities and differences between sounds and sound sequences; these provide the bases for grouping sounds into classes and sequences into structures.

5. The aim of therapy, therefore, is to facilitate cognitive reorganization of the child's phonology and his or her phonological strategies for perceptual, organizational, and production processing.

The following *principles of phonological therapy* are the modus operandi (operational policy), often unstated, of phonological therapy (see Bernhardt, 1992; Bernhardt & Gilbert, 1992; Gierut, 1989, 1990, 1991, 1992; Gierut & Morisette, 1996):

1. The treatment is based on a phonological assessment, and the aims are defined by the phonological assessment.
2. Therapy is based on the principle that there are regularities in the child's pronunciation patterns (i.e., "order in disorder").
3. Therapy is based on the principle that the principal function of phonological organization is communicative (i.e., differences in sounds and sequences signal meaning differences).
4. Therapy aims to facilitate change in the child's pronunciation patterns in order to build up a more adequate system of sound contrasts and sound structures.
5. Therapy is designed to make maximally effective use of the organization of phonological patterning in the target system by introducing and establishing changes in the child's patterns through use of natural classes of contrastive phones and structures.

These philosophical premises and principles form the basis for an action plan for formulating treatment aims that has been developed from a phonological assessment. The plan is to identify communicative inadequacies in the child's pronunciation patterns and then to develop a principled progression of treatment aims that focus on phonological outcomes (stability, system expansion, and structural extension), bearing in mind that the primary objective of treatment is to change patterns of pronunciation in order to enhance communicative adequacy.

To put this action plan into operation, two fundamental tendencies in pronunciation development need to be recognized: (a) the tendency to establish rule-governed or systematically patterned speech production and (b) the tendency to function initially with a simple sound system and gradually to increase its complexity, building upon and extending existing abilities.

In working through the action plan as the basis for formulating treatment aims for individual children, one should apply the following decision-making principles for treatment planning:

1. Variability should be targeted to establish stable and accurate realizations.
2. The system of contrasts should be expanded to increase communicative adequacy.

3. New contrasts should be introduced first in well-established structures.
4. The phonotactic potential should be extended to increase communicative adequacy.
5. New structures should be introduced, using well-established consonants.
6. Where possible, the treatment program should follow the normal developmental sequence.
7. Where appropriate, the patterns that should be targeted first are those that are (a) most different from the normal sequence of development and (b) most destructive of communicative adequacy.

Bernhardt and Gilbert (1992) stated almost verbatim Principles 4 and 5 in the rationale for one of their treatment aims.

There is a noteworthy omission from our set of principles: a guideline that is often invoked in treatment planning, namely the child's stimulability for target sounds absent from his or her inventory; (e.g., Bernhardt, 1992; Powell, 1993). Although stimulability can be a factor in deciding what to treat, it is viewed in this framework as a technique of diagnostic therapy that provides information as to the type of treatment procedures needed to establish whether articulation therapy is required before phonological therapy can commence (see Grundy & Harding, 1995).

In implementing phonological therapy, one must identify the nature of the change being sought as well as the specific treatment targets. Clinical experience indicates that four basic types or mechanisms of phonological change can be induced by phonological therapy:

1. *Stabilization* is a mechanism whereby a variable pronunciation pattern is resolved into a stable pattern. Stabilization is therefore sought where there is instability/variability. Stabilization establishes new contrasts by positively stimulating progressive change in variable patterns.
2. *Destabilization*, which involves the disruption of a stable pattern to promote variability, is indicated where there is inappropriate stability. Destabilization leads eventually to potential progressive change when the resultant variability is ultimately resolved by stabilization.
3. *Innovation* involves the introduction of a new pattern, which will lead to progressive change by destabilization of existing patterns and/or stabilization of the new pattern.
4. *Generalization* involves the transfer of a pronunciation pattern from one context to another. This mechanism is indicated when an actual or potential target is accurately realized in one context that should be occurring in another context, most often another position in structure.

Finally, in planning phonological therapy, one must consider the types of treatment techniques to be employed. The primary strategy is to control the child's linguistic environment such that it promotes and facilitates the phonological changes that have been identified as treatment targets. It must be assumed that phonological development is sensitive to input (Gierut & Morisette, 1996; Ingram, 1986). There are, however, two basic types of techniques that can structure therapeutic input: metalinguistic and manipulative techniques. *Metalinguistic techniques* provide a child with information about phonological functioning "virtually directly." This could be called a system-based approach because it reveals the system "at work" through discrimination of minimal pairs, minimal-pair-contrast therapy in production, and homophony confrontation. *Manipulative techniques* expose a child to increased numbers of a selected target type. This could be called a word-based approach because the child is required to pay attention to and learn words containing the target type through "auditory bombardment" with a slight amplification (Hodson & Paden, 1991), word lists, and sentences and stories that are "phonologically loaded." The types of techniques chosen are dependent upon the findings of the phonological assessment and the aims of the phonological treatment plan.

Case Study

The following case study exemplifies the evolution of a treatment program for a child with a severe developmental phonological disorder. C had received 10 months of weekly speech therapy before he was referred to a specialist clinic at the age of 5:10. Over the previous period of therapy, no change had occurred in his pronunciation patterns. The first full phonological assessment at 5:10 revealed an extremely restricted and asymmetrical consonant system that was also asymmetrically distributed (Appendix 4–I). In syllable-initial word-initial (SIWI) position, the consonants were [b d n w l]; in syllable-initial within-word (SIWW) position, the consonants were [b n]; in syllable-final word-final (SFWF) position, only [n] occurred. There were, however, an appreciable number of marginal phones. These were realizations that occurred only once or twice in the data sample. They gave the impression of variability, especially in SIWI position. They included [p g f v]. It was also noteworthy that [m] occurred as a marginal phone in SIWW position.

The primary treatment aim for C at this stage was: system expansion through the process of innovation. The specific aims were:

- *in SIWI position*—to introduce the plosive/fricative contrast using [d] versus [f]. This particular pair was chosen for four reasons (see Edwards, 1983):
  1. [f] occurred as a marginal phone matching the target /f/ correctly on one occasion.

2. The realization of target /f/ as an alveolar plosive is developmentally atypical; Ingram (1976) called it *tetism*. Furthermore, this pattern is part of a systematic sound preference for [d] that results in multiple losses of phonological contrasts.
3. [f] is often the first fricative to be established in normal speech development.
4. This pair of contrasts involved the voiced/voiceless contrast, which was absent from C's speech. Perhaps it would be possible to induce the development of this contrast indirectly.

- *in SIWW position*—to introduce/stabilize [m]; once again, this was a marginal phone with one correct match. Also, in establishing [m], a more symmetrical system would be created.
- *in SFWF position*—through auditory discrimination, to target the contrasts between [n k] and zero. This was intended:
  1. to begin to replace SFWF zero realizations with new accurate matches
  2. to introduce the velar place of articulation, on the basis of the observation that velars often emerge first in word-final position in normal speech development (Ingram, 1974)
  3. to provide another opportunity to focus on the voiced/voiceless contrast indirectly

Two aspects of this plan require further comment. First, the decision to target marginal phones might be termed "the clutching at straws" principle. Marginal phones are, in effect, spontaneous evidence of stimulability. Bernhardt and Gilbert (1992, pp. 140–141) adopted the very same principle. Second, the aim of inducing the development of the voiced/voiceless contrast indirectly is based on clinical experience, which has shown that direct targeting of this contrast is frequently unsuccessful and that apparently spontaneous emergence occurs when it is targeted indirectly. This could be further evidence of the principle of laryngeal-supralaryngeal cyclicity (Gierut & Morisette, 1996). On the other hand, it is interesting that this should be proposed as a principle; it is my own long-standing practice, on the basis of the phonetic nature of the "voiced/voiceless" contrast in English (see Grundy, 1995b), to seek an indirect method of introducing this contrast. Perhaps a hierarchy of indirect and direct principles would be useful.

C benefited from the availability of intensive individual therapy sessions, three to four times per week, for a period of 3 months. During this period, SFWF aims were modified to include more and different types of targets. This was in response to the apparently spontaneous emergence of new consonants in this position. These were [ʃ d]. First, [ʃ] was added to the range of contrasts because it provided further opportunities to focus on both the plosive/fricative and the voiced/voiceless contrasts. Subsequently, [t] was added—the voiceless alveolar plosive being selected so as not to reinforce the dominance of [d], though in a different word position. During the following 2 months, C had less frequent therapy, one to two sessions per week. New aims were identified that involved generalization of two of the consonants introduced in therapy. These were the transfer of [f] to SFWF position and of [k] to SIWI position.

At 6:3, C was reassessed fully (see Appendixes 4–F and 4–H). He had made 12 months' progress in the development of his pronunciation patterns. The range of consonants had expanded along intended lines. Major changes had occurred in SFWF position, as revealed numerically by the phonological performance indicators (see Appendix 4–G). These showed not only new consonant types but noticeable destabilization. Voiceless cognates of the previously dominant voiced plosives were emerging, most notably [p t k] in SFWF position. Although therapy activities had concentrated on auditory discrimination in SFWF position, the consonants targeted [t k f ʃ] were now being produced. There was also evident generalization of [m] to SIWI and SFWF positions and of [ʃ] to SIWW position.

Unfortunately, there was also an increase in the occurrence of [n] in SIWW position for almost all target types. Because these realizations replaced zero, this change could be interpreted as progressive. But it increased the dominance of a systematic sound preference and required remedial attention.

Treatment aims were revised and expanded on the basis of this assessment. System expansion remained a primary aim, but treatment now needed to focus on the processes of generalization and stabilization. Specific aims were:

- *in SIWI position*—to target the [d] versus [k] contrast in order to reinforce the generalization of [k] from SFWF position and to stabilize accurate realizations. This target also provided another opportunity to focus indirectly on the voiced/voiceless contrast.
- *in SFWF position*—to stabilize the production of [f t k] and of [s], which had emerged as a marginal phone with one accurate match. In addition, auditory discrimination exercises focused on [b d g] and later [l] in contrast with ø. Collectively, these two aims also targeted the voiced/voiceless contrast.

After 2 additional months, new aims were added to the program:

- *in SIWI position*—to target [s] through generalization from SFWF, where it had been established. This aim was developmentally appropriate, and the realization of /s/ as [n] was one of the most atypical patterns in the data.
- *in SFWF position*—to target the contrast [n] versus [g] in order to generalize the alveolar/velar contrast and to promote symmetry.
- *in SIWW position*—to destabilize and, if possible, eradicate the dominance of [n]. It was decided to target plosives and fricatives in CVCV structures, using

the previously successful approach of introducing reduplication (Grunwell, 1992b). The first targets were [p b], on the basis that this would involve stabilization; stimuli were selected to present sequences of voiced or voiceless targets only. Subsequently, generalization was sought by targeting [t d k g]. This aspect of the treatment program was aimed at one of the most different and destructive patterns in C's speech, the systematic sound preference for [n] in SIWW position.

At 6:8, C was reassessed again (see Appendixes 4–H and 4–J). As before, he had made 12 months' progress in the development of his pronunciation patterns. His system was now normal but delayed. His patterns were matched chronologically and were symmetrical both phonetically and distributionally. The delay was evidenced in the variability of the realizations of targets /ʃ/ and /r/ and the absence of affricates. There were also the typical child realizations of /θ/ → [f] and /ð/ → [d] or [v]. It is noteworthy that clusters had been established spontaneously in both initial and final positions, except for obstruent +/r/ in SIWI position.

The final phase of the treatment program had limited aims designed to assist C achieving completely normal pronunciation patterns. The aims were:

- to stabilize [ʃ] in SIWI and SIWW positions; then to introduce the affricates [ʧ ʤ], in SFWF first because the realizations were more progressive in this position
- to introduce the /w/ versus /r/ contrast in SIWI position; then to generalize the use of [ɹ] to the obstruent +/r/ clusters

These aims were accomplished successfully during a further month of individual therapy sessions three to four times a week.

At the outset of this study, C had extremely disordered and inadequate pronunciation patterns. Furthermore he was 5:10, at which age phonological development is normally complete. Within 12 months, through a program of intensive speech therapy, he had established developmentally normal and communicatively adequate speech.

CONCLUSION

Applying phonological techniques to the analysis of disordered child speech allows us to discern the systematic patterns in these data: the order in disorder. It also allows us to identify how these patterns are disordered. As we have seen in this chapter, there are two fundamental aspects of this disorder. Disordered speech patterns fail to satisfy the functional requirements of phonology in that they do not adequately signal meaning differences. As a consequence, speakers with disordered speech cannot make themselves understood. Disordered speech patterns also fail to comply with the organizational characteristics of phonology; they tend to be uneconomical, asymmetrical, and variable. The assessment procedures used in this chapter are based on a selection of phonological techniques. Over many years, they have been shown to be feasible as routine clinical assessment procedures. It must be acknowledged, however, that some phonological patterns are not easily described within this framework. Vowels are ignored; yet in the assessment of some children's speech disorders, disordered use of vowels is an important factor (see Grunwell, 1995, for a review of recent studies of disordered vowels). Further systematic investigation of vowel disorders is required. Patterns involving interactions between consonants, such as consonant harmony or assimilation, also have been reported (see, e.g., Grunwell, 1992a; Leonard, 1985). Although the occurrence of such patterns appears to be infrequent, their nature needs to be investigated further, especially in regard to effective treatment techniques.

Phonological analysis and assessment have been used in this chapter as descriptive procedures. The future development of these techniques could lead to their being employed as diagnostic and predictive procedures. The differential diagnoses of developmental speech disorders are generally based on nonlinguistic data relevant to the overall clinical management of the child. In Grunwell (1990), for example, each chapter addresses the speech patterns of a different client group: children with hearing impairment, children with neurological disorders, and so on. What studies demonstrate collectively, however, is that there is order in all types of disordered speech, whatever the etiology. It may be possible, therefore, to develop a typology of phonological disorders, which could also include an indicative measure of severity, based on the phonological characteristics of the speech patterns (see Shriberg, Chapter 5). Its predictive dimension would be the measure of severity and its implications for response to treatment. The procedures employed in this chapter apply concepts that could be developed in this direction, such as contrastive assessment and phonological performance indicators.

To realize this goal, clearly more longitudinal studies of children with disordered speech development are required. These studies need to cover the whole spectrum of developmental speech disorders, not just developmental phonological disorders. Ideally, we also need a cross-linguistic dimension. There are few studies of languages other than English (see Grunwell, 1996, for a review, and Ingram, Chapter 2); more are needed. There is much that we still need to discover about disordered phonologies.

REFERENCES

Bedore, L.M., Leonard, L.B., & Gandour, J. (1994). The substitution of a click for sibilants: A case study. *Clinical Linguistics and Phonetics, 8,* 283–293.

Bernhardt, B. (1992). The application of nonlinear phonological theory to intervention with one phonologically-disordered child. *Clinical Linguistics and Phonetics, 6,* 283–316.

Bernhardt, B., & Gilbert, J.G. (1992). Applying linguistic theory to speech-language pathology: The case for non-linear phonology. *Clinical Linguistics and Phonetics, 6,* 123–145.

Crystal, D. (1981). *Clinical linguistics.* New York: Springer-Verlag.

Crystal, D. (1982). *Profiling linguistic disability.* London: Edward Arnold.

Crystal, D. (1992). *Profiling linguistic disability* (2nd ed.). London: Whurr.

Duckworth, M., Allen, G., Hardcastle, W., & Ball, M. (1990). Extensions to the International Phonetic Alphabet for the transcription of atypical speech. *Clinical Linguistics and Phonetics, 4,* 273–280.

Edwards, M.L. (1983). Selection criteria for developing therapy goals. *Journal of Childhood Communication Disorders, 7,* 36–45.

Gierut, J.A. (1989). Maximal opposition approach to phonological treatment. *Journal of Speech and Hearing Disorders, 54,* 9–19.

Gierut, J.A. (1990). Differential learning of phonological oppositions. *Journal of Speech and Hearing Research, 33,* 540–549.

Gierut, J.A. (1991). Homonymy in phonological change. *Clinical Linguistics & Phonetics, 5,* 119–137.

Gierut, J.A. (1992). The conditions and course of clinically-induced phonological change. *Journal of Speech and Hearing Research, 35,* 1049–1063.

Gierut, J.A., & Morisette, M.L. (1996). Triggering a principle of phonemic acquisition. *Clinical Linguistics and Phonetics, 10,* 15–30.

Grundy, K. (Ed.). (1995a). *Linguistics in clinical practice.* London: Whurr.

Grundy, K. (1995b). Metaphon: Unique and effective? *Clinical Linguistics and Phonetics, 9,* 20–24.

Grundy, K., & Harding, A. (1995). Developmental speech disorders. In K. Grundy (Ed.), *Linguistics in clinical practice* (2nd ed., pp. 329–357). London: Whurr.

Grunwell, P. (1975). The phonological analysis of articulation disorders. *British Journal of Disorders of Communication, 10,* 31–42.

Grunwell, P. (1981a). The development of phonology: A descriptive profile. *First Language, 3,* 161–191.

Grunwell, P. (1981b). *The nature of phonological disability in children.* London: Academic Press.

Grunwell, P. (1982). *Clinical phonology.* London: Croom Helm.

Grunwell, P. (1983, August). Phonological therapy: Premises, principles and procedures. In *Proceedings of the 11th International Association of Logopedics and Phoniatrics Congress,* Edinburgh.

Grunwell, P. (1985). *Phonological assessment of child speech (PACS).* Windsor, UK: NFER-Nelson.

Grunwell, P. (1987). *Clinical phonology* (2nd ed.). London: Croom Helm.

Grunwell, P. (1988a). Comment on "Helping the development of consonant contrasts." *Child Language Teaching and Therapy, 4,* 57–59.

Grunwell, P. (1988b). Phonological assessment, evaluation and explanation of speech disorders in children. *Clinical Linguistics and Phonetics, 2,* 221–252.

Grunwell, P. (Ed.). (1990). *Developmental speech disorders.* Edinburgh, Scotland: Churchill Livingstone.

Grunwell, P. (1992a). Assessment of child phonology in the clinical context. In C.A. Ferguson, L. Menn, & C. Stoel-Gammon (Eds.), *Phonological development: Models, research, implications* (pp. 457–483). Timonium, MD: York.

Grunwell, P. (1992b). Principled decision-making in the remediation of children with phonological disability. In P. Fletcher & D. Hall (Eds.), *Specific speech and language disorders in children* (pp. 215–240). London: Whurr.

Grunwell, P. (1992c). Processes of change in developmental speech disorders. *Clinical Linguistics and Phonetics, 6,* 101–122.

Grunwell, P. (1994). Phonological therapy: The linguistic challenge to facilitate change. In R. Aulanko & A-M. Korpijaakko-Huuhka (Eds.). *Proceedings of the Third Congress of the International Clinical Phonetics and Linguistics Association*,(pp. 43–58). Helsinski: University of Helsinki Department of Phonetics.

Grunwell, P. (1995). Changing phonological patterns. *Child Language Teaching and Therapy, 11,* 61–78.

Grunwell, P. (1996). Natural phonology. In M. Ball & R. Kent (Eds.), *The new phonologies.* San Diego: Singular.

Grunwell, P., & Dive, D. (1988). Treating "cleft palate speech": Combining phonological techniques with traditional articulation therapy. *Child Language Teaching and Therapy, 4,* 193–210.

Grunwell, P., & Harding, A. (1995). *PACS TOYS.* Windsor, UK: NFER-Nelson.

Grunwell, P., March, E., & Russell, J. (1990). Facilitating speech development: A case study. *Child Language Teaching and Therapy, 6,* 113–126.

Grunwell, P., & Russell, J. (1990). A phonological disorder in an English-speaking child: A case study. *Clinical Linguistics and Phonetics, 4,* 29–38.

Grunwell, P., Yavas, M., Russell, J., & Le Maistre, H. (1988). Developing a phonological system: A case study. *Child Language Teaching and Therapy, 4,* 142–153.

Halle, M., & Stevens, K.N. (1979). Some reflections on the theoretical basis of phonetics. In B. Lindblom & S. Ohman (Eds.), *Frontiers of speech communication research* (pp. 335–349). London: Academic Press.

Henderson, E.J.A. (1971). Structural organisation of language: Phonology. In N. Minnis (Ed.), *Linguistics at large* (pp. 35–53). London: Paladin.

Hodson, B.W., & Paden, E.P. (1983). *Targeting intelligible speech.* San Diego: College Hill.

Hodson, B.W., & Paden, E.P. (1991). *Targeting intelligible speech* (2nd ed.). Austin, TX: Pro-Ed.

Ingram, D. (1974). Fronting in child phonology. *Journal of Child Language, 1,* 233–242.

Ingram, D. (1976). *Phonological disability in children.* London: Edward Arnold.

Ingram, D. (1986). Explanation and phonological remediation. *Child Language Teaching and Therapy, 2,* 1–19.

Lancaster, G., & Pope, L. (1989). *Working with children's phonology.* Oxford, UK: Winslow.

Leonard, L.B. (1985). Unusual and subtle behaviour in the speech of phonologically disordered children. *Journal of Speech and Hearing Disorders, 50,* 4–13.

Powell, T.W. (1993). Phonetic inventory constraints in young children: Factors affecting acquisition patterns during treatment. *Clinical Linguistics and Phonetics, 7,* 45–57.

Powers, M.H. (1959). Functional disorders of articulation. In L.E. Travis (Ed.), *Handbook of speech pathology* (pp. 708–768). London: Peter Owen.

Powers, M.H. (1971). Functional disorders of articulation. In L.E. Travis (Ed.), *Handbook of speech pathology and audiology* (pp. 837–875). New York: Appleton Century Crofts.

Stoel-Gammon, C., & Dunn, C. (1985). *Normal and disordered phonology in children.* Baltimore: University Park Press.

APPENDIX 4–A

PACS TOYS Word List A: Stephen

PACS TOYS
SCREENING ASSESSMENT

Word List A – Alphabetical

Name STEPHEN Chronological Age 3:3 Date 11/94 Tester AH

apple	ˈabl	fork	fɔk	sand	sand
badge	dads [CH] bads	glove	sʌv	scissors	ˈsɪsəs
brush	gɾʌs	go	gəʊ	sheep	ʧip
bucket	ˈbʌkɪt	hand	ʔand	shoes	suz
bus	bʌs	horse	ˈɔsɪ	snake	neɪk
car	k̿ɑ	jam/jar	sam	soap	səʊp
driver	ˈgɾaɪvə	knife	naɪf	sock	sɒt
caravan	ˈdeɪv̥an	letter	ˈlɛtə	spade	peɪd
case	geɪs	stamp	damp	thumb	vwʌm
chair	sɛə	nose	nəʊs	tiger	ˈkaɪgə [CH]
cheese	siz	picture	ˈb̥ɪʔsə	toe	dəʊ
dinosaur	ˈsaɪnəsɔ [CH]	house	ʔaʊs	torch	ʃjɔʔs
doll	dɔ	door	dɔ	trousers	ˈtɾaʊzəz
girl	gɜ	roof	ˈʋufɪz	van	van
mouth	maʊf	pig	bɪg pɪg	washing machine	ˈwɒsɪn əsin
elephant	ˈɛlɪfant	plaster	ˈzaʔzə [CH]	watch	wɒʔs
feather	ˈfɛfə [CH]	purse	b̥ɜs	whistle	wɪs̪
fire engine	ˈfaɪjə ɛndɪn	money	ˈmʌnɪz	yes	jɛ
ladder	ˈladə	rabbit	ˈlabɪt	zip	sɪp
flower	ˈsaʊwə	ring	wɪŋ̃		

CH indicates CONSONANT HARMONY

Additional target words	
boat	bəʊt
digger	NR
Mickey Mouse	maʊs
plane	sweɪn
straw	swɔ
Thomas	NR
Tank Engine	ˈdaŋg ɛndɪn

Additional transcription

three	twi
work	vɜk
wash	jɒs
two	d̥u

Appendix 4–B

PACS Phoneme Realization Chart

Phoneme Realizations

Name STEPHEN

	SIWI			SIWW			SFWW			SFWF			
	CORRECT	ZERO	INCORRECT	CORRECT	ZERO	INCORRECT	CORRECT	ZERO	INCORRECT	CORRECT	ZERO	INCORRECT	
m	m III	I								m II			m
n	n II			n II			n II			n 卌 I			n
ŋ										n I		ŋ̃ I	ŋ
p	p I		b̥ II b I			b I				p III			p
b	b IIII		d I	b I									b
t			k I d III ʃi I	t I		z I				t III			t
d	d II		s I	d I						d I			d
tʃ			s II			s I						ʔs II	tʃ
dʒ			s I			d II						ds II	dʒ
k			kʷ I d I g I	k I					ʔ I	k III		t I	k
g	g II			g I						g II			g
f	f III			f II						f I			f
v	v I			v I		v̥ I				v I			v
θ			vw I									f I	θ
ð						f I							ð
s	s IIII			s II		s̪ I			ʔ I	s 卌	I		s
z			s I	z I		s I				z 卌		s II	z
ʃ			tʃ I s I			s II						s II	ʃ
ʒ													ʒ
w	w III		v I j I	w I									w
r			ʋ I l I w I		I								r
l	l II			l I						l I	III		l
j	j I			j I									j
h			ʔ II ∅ I										h

APPENDIX 4–C

PACS Cluster Realization Chart

Cluster Realizations

Name STEPHEN

	SIWI			SIWW		
Cluster	1	2	3	1	2	3
p r						
l			zı swı			
j						
b r			grı			
l						
j						
t w						
r	ı					
j						
d w						
r			grı			
j						
k w						
r						
l						
j						
g w						
r						
l			sı			
j						
f r						
l			sı			
j						
θ w						
r			twı			
j						
s p			pı			
t			dı			
k						
m						
n			nı			
w						
l						
j						
ʃ r						
m j						
n						
v						
l						
h						
sp r						
l						
j						
st r			swı			
j						
sk w						
r						
l						
j						

−CCC	SFWW			SFWF		

	SFWW			SFWF		
Cluster	1	2	3	1	2	3
m p				ı		
d						
f						
θ						
z						
n t				ı		
d				ıı		
tʃ						
dʒ						
θ						
s						
z						
ŋ k						ŋgı
d						
z						
p t						
θ						
s						
b d						
z						
t θ						
s						
d z						
tʃ t						
dʒ d						
k t						
s						
g d						
z						
f t						
θ						
s						
v d						
z						
θ t						
s						
ð d						
z						
s p						
t						
k						
z d						
ʃ t						
ʒ d						
l m						
n						
p/b						
t						
d						
k						
tʃ/dʒ						
f						
v						
θ						
s						
z						

APPENDIX 4–D

PACS TOYS Extended Phoneme Realization Chart

Extended Phoneme Realization Chart

Name STEPHEN Chronological Age 3:3 Date 11/94 Tester AH

	SIWI					SIWW					SFWF				
	✓	Incorrect				✓	Incorrect				✓	Incorrect			
Target Phoneme	Correct	Almost Mature	Develop-mentally Immature	Atypical	Other	Correct	Almost Mature	Develop-mentally Immature	Atypical	Other	Correct	Almost Mature	Develop-mentally Immature	Atypical	Other
m	|||			ø|							||				
n	||					||					卌|				
ŋ												ŋ̃|			n|
p	|	b̥||	b|					b|			|||				
b	||||		d|			|									
t			d|||	ʃj|	k|	|				z|	|||				
d	||				s|	|					|				
ʧ					s||					s|					ʔs||
ʤ					s|			d||					ds||		
k		k⁼|	d' g'			|					|||		t|		
g	||					|					||				
f	|||					||					|				
v	|					|	v̥|				|				
θ				vw|									f|		
ð								f|						
s	||||					||					卌				ø|
z				s|		|		s|			卌		s||		
ʃ			s|		ʧ|			s||					s||		
ʒ															
w	|||			v| j|		|									
r			υ| l| w|							ø|					
l	||					|					|		ø||		
j	|					|									
h		ʔ|| ø|													

Source: Copyright © 1995, Pamela Grunwell and Anne Harding.

APPENDIX 4–E

PACS TOYS Contrastive Phones Chart

Contrastive Phones Chart

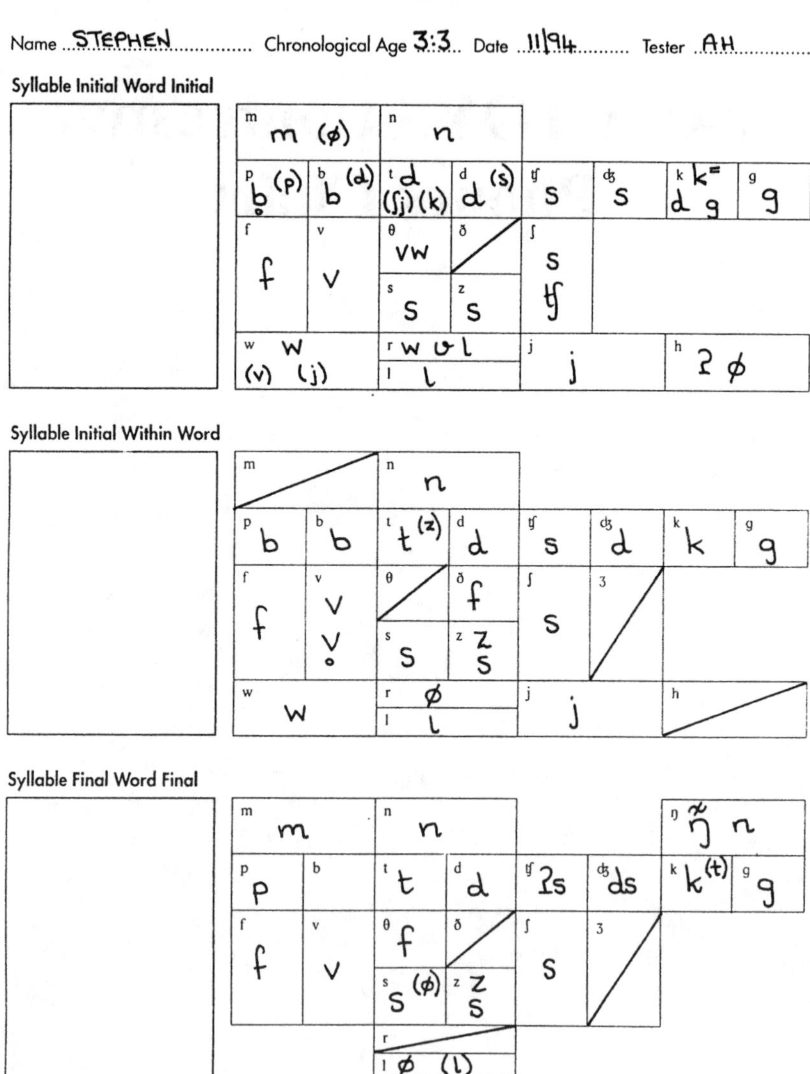

APPENDIX 4–F

PACS Contrastive Assessment: C 6:3

Systems of Contrastive Phones and Contrastive Assessments

Name C 6:3

Syllable Initial Word Initial

Target	Realizations
m	m 10/10
n	n 4/5, d 1/5
p	b 9/9
b	b 16/17, f 1/17
t	d 7/10, t' g' k'
d	d 11/11
tʃ	d' w' b'
dʒ	n 2/4, b' d'
k	k 5/12, d 5/12, b' n'
g	d 6/8, k' b'
f	f 7/14, fd 3/14, d 2/14, w', b'
v	w', d'
θ	n', d'
ð	n'
ʃ	n', ʃb', b', w'
s	n 10/11, d'
z	n', w'
w	w 16/16
r	w 4/4
l	l 10/11, n'
j	j 1/3, ∅ 2/3
h	∅ 5/7, ʔ 2/7

Syllable Initial Within Word

Target	Realizations
m	m 5/7, n', b'
n	n 7/7
p	p 3/10, n3, m', b2, j'
b	b 8/9, n1
t	n 10/10
d	n 4/6, l' j'
tʃ	n 2/2
dʒ	w'
k	n 2/2
g	n' k', l' j'
f	n', j'
v	n', j', w'
θ	n'
ð	n', l'
ʃ	ʃ 2/3, j'
ʒ	n', l'
s	n 3/3
z	n 2/3, w'
w	w 3/4, m'
r	n 5/7, w' j'
l	l 5/8, w2 j'
j	j'
h	n'

Syllable Final Word Final

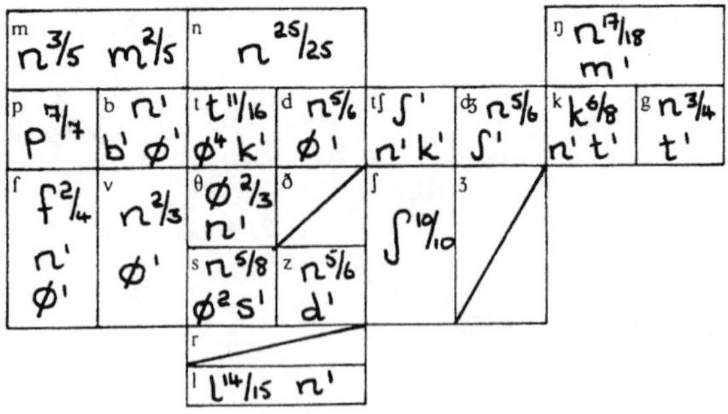

Target	Realizations
m	n 3/5, m 2/5
n	n 25/25
ŋ	n 17/18, m'
p	p 7/7
b	n', b' ∅'
t	t 11/16, ∅4 k'
d	n 5/6, ∅'
tʃ	ʃ', n' k'
dʒ	n 5/6, ʃ'
k	k 6/8, n' t'
g	n 3/4, t'
f	f 2/4, n', ∅'
v	n 2/3, ∅'
θ	∅ 2/3, n'
ð	
ʃ	ʃ 10/10
ʒ	
s	n 5/8, ∅2 s'
z	n 5/6, d'
r	
l	l 14/15, n'

APPENDIX 4–G

Phonological Performance Indicators: C 5:10 Compared with C 6:3

	5:10			6:3		
	SIWI	*SIWW*	*SFWF*	*SIWI*	*SIWW*	*SFWF*
No. targets attempted	21/	23/	18/	22/	23/	18/
No. possible	/22	/23	/20	/22	/23	/20
No. different Cs	10	8	4	14	9	11
No. stable correct matches	2	0	1	3	2	3
No. stable mismatches (errors)	2	7	8	3	7	0
No. variable matches (errors & correct)	17	16	9	16	14	15
No. variable matches involving correct	6	4	1	6	6	7
SFWF only						
No. stable zero realizations			2			0
No. variable zero realizations			9			7
No. variable zero realizations involving correct matches			1			4

Note Marginal phones are included

Key

SIWI Syllable-Initial Word-Initial
SIWW Syllable-Initial Within-Word
SFWF Syllable-Final Word-Final
No. Number

Appendix 4–H

PACS Developmental Assessment and Reassessment: C

Developmental Assessment

Name ....C........................ Chronological Age 5:10 / 6:3 / 6:8 .... Date .... Tester ....

Stage		Labial	Lingual	Protowords and First Words
Stage I (0;9 – 1;6)	Nasal			Show phonetic variability and all phon processes. *Examples*
	Plosive			
	Fricative			
	Approximant			

Stage	Sounds	Processes	Patterns	Age
Stage II (1;6 – 2;0)	m, n; p b, t d; w, l, j	Reduplication Consonant Harmony FINAL CONS. DELETION CLUSTER REDUCTION	FRONTING STOPPING GLIDING C.S. VOICING	5:10
Stage III (2;0 – 2;6)	m, n, (ŋ); p b, t d, (k g); w, (h)	Final Cons. Deletion CLUSTER REDUCTION	Fronting STOPPING GLIDING C.S. VOICING	
Stage IV (2;6 – 3;0)	m, n; p b, t d, k; ʃ, ʃ; w, (l), j	Final Cons. Deletion CLUSTER REDUCTION	STOPPING /v ð z tʃ ʤ/ FRONTING /ʃ/→[s] GLIDING C.S. Voicing	6:3
Stage V (3;0 – 3;6)	m, n, ŋ; p b, t d, (tʃ), k g; f, s, (ʃ); w, l, j, h	Clusters used: obs. + approx. /s/ + cons.	STOPPING /v ð z/ FRONTING /ʃ tʃ ʤ/ GLIDING /θ/→[f]	
Stage VI (3;6 – 4;6)	m, n, ŋ; p b, t d, k g; f v, s, z, ʃ; w, l, j, h	Clusters used: obs. + approx. /s/ + cons.	/ð/→[d] or [v] PALATALIZATION /ʃ tʃ ʤ/ GLIDING /θ/→[f]	6:8
Stage VII (4;6 <)	m, n, ŋ; p b, t d, tʃ ʤ, k g; f v, θ s, ð z, ʃ (ʒ); w, l, r, j, h	Clusters used: obs. + approx. /s/ + cons.	/ð/→[d] or [v] /r/→[w] or [ʋ] /θ/→[f]	

Comments and Notes ______________________________

APPENDIX 4–I

PACS Contrastive Assessment: C 5:10

Systems of Contrastive Phones and Contrastive Assessments

Name C 5:10

Syllable Initial Word Initial

Sound	Realisation
m	b
n	d (b)
p	b (p)
b	b (v)
t	d (b)
d	d
tʃ	b (v) (d)
ʤ	n b
k	d (n)(b)(g)
g	d (g)(b)
f	d (v) (b) (f)
v	w (d)
θ	n d
ð	/
ʃ	n (w) (b)
s	n (d)
z	n v
w	w
r	w (t) (ø)
l	l (d)
j	ø
h	ø (d) (n)

Syllable Initial Within Word

Sound	Realisation
m	b (m) (n)
n	n ø
p	b ø (n)
b	b (j) (l) (ʔ) (ø)
t	n ø
d	n ø (l)
tʃ	n (j)
ʤ	w
k	n d ʔ
g	n ø
f	ø
v	n (j)
θ	ø
ð	ø ʔ
ʃ	j n
ʒ	ø ʔ
s	n
z	ø (n)
w	ø
r	ø j (w)
l	l ø w ʔ
j	ø
h	ø

Syllable Final Word Final

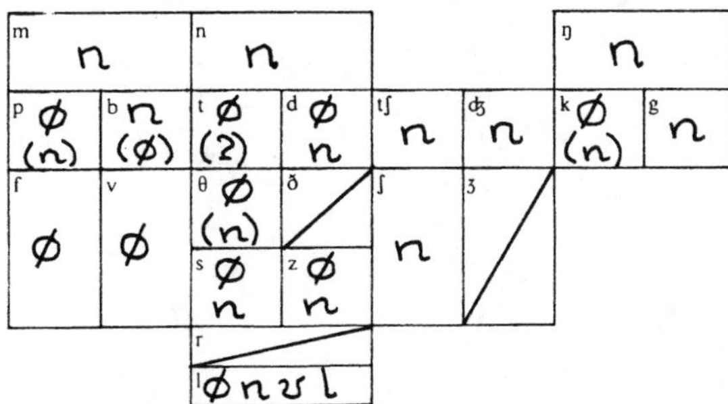

Sound	Realisation
m	n
n	n
ŋ	n
p	ø (n)
b	n (ø)
t	ø (ʔ)
d	ø n
tʃ	n
ʤ	n
k	ø (n)
g	n
f	ø
v	ø
θ	ø (n)
ð	/
ʃ	n
ʒ	/
s	ø n
z	ø n
r	/
l	ø n ʊ l

Appendix 4–J

PACS Contrastive Assessment: C 6:8

Systems of Contrastive Phones and Contrastive Assessments

Name ......C 6:8......

Syllable Initial Word Initial

Target	Realisation
m	m
n	n
p	p
b	b
t	t
d	d
tʃ	t
ʤ	d(t)
k	k
g	g
f	f
v	v
θ	f
ð	d
ʃ	ʃ s
s	s
z	s
w	w
r	ʋ (w)
l	l
j	j
h	h

Syllable Initial Within Word

Target	Realisation
m	m
n	n
p	p
b	b
t	t
d	d
tʃ	f ʃ s
ʤ	d
k	k
g	g
f	f
v	f (v)
θ	f
ð	v
ʃ	ʃ s
ʒ	j
s	s
z	z
w	w
r	wj (ɹ)
l	l
j	j
h	h

Syllable Final Word Final

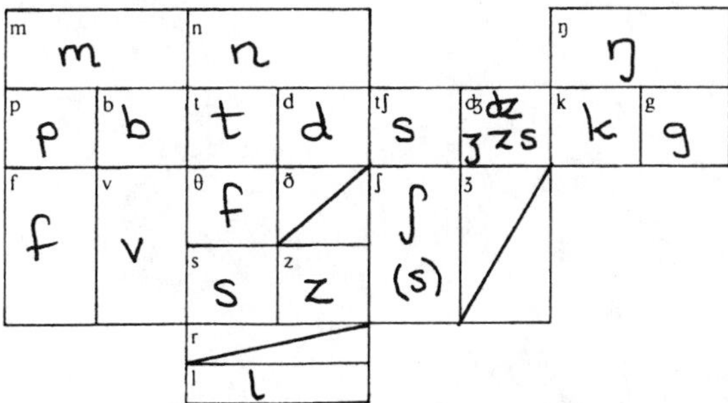

Target	Realisation
m	m
n	n
ŋ	ŋ
p	p
b	b
t	t
d	d
tʃ	s
ʤ	dz ʒ z s
k	k
g	g
f	f
v	v
θ	f
ð	/
ʃ	ʃ (s)
ʒ	/
s	s
z	z
r	/
l	l

CHAPTER 5

Developmental Phonological Disorders: One or Many?

Lawrence D. Shriberg

For the past 20 years, I have had the privilege of studying a compelling public health problem—childhood speech disorders. The challenge to add new and useful information to our knowledge base has been at times exhilarating and at times frustrating, but always interesting. I assume that other authors in this volume share similar histories.

My initiation occurred in 1975, when Joan Kwiatkowski, an instructor on our faculty, invited me to observe some preschool children she was working with in a summer program. In the classificatory term of the times, each of these children had "multiple articulation errors"; most also had some degree of language delay. More colloquially, these children were called "tough artic kids"! My previous work with older children who had /r/ and /s/ distortions left me unprepared for these children's severe speech involvements. When I could finally understand enough of what they were saying, I was impressed by their individual differences. Each child was severely speech involved, yet each also seemed to have a distinctive speech error pattern. As with many significant first-time experiences, my memories of these children remain vivid. Their pronounced speech, educational, and psychosocial needs set benchmarks that continue to motivate my research activities.

At some point, when Joan, some graduate students, and I had begun our studies of these children, we began to question the concept of a *functional* articulation disorder. Rather than working within the prevailing division between "organic" and "functional" disorders, it seemed more useful to focus on developmental and phonological issues in these children. We preferred the term *developmental phonological disorder* to the then-prevalent term *functional articulation disorder* (Shriberg, 1980a). But this shift in emphasis did not change the central fact that these children's speech delays were of unknown origin. The long-term goals of our developing research program began to converge on etiologic classification: Are there subtypes of developmental phonological disorders, each with its own etiology, error pattern, and course of normalization? Pursuit of this question generated many methodological needs, including the need for new measures and a sufficient database.

The following pages are a condensed progress report to acquaint readers with my past, present, and future research. I first discuss conceptual frameworks and then applied issues in assessment and treatment. Crystal ball gazing and wish listing are interleaved within these contexts. Literature citations are used liberally to point the interested reader to places for more detail.

THEORETICAL PERSPECTIVES

Three Populations of Childhood Speech Disorders

Figure 5–1 is an overview of the current scope of practice in childhood speech disorders. This scope of practice stands in stunning contrast to clinical responsibilities of 20 years ago. Contemporary practitioners and service providers must meet the needs of three populations of children. The primary variable differentiating the three groups is the degree to which they have medical, educational, psychosocial, or sociolinguistic needs in addition to their speech needs. It is useful to introduce the three populations in the chronological order in which they have been studied, both by the discipline and in our research activities.

Residual Errors

The population with childhood speech disorders that we first studied consisted of children with what we term *residual errors* (Shriberg, 1980a; Shriberg, Austin, Lewis, McSweeny, & Wilson, in press b). The concept of residual errors follows from the sociobiological perspective of a developmental period for speech-sound acquisition that normally terminates at approximately 9 years of age (Locke, 1994; Shriberg, Gruber, & Kwiatkowski, 1994). At the end of this period, some children retain certain speech-sound errors, typically speech-sound distortions of English fricatives/affricates and/or liquids. Such errors may be regarded as the "residuals" of the period in which one developmental task is to acquire full allophonic mastery of all consonants and vowels/diphthongs of the ambient language.

From a scope-of-practice perspective, it is important to underscore what has happened to children with only residual distortion errors during the past several decades. Two decades ago, the assumption was that all articulation errors were potentially handicapping to speakers. That is, even one speech-sound distortion might distract listeners from the speaker's message—much as a minor orofacial or cosmetic difference might be a visual distraction. Accordingly, services for speech-sound distortions were routinely provided to children in public school settings, and considerable research resources were focused on procedures to assess and treat children with these articulation errors. We, too, found it challenging to find ways

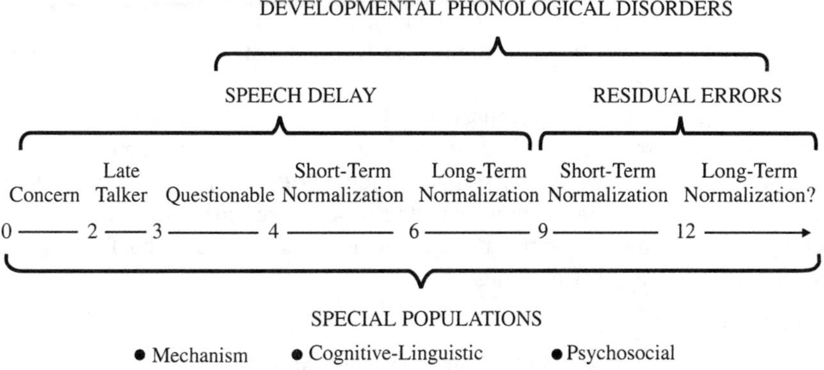

Figure 5–1 The Three Populations of Childhood Speech Disorders

to try to help speech-language pathologists evoke correct /r/ and /ɝ/ sounds from older children with persisting distortions. In one study of 65 children, we described an eight-step response evocation procedure that evoked correct /ɝ/ from 70% of children within 6 minutes; another approximately 10% of children emitted correct /ɝ/s in subsequent sessions that trained program step failures (Shriberg, 1975b). In a later study, we described a "ventriloquist stick" technique to evoke correct /ɝ/ from children with persistent /ɝ/ and /r/ distortions (Shriberg, 1980b).

More recently, three factors have militated against this type of research and the routine provision of public school speech services for children with only distortion errors. First is the issue of the importance of such errors in a child's development of speech and language. Unlike phoneme deletions and phoneme substitutions, phoneme distortions have not been associated with deficits in the phonological skills underlying reading, writing, and other verbal skills. Second is the issue of the sociolinguistic consequences of distortions such as dentalized and lateralized lisps and derhotacized consonant and vowel sounds. Their consequences have not been associated with intelligibility deficits, and in the current pluralistic culture, they may not be associated with unfavorable stereotypes. In fact, close listening to the speech of broadcasters and celebrities suggests that at least some types of speech distortions may be favored for their distinctive quality.

Third, even if distortion errors may be attested as handicapping, they are viewed as lower priority needs at a time when special educational resources are severely taxed. Thus, although included in the scope of practice in Figure 5–1, speech services for children with residual errors may increasingly be more difficult to fund from public sources. For children with residual errors that do not normalize by 12 years of age (*short-term* normalization), alternative services in the private sector are increasingly the only option, and for an undocumented percentage of adults not experiencing *long-term* normalization, speech-sound distortions may persist unchanged for a lifetime.

Interestingly, it is the theoretical significance of residual errors that is of contemporary interest, rather than their importance as a public health concern. Later we will have more to say about possible etiologic origins of residual errors. Here we will just underscore the theoretical puzzle posed by residual errors: Why might a child correctly acquire everything else about the ambient language but fail to learn how to articulate one or two sounds?

Speech Delay

The second population with childhood speech disorders, also subsumed by the term *developmental phonological disorders* in Figure 5–1, consists of children who have what we term *speech delay* (Shriberg, 1980a). This classificatory label, too, is referenced to the developmental period for speech acquisition. Children meeting criteria for speech delay have persisting deletion and substitution errors not observed in typically speaking children of the same chronological age. As suggested above, if there were one core developmental phonological disorder, speech delay and residual errors might just represent different levels of severity of expression of the disorder. Unlike children with residual errors, however, a significant percentage of children with speech delay appear to have associated cognitive-linguistic, learning, and other special educational needs. It was the significance of these needs, also recognized in the Education of All Handicapped Children Act of 1975 (see U.S. Education Department, 1992), that motivated the considerable research effort over the past 20 years to describe and treat speech delay.

Ingram's (1976) influential synthesis and conceptual frameworks by others provided developmental ties among cognitive-linguistic processes. Speech delay can be referenced to several subperiods, phases, or stages within the period of development from birth to approximately 9 years. Again, because children with speech delay typically, but not invariably, have some other developmental involvements—most often language delays or later reading or other learning delays—delayed speech is a public health concern throughout the developmental period. Let us look briefly at each age period.

As indicated in Figure 5–1, there is concern about any notable delay from the landmarks of speech development from 0 to 2 years of age, as addressed in earlier chapters in this volume. Of signal interest are Oller's emerging data indicating that children who are late canonical babblers are at risk for later verbal development (Oller, Eilers, Steffens, Lynch, & Urbano, 1994). The second period of concern about speech delay occurs from 2 to 3 years, with a significant percentage of children termed *late talkers* later having clinically notable speech-language delays (Paul, 1993). The third period is from 3 to 4 years, a period of large individual differences in speech development. As shown in Figure 5–1, we find it appropriate to describe children at the low end of the normal distribution during this period as having *questionable speech delay*. Fourth is the period from 4 to 9 years, when children may fall into two groups: *speech delay* or *questionable residual errors* (not shown in Figure 5–1). Finally, as described later, subtypes of residual errors describe the error types and error histories of persons who have retained speech errors past 9 years of age.

The course of normalization of a disorder can provide important information for purposes of classification, as well as for clinical-prognostic purposes. In several follow-up studies, we have found that approximately 75% of children with speech delay normalize their speech errors by 6 years of age (termed *short-term normalization*; Shriberg, 1994; Shriberg, Gruber, & Kwiatkowski, 1994; Shriberg, Kwiatkowski, & Gruber, 1994). Of the remaining 25% of children, most normalize by 9 years of age (long-term normalization), but some continue to manifest one of the three types of residual error patterns described below. Children in the latter two groups especially may have other special educational needs throughout early and later primary grades (Shriberg & Kwiatkowski, 1988).

Special Populations

The third category of childhood speech disorders in Figure 5–1 is termed *special populations* (see Bernthal and Bankson's, 1994, use of this term to organize an edited text on this topic). In contrast to children with speech-language delay as their primary need, the primary needs of children in special populations are typically in other health or educational areas (e.g., tracheostomy, traumatic brain injury, behavioral disorders). We have found it useful to subgroup children in these populations by etiology in three domains: speech-hearing mechanism, cognitive-linguistic processes, and psychosocial processes (Shriberg & Kwiatkowski, 1982, 1994; Shriberg, Kwiatkowski, Best, Hengst, & Terselic-Weber, 1986). Speech-language pathologists working with these children need to be well trained to understand relevant aspects of their primary needs, as well as to meet speech needs. As illustrated in Figure 5–1, the speech involvements in these special populations may originate and persist over varying age ranges within the birth to 9-year period for normal speech acquisition, as well as in any time period beyond 9 years.

In the context of emerging trends in health care, the needs of special populations have redefined the clinical landscape. Speech-language pathologists must be able to apply their knowledge of phonological and speech-motor development to an ever-widening array of clinical responsibilities. It is for these reasons that we currently prefer the term *childhood speech disorders*—in contrast to terms such as *articulation disorders, phonological disorders*, or *articulation/phonological disorders*—as the most useful cover term for the three populations of children studied and served by the discipline of communicative disorders.

Etiologic Classification of Childhood Speech Disorders

For all but the most general purposes, the disorders of children in the three population groups depicted in Figure 5–1 require further categorization using some type of classification system. In contrast to other options, we favor a medical model approach to classification in which the categories are based on the putative etiology of the disorder (Shriberg, 1982b). We think that such a system provides the most useful organization of disorders—for research, for training programs in communicative disorders, and for clinical practice. A system developed for these three needs, termed the *Speech Disorders Classification System (SDCS)*, is shown in Figure 5–2. The SDCS was first described in Shriberg (1993), updated in Shriberg (1994), and finalized in Shriberg et al. (in press b).

The eight boxes in the top two rows of Figure 5–2 indicate the major descriptive classifications in the SDCS system. The box in the upper row titled *developmental phonological disorders* is the classification suggested previously as useful to underscore the developmental component in speech delay and residual errors. In turn, two subordinate descriptive classifications—*speech delay* and *residual errors*—each subsume putative etiologic subtypes. The following discussion provides a description of each of the remaining boxes in Figure 5–2 and highlights emerging research findings.

Normal or Normalized Speech Acquisition

The upper leftmost box in Figure 5–2 includes two descriptive classifications. Speakers with normal speech at assessment and no history of speech delay are classified as *normal speech acquisition (NSA)*. The SDCS determines what is normal using a table of reference data (Shriberg, 1993; Shriberg et al., in press b). Speakers who meet age-based criteria for normal speech but who have documented histories of earlier speech delay (see below) are classified as *normalized speech acquisition (NSA-X)*. The "X" is a place holder for the age at which a person has normalized speech. For example, "NSA-6" indicates speech normalization at age 6. Accurate speech histories and classification are central in some research designs, such as emerging studies using behavioral and molecular genetics techniques with children with speech disorders and their nuclear and extended families.

Nondevelopmental Speech Disorders

Nondevelopmental speech disorders is an appropriate classification for all speech disorders that occur after the developmental period for speech, nominally 9 years of age. The classification includes the full scope of adult speech disorders, including those due to trauma, disease, and various physical and emotional illnesses. The study and treatment of adult-onset speech disorders differs from developmental phonological disorders in the need for attention to factors associated with growth and development.

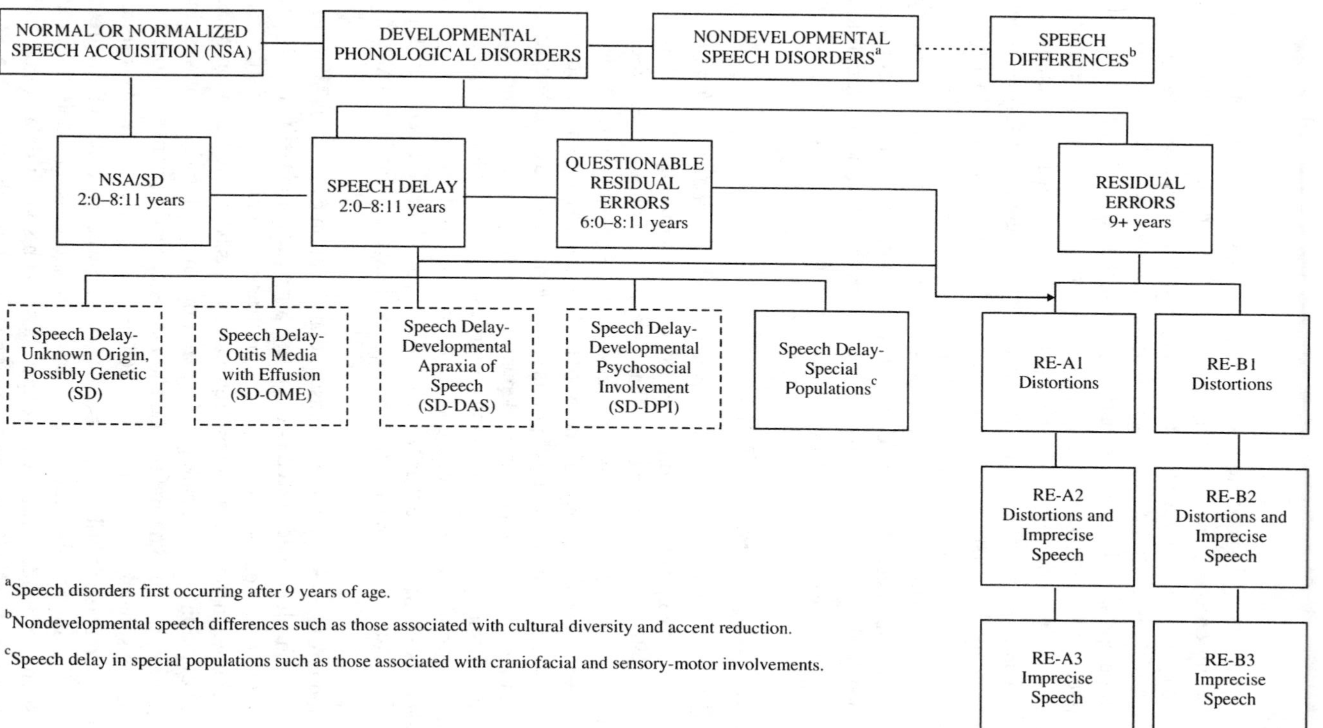

[a]Speech disorders first occurring after 9 years of age.

[b]Nondevelopmental speech differences such as those associated with cultural diversity and accent reduction.

[c]Speech delay in special populations such as those associated with craniofacial and sensory-motor involvements.

Figure 5–2 The Speech Disorders Classification System

Speech Differences

The upper rightmost classification is a category for speakers with nondevelopmental *speech differences*. This category includes all speech and prosody-voice differences that speakers might elect to modify, such as those associated with mastery of English as a second language. As indicated by the dashed line to this category, competent speech-language pathologists make clear classification distinctions between speech disorders and speech differences. For example, the speech and prosody-voice patterns of children speaking African American Vernacular English (AAVE) reflect phonological difference, not phonological disorder. When speech-language pathologists are called upon to develop programs to modify speech differences, however, some of the instructional techniques they use are similar to those used to modify speech disorders. Therefore it is important formally to tie the instructional needs of children in this population with those of children who have speech disorders. As reviewed elsewhere in this volume, multicultural and diversity issues warrant full integration into the research agenda of our discipline.

Normal Speech Acquisition/Speech Delay

The need for a classification termed *normal (or normalized) speech acquisition/speech delay (NSA/SD)* is familiar territory in epidemiologic research. Although service delivery systems require that persons be dichotomized as either normal or disordered, it is inappropriate to classify the status of some children as either normal or affected (i.e., speech delayed). If the underlying trait is continuously distributed in a population, cutoff points between normal and disordered must be arbitrary and may differ significantly depending on the purpose for the dichotomy. From this perspective, we have found it more useful to trichotomize speakers, providing a category for speakers whose status is intermediate between normal and disordered (i.e., NSA/SD). Note that NSA/SD also is coded for children who, after having a speech delay, are almost but not yet normalized (i.e., neither NSA-X nor SD).

Sample support for NSA/SD as a necessary classification category is shown in Figure 5–3, which plots speech trends over age for children classified as NSA, NSA/SD, and SD. Notice that at each age, the trend for children classified as NSA/SD falls between the trends for children classified as NSA and SD. Moreover, the standard deviation bars indicate good separation among the distributions for each classification group. The metric used to assess speech in conversation, the Percentage of Consonants Correct-Revised (PCC-R), scores all distortion errors as phonemically correct (see Shriberg, Austin, Lewis, McSweeny, & Wilson, in press a). Thus these data support the view that children with speech-sound deletions and substitutions can be divided into two groups: those with speech delay (SD) and those whose error patterns fall between normal speech and speech delay (NSA/SD).

Five Subtypes of Speech Delay

As introduced above, *speech delay* was suggested as an appropriate nosological term for the estimated 2% to 3% of preschool children with a developmental phonological disorder of unknown origin (Shriberg & Kwiatkowski, 1994). The SDCS classifies a child as *speech delayed (SD)* when certain age-inappropriate speech-sound deletions and/or substitutions occur reliably in a conversational speech sample. Is there just one core form of SD? Or, alternatively, are there subtypes of SD based on differing etiologies? As indicated in the title of this chapter and the following brief discussion, this is the research question we continue to pursue.

The boxes subsumed by speech delay in Figure 5–2 comprise four putative etiologic subtypes of developmental phonological disorders. Biolinguistic and sociolinguistic distinctions associated with each proposed subtype are viewed as central to an eventual account of the origin and course of childhood speech disorders. Rationale for each subtype and preliminary estimates of epidemiologic and other nonspeech data (prevalence, gender ratio, language status, speech-sound normalization history, residual error status, and familial aggregation) are provided in Shriberg (1994). Following are brief comments on each proposed subtype.

Speech Delay. The common or most prevalent subtype of speech delay is simply termed *speech delay (SD)*. Preliminary estimates, based solely on our clinical studies, are that this form of SD occurs in perhaps 60% of preschool children identified as having a speech disorder of unknown origin. Among other speculations about possible etiologic origins, there is emerging support for the heritability of SD. The primary evidence to date for genetic transmission is the high prevalence of verbal trait deficits in nuclear and extended families of children with speech-language disorders (familial aggregation). Studies have reported that 20% to nearly 80% of affected children have at least one affected nuclear family member (see Felsenfeld, McGue, & Broen, 1995; Lahey & Edwards, 1995). Our own finding is that 56% of 84 children with SD had one or more family members with "the same speech problem" (as reported by caregivers; Shriberg & Kwiatkowski, 1994). In collaboration with colleagues at two other centers, behavioral and molecular genetics studies are in progress to assess possible modes of genetic transmission of SD and to search for candidate genes.

The concept of a speech *delay* is a central assumption in our genetics studies, as well as in studies of the other proposed subtypes of SD. To test support for this concept, we compared the course of normalization of 10 SD children followed longitudinally to cross-sectional data on normal speech acquisition reported in Smit, Hand, Freilinger, Bernthal, and Bird (1990). Following Bishop and Edmundson's (1987) lucid discussion of this topic, we reasoned that support for delay would

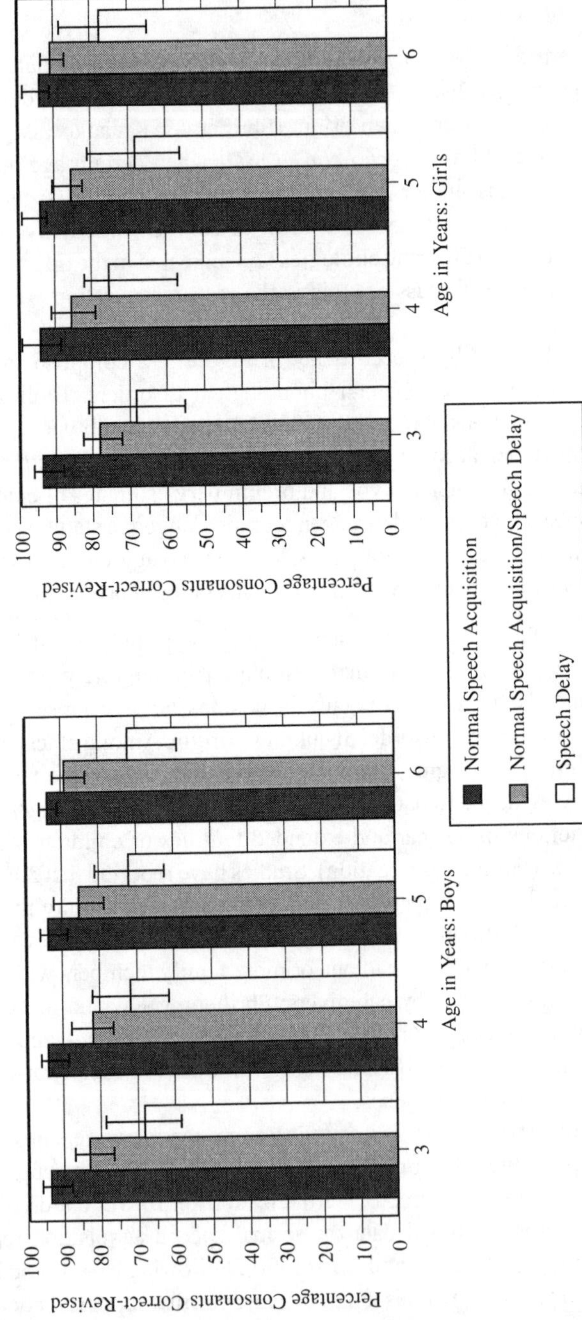

Figure 5–3 Age Trends (Means, Standard Deviations) for 3- to 6-Year-Old Boys and Girls Classified by the SDCS as Having Normal or Normalized Speech Acquisition (NSA), Intermediate Status (NSA/SD), or Speech Delay (SD)

be gained if the SD children had the same course of normalization as children with normal speech acquisition but achieved mastery at later ages.

The data in Figure 5–4 and associated analyses were viewed as strong support for the construct of speech delay (Shriberg, Gruber, & Kwiatkowski, 1994; see Figures 5 through 7, pp. 1167–1168). The unfilled circles are mean PCC scores (divided into the Early-8, Middle-8, and Late-8 consonants; Shriberg, 1993) for the children with normal speech acquisition; the filled circles are mean PCC scores for the children with SD. The ages of the SD children have been shifted leftwards to allow visual and statistical comparison. As attested by statistical findings, the acquisition trends for the two groups are well described by one function. For this proposed subtype of speech delay, SD, the research challenges are to explicate the underlying neurolinguistic processing deficits and eventually the sociobiological origins of those deficits.

Detailed information on the speech characteristics of SD also provides benchmarks for diagnostic classification of the other forms of SD described below. The subtypes view of SD would be supported if each subtype had at least one unique speech characteristic in addition to the general pattern of speech delay. As described next, such speech characteristics could function as diagnostic markers for each of the subtypes.

Speech Delay-Otitis Media with Effusion. A second possible cause of speech delay is processing deficits associated with fluctuant conductive hearing loss due to recurrent otitis media with effusion (OME). Criteria for recurrent OME vary considerably in the research literature. In our studies, children must have had at least six episodes of OME in the first 3 years of life to be classified as having recurrent involvement (Shriberg, 1987; Shriberg & Flipsen, 1996; Thielke & Shriberg, 1990). Many children referred to our speech clinic for suspected speech delay have had nearly continuous OME during some period of the first 3 years of life and beyond. Typically, the case histories of such children include ample evidence of fluctuant hearing loss in one or both ears. A preliminary estimate, based solely on our clinical referrals, is that this proposed form of speech delay, which we term *speech delay-otitis media with effusion (SD-OME)*, is found in approximately 30% of preschool children referred for speech delay of presently unknown origin (Shriberg, 1994; Shriberg & Kwiatkowski, 1994; see Shriberg, Aram, & Kwiatkowski, in press, for a description of local ascertainment procedures).

Shriberg (1987) is an anecdotal account of a series of studies attempting to determine diagnostic markers for SD-OME; retrospective and prospective studies with several hundred children are in progress. To date, the quest for a diagnostic marker for SD-OME has isolated several speech error targets and error types that differ from those observed in SD (Shriberg & Flipsen, 1996). Briefly, they focus on differences in these children's place/manner errors on nasals, stops, and glides;

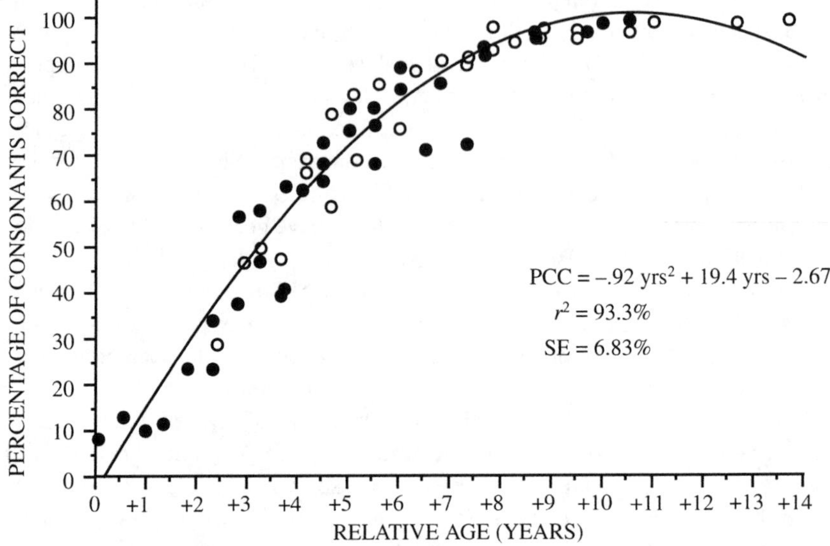

Figure 5–4 Age-Adjusted Plot of Speech Acquisition and Speech Normalization in Children with Normal (Unfilled Circles) and Delayed (Filled Circles) Speech. *Source*: Reprinted with permission from L.D. Shriberg, F.A. Gruber and J. Kwiatkowski, *Journal of Speech and Hearing Research,* Vol. 37, p. 1168, © 1994, American Speech-Language-Hearing Association.

place of production of fricatives; frequency of errors on rhotics; and deletions of certain sounds in certain word positions. Among these candidates (see later discussion of non-natural sound changes), we hope to cross-validate at least one or more speech characteristics associated with a history of early recurrent OME. The availability of such markers would, in turn, permit studies to model the processes by which significant fluctuant hearing loss affects speech acquisition in some children.

Speech Delay-Developmental Apraxia of Speech. The third suspected subtype of a developmental speech delay shown in Figure 5–2 is a form that resembles acquired apraxia of speech in adults. Consistent with the classification format in the SDCS, we term this form *speech delay-developmental apraxia of speech (SD-DAS)*. Using samples of children referred for speech delay of unknown origin as the denominator (350 children; see Kwiatkowski & Shriberg, 1993), we estimated that children with this suspected form of speech delay constituted 3% to 5% of our clinical sample. In Shriberg, Aram, and Kwiatkowski (in press), we attempted a broad review of the DAS literature. Although the prevailing notion is that this childhood speech disorder has its origin in speech-motor processing deficits, attempts to date to document a specific disorder of *praxis* as the origin of SD-DAS have been unsuccessful.

Our studies of suspected SD-DAS have involved 53 children, including speech samples collected by research colleagues at five other clinical research sites. We have found that approximately half of these children with suspected DAS have inappropriate sentential stress. The specific pattern is one of excessive-equal stress. We suggest that this prosodic difference in stress can be used as a diagnostic marker for at least a subgroup of children with suspected SD-DAS. Inappropriate stress of the type coded in these studies is seldom observed in children acquiring speech normally or with SD (Shriberg, Kwiatkowski, Rasmussen, Lof, & Miller, 1992). Studies in process are exploring alternative processing loci for the observed inappropriate stress (Velleman & Shriberg, 1996) and comparing these children's speech and prosody profiles to profiles of adults with apraxia of speech (Odell & Shriberg, 1996). The reported family histories in SD-DAS studies (Hall, Jordan, & Robin, 1993) suggest that this prosodic diagnostic marker might also serve as a phenotype marker. That is, inappropriate stress may be the behavioral expression (i.e., the phenotype) of SD-DAS as a genetically transmitted disorder.

Speech Delay-Developmental Psychosocial Involvement. The fourth type of speech delay, *speech delay-developmental psychosocial involvement (SD-DPI)*, is the most speculative of the SD subtypes in the SDCS. The proposal that psychosocial issues can be causally sufficient for speech delay is predicated on the observations of pioneer speech pathologists such as Charles Van Riper, Wendell Johnson, and Muriel Morley. In a variety of sources, each of these perceptive clinical researchers has reported psychosocial needs in some children with speech delay. These observations are supported in several surveys and follow-up studies (Shriberg & Kwiatkowski, 1988, 1994) documenting psychosocial needs in some children with SD. Solely on the basis of our local data, we believe that children with SD-DPI make up some percentage of the remaining approximately 7% of children with speech delay of unknown origin (i.e., SD: 60%; SD-OME: 30%; SD-DAS: 3%; SD-DPI [and others]: 7%).

To date, we have only preliminary proposals for diagnostic markers for children with SD-DPI. A leading candidate is in the prosody-voice domain, which provides considerable information on affective states and traits. What strikes us in some children is their moment-to-moment variability in prosody-voice domains, as well as their retest variability on indices of segmental competence. Also, some children with SD seem to have considerable difficulty with the types of dyadic activities that most children like and learn from. As with each of the other proposed subtypes, eventual validation of a subtype of speech delay associated with psychosocial issues would assumedly have useful implications for the form and content of treatment.

Speech Delay/Special Populations. We offer only a few comments here on research and clinical trends for children with speech delay in special populations. As suggested in Figure 5–1 and discussed previously, the needs of children in these populations demand ever-increasing clinical competencies. Including this classification within developmental phonological disorders emphasizes two considerations: (a) that children with other disorders have developmental speech needs in addition to their unique speech involvements and (b) that clinical decision making with these children is informed by findings in other forms of childhood speech disorders. The proposal to subsume these forms of developmental phonological disorders within childhood speech disorders encourages clinical-research rapprochement among *all* types of speech disorders in children.

Questionable Residual Errors

In addition to SD or NSA/SD, there is one other classification for children with developmental speech disorders that can occur during the period from 6 to 9 years of age. The classification termed *questionable residual errors* (QRE) is used for children who have one or more speech sound distortions or common substitutions (e.g., distortions of fricatives or liquids; substitutions of /θ/ for /s/ or /w/ for /r/), but do not otherwise meet criteria for SD or NSA/SD. Some children with QRE could be children who normalized from SD or NSA/SD status, or as indicated in Figure 5–2, they could have no such history. Such errors *may* normalize by 9 years of age, or they could persist. The following section provides additional information on the concept of residual errors.

Residual Errors

The SDCS posits temporal, historical, and conceptual distinctions between *residual errors (RE)* and speech delay, as well as differences among several subforms of RE. As introduced earlier, research interest in RE will be important to efforts to assemble a coherent account of the origins and nature of all childhood speech disorders.

If 9 years is taken as the end point for the developmental period, the term *speech delayed* is a misnomer for persons who retain errors past this age. The SDCS first divides such speakers on the basis of their speech histories. Children or adults who have histories of SD are classified as *Residual Errors-A* (RE-A) whereas children or adults with speech errors but no history of speech delay are classified as *Residual Errors-B* (RE-B). Acoustic studies in process are attempting to determine if there are differences in the residual speech-sound distortions of teenage children who meet criteria for RE-A, compared to errors on the same sounds for children classified as RE-B. The possibility that they might differ follows from a long-held proposal that the causal origins of RE-B differ from those of RE-A (Shriberg, 1975a, 1994). Essentially, the assumption is that the fricative and liquid distortions of RE-B children (i.e., children without histories of speech delay) occurred in response to environmental situations, whereas the same errors in RE-A children are the residuals of speech delay due to nonenvironmental (i.e., genetic) origins.

The three numbered subtypes in Figure 5–2 can be used to further classify error patterns. RE-A1 and RE-B1 are for residual common distortion errors (e.g., dental /s/, lateral /s/, derhotacized /r/, velarized /l/; see Shriberg, 1993, Appendix). RE-A2 and RE-B2 are for residual common distortions and imprecise speech (i.e., speech-sound omissions and substitutions). RE-A3 and RE-B3 are for imprecise speech alone. Reference data provided in Shriberg et al. (in press b) suggest that the RE-2 and RE-3 forms of residual errors have low prevalence in normal adult populations. Note that decreased articulatory precision as it may occur in special populations in adults (e.g., traumatic brain injury) would be classified as a nondevelopmental speech disorder.

ASSESSMENT OF CHILDHOOD SPEECH DISORDERS

One consequence of the considerable activity in childhood speech disorders during the past 20 years is a profusion of assessment approaches for children with SD. Indeed, the chapters in this volume illustrate the diversity of theoretical positions, each requiring specific assessment stimuli and analytic procedures. In contrast, there are few guidelines for speech assessment of children with SD in many special populations. The following discussion reflects some of the assessment topics our group has studied over the past two decades. Associated issues will be important as measures are developed for children included in the contemporary scope of practice.

Conversational Speech Sampling

One of the most extensively studied questions in childhood speech disorders concerns the potential influence of sampling mode. A position we have advocated is that conversational speech samples provide the only source for valid, integrated analysis of phonetic, phonologic, prosodic, and language variables. All of the findings reported above have been based on information taken from a 5- to 10-minute conversational speech sample. Methodological studies have focused on development of protocols for effective and efficient conversational speech sampling, including attention to audio-recording issues, and empirical studies of the representativeness and stability of various structural statistics in conversational speech (Morrison & Shriberg, 1992; Shriberg, 1982a, 1986, 1993; Shriberg et al., in press a; Shriberg & Kwiatkowski, 1985).

An observation about conversational speech sampling to highlight is simply that in most situations, it works. In the face of the many words of concern that have been written about constraints on conversational speech sampling for clinical and research decision making, we continue to find this mode of assessment valid, reliable, and efficient for all but a small number of children with limited intelligibility or productivity (see Morrison & Shriberg, 1994). That is not to minimize the skills needed to obtain technically adequate and linguistically rich conversational speech samples. Experience with hundreds of conversational speech samples obtained by student clinicians, speech-language pathologists, and colleagues elsewhere suggests that the crucial factor underlying productivity is the examiner's skill in evoking and glossing speech. Conversational speech sampling is not a sufficient assessment approach for all children or all clinical-research questions, however. For example, the assessment of children in special populations typically requires information from a variety of speech tasks to assess thoroughly articulatory capacity and phonological status.

Phonetic Transcription

When we began to listen to the speech of children with speech delay, it was clear that clinical research with these children would require more skills in scoring and transcribing speech than had been needed when working with children with residual errors. In the course of our work, we found it necessary to study procedures for (a) narrow phonetic transcription (Shriberg, 1972, 1986; Shriberg & Kent, 1982), (b) phonetic transcription by consensus (Shriberg, Kwiatkowski, & Hoffmann, 1984), (c) selecting and training persons to do research transcription (Shriberg, Hinke, & Trost-Steffen, 1987), (d) computerized reliability assessment (Shriberg & Olson, 1988), and (e) using caregivers as an aid in glossing their children's speech (Kwiatkowski & Shriberg, 1992). Shriberg and Lof (1991) and McSweeny and Shriberg (1995) provided information on the reliability of narrow and broad phonetic transcription of children with typically developing and disordered speech.

We estimate that the research activities cited above have pushed to the limits the capacity of motivated people to transcribe speech samples that range from normal to mildly disordered to substantially unintelligible. Among the specific findings, guidelines, recommendations, and conclusions reported in the above citations, one conclusion and some comments are highlighted.

The primary conclusion is that the validity and reliability of phonetic transcription remain significant constraints on all reported findings in the childhood speech disorders literature (see Kent, 1996). Despite continuous efforts to upgrade interjudge reliability in our data, broad transcription agreement commonly reaches into the 90% range, and narrow phonetic transcription agreement percentages typically are in the 70% range. Moreover, reliability estimates for specific diacritic symbols (for example, the symbol for devoicing [̥]) indicate that such data may not be adequate for some clinical and research questions in childhood speech disorders.

Lowered reliability findings make it mandatory that researchers estimate and present reliability data at the level at which data are used to draw conclusions about phenomena (see Shriberg, 1972). Moreover, reliability estimates should be considered closely when evaluating supposed changes in speech occurring within or across speakers (i.e., effect size). We recently assembled standard error-of-measurement data on nine speech metrics, using transcriber agreement coefficients as the estimate of measurement error (Shriberg et al., in press a). Such data allow close evaluation of the reliability of the test scores derived from phonetic transcription, rather than the reliability of transcribers (as typically estimated by point-to-point percentage of agreement).

A final comment here underscores the potential of microcomputer-based acoustic displays to improve the validity and reliability of phonetic transcription. Information from wave form and spectral displays should markedly increase the accuracy of perceptual decisions, such as decisions about speech-sound deletions (presence/absence of energy), substitutions (voicing, place, and manner information), and distortions (information on place, manner, timing, duration, and force). Until automated phonetic transcription is feasible using speech recognition processors, acoustic-aided auditory transcription procedures have promise to upgrade information from this core assessment task.

Prosody-Voice Coding

A third methodological need to underscore is the need for means to assess suprasegmental characteristics of children's speech. There is a need to develop theoretically sound, clinically relevant, and methodologically efficient procedures to assess prosody and voice. Our interests, again, focus on their potential as diagnostic markers. A procedure developed for these purposes requires a trained person to code seven prosody-voice variables for each codable utterance in a conversational speech sample (Shriberg, Kwiatkowski, & Rasmussen, 1990).

Exhibit 5–1 is a list of the 31 exclusion codes (used to exclude utterances from prosody-voice coding) and the 32 prosody-voice codes used in the prosody-voice procedure. Coding categories were developed after listening to conversational speech samples reflecting a wide range of speech disorders, including children and adults from many special populations (e.g., craniofacial disorders, cognitive disorders, neuromotor disorders, psychiatric disorders). Exemplars for each code were assembled on audiocassette training tapes.

A methodological conclusion from reliability studies with this instrument is quite similar to those suggested above for phonetic transcription. Although interjudge and intrajudge agreement percentages for prosody-voice variables are acceptable at the level of "broad" coding (e.g., appropriate vs. inappropriate), agreement at more narrow levels of coding may not be adequate for certain clinical research questions. And for speakers with only mild involvement in certain prosody-voice

Exhibit 5–1 Exclusion Codes and Prosody-Voice Codes Used in the Prosody-Voice Assessment Procedure

Exclusion Codes

Content/Context			Environment			Register			States		
C1	Automatic Sequential	____	E1	Interfering Noise	____	R1	Character Register	____	S1	Belch	____
C2	Back Channel/Aside	____	E2	Recorder Wow/Flutter	____	R2	Narrative Register	____	S2	Cough/Throat Clear	____
C3	I Don't Know	____	E3	Too Close to Microphone	____	R3	Negative Register	____	S3	Food in Mouth	____
C4	Imitation	____	E4	Too Far from Microphone	____	R4	Sound Effects		S4	Hiccup	____
C5	Interruption/ Overtalk	____				R5	Whisper	____	S5	Laugh	____
C6	Not 4 (+) Words	____							S6	Lip Smack	____
C7	Only One Word	____							S7	Body Movement	____
C8	Only Person's Name	____							S8	Sneeze	____
C9	Reading	____							S9	Telegraphic	____
C10	Singing	____							S10	Yawn	____
C11	Second Repetition	____									
C12	Too Many Unintelligibles	____									

continues

Prosody-Voice Codes

Prosody

Phrasing			Rate			Stress		
1	Appropriate	____	1	Appropriate	____	1	Appropriate	____
2	Sound/Syllable Repetition	____	9	Slow Articulation/Pause Time	____	13	Multisyllabic Word Stress	____
3	Word Repetition	____	10	Slow/Pause Time	____	14	Reduced/Equal Stress	____
4	Sound/Syllable and Word Repetition	____	11	Fast	____	15	Excessive/Equal/Misplaced Stress	____
			12	Fast/Acceleration	____			
5	More than One Word Repetition	____				16	Multiple Stress Features	____
6	One Word Revision	____						
7	More than One Word Revision	____						
8	Repetition and Revision	____						

Voice

Loudness			Pitch			Quality: Laryngeal Features			Quality: Resonance Features		
1	Appropriate	____	1	Appropriate	____	1	Appropriate	____	1	Appropriate	____
17	Soft	____	19	Low Pitch/Glottal Fry	____	23	Breathy	____	30	Nasal	____
18	Loud	____	20	Low Pitch	____	24	Rough	____	31	Denasal	____
			21	High Pitch/Falsetto	____	25	Strained	____	32	Nasopharyngeal	____
			22	High Pitch	____	26	Break/Shift/Tremulous	____			
						27	Register Break	____			
						28	Diplophonia	____			
						29	Multiple Laryngeal Features	____			

domains, such as speakers with mild differences in laryngeal quality, agreement may not be high even at the level of appropriate vs. inappropriate. As above, methodological solutions to such problems also include the use of acoustic-aided perceptual procedures, guided by database information to anchor coding criteria.

Reliability constraints notwithstanding, prosody-voice profiles seem to have promise for questions about processing deficits underlying speech disorders. In Shriberg and Widder (1990), speech and prosody-voice profiles were inspected for 40 noninstitutionalized adults with mental retardation. Extensive utterance-to-utterance variability on certain prosody-voice and paralinguistic variables was interpreted as more consistent with cognitive resource allocation deficits than with speech-motor constraints. More recently, assessment of stress was central in the study of children with suspected SD-DAS described previously.

Phonological Analysis

Our early reading of Stampe's (1973/1979) natural process theory was that it provided exactly the link between linguistic competence models and relevant psycholinguistic constructs needed for research on the etiologic subtypes of speech delay (Shriberg & Kwiatkowski, 1978). Stampe's view that certain speech-sound changes are *natural* because they reflect "hard-wired" perceptual, cognitive, or production processes offered a theoretical base for studies in etiologic subtypes. We reasoned that if the core sound changes of speech delay could be accounted for by a set of natural phonological processes, then all remaining *non-natural* sound changes might reflect deficits in certain perceptual, cognitive, or speech-motor processes (Shriberg & Kwiatkowski, 1980). Specifically, each sound change not accounted for by a natural phonological process might be a potential diagnostic marker for a subtype of speech delay. For example, if fronting of consonants is natural, backing must be non-natural. Children who back consonants may do so because of some type of perceptual, cognitive, or speech-motor processing deficit associated with one or more etiologic subtypes (e.g., SD-OME, SD-DAS, SD-DPI).

For our specific goals, this perspective on natural phonological processes has been useful. Using a computer-aided procedure that classifies children's sound changes into eight natural processes, we have reported that approximately 92% of the sound changes of children with speech delay meet criteria for one of the eight natural processes (Shriberg, 1991; Shriberg & Kwiatkowski, 1983; Shriberg et al., 1986). We continue to mine the remaining 8% of non-natural sound changes (e.g., initial-consonant deletion, backing, certain uncommon place and manner substitutions), as well as prosody-voice variables, for potential diagnostic markers of etiologic subtypes of speech delay. Analyses termed *speech profiles* and *prosody-voice profiles* provide detailed information on a speaker's productive speech (Shriberg, 1993). New perspectives from this work include the development of alternatives to the Percentage of Consonants Correct metric for certain research and applied questions (Shriberg et al., in press a).

In comparison to procedures reported by other colleagues over the past 20 years, our linguistic procedures to identify speech disorders have remained "surfacy." That is, to date, we have not incorporated analyses that purport to describe a child's underlying representations of words or sounds. In part, this is due to a certain frustration with the changing landscape of linguistic theory and analysis procedures. Each new theoretical view has been welcomed with excitement for its potential to describe phonological disorder and pinpoint treatment targets. Yet the need remains for researchers to conduct programmatic studies that bring these theories fully into practice. Lahey (1990) appeared to share this perspective in a useful discussion of measurement issues in the identification of children with language disorders. Our rationale for speech assessment is consistent with each of the points Lahey made in the following paragraph on language assessment:

> The perspective taken here is that, even within a mentalistic view of language, identification of a language disorder should be based on differences in language behaviors (e.g., the production and comprehension of units of connected language) and not on inferences about the nature of the underlying system based on these performance variables. One reason to focus on performance is the practical consideration that there is no agreed-upon way to describe the underlying system and, thus, no way that a description of the expected system could be used as a comparison. More important is the fact that we are interested not only in children who have deficits in their underlying knowledge of language but also in those who might have difficulty in accessing or using that knowledge. (pp. 613–614)

Certainly for other purposes, such as for theory testing, clinical prediction decisions, and clinical treatment questions, alternative phonological analysis procedures have demonstrated considerable utility.

One construct that has become quite important in all areas of developmental linguistics is phonological awareness. Procedures to characterize children's phonological awareness have been associated with compelling construct and predictive validity (Hodson, 1994). In addition to its potential as a phenotype marker for reading disability and as a predictive marker for normalization outcomes, phonological awareness may have potential as a diagnostic marker for subtypes of speech delay. For example, we are currently studying phonological awareness profiles for children with suspected SD-OME compared to children with SD.

TREATMENT OF CHILDHOOD SPEECH DISORDERS

At the center of research in childhood speech disorders is the speech clinic. In our clinic, preschool children with speech delay are seen twice weekly for one to two semesters of intervention. In our prior work, we have studied alternative instructional structures of treatment (Shriberg & Kwiatkowski, 1982), compared tabletop therapy to computer-aided therapy (Shriberg, Kwiatkowski, & Snyder, 1989, 1990), and examined processes and strategies associated with speech-sound normalization (Shriberg & Kwiatkowski, 1988, 1990). Recent consolidation of what we have learned from these studies proposes that intervention can be modeled as a two-parameter system termed the *capability-focus framework*. We conclude with a brief review of this perspective.

THE CAPABILITY-FOCUS FRAMEWORK

In our efforts to understand the "big picture" of successful treatment, we have been struck by clinicians' concerns about whether a child is "attentive," "motivated," "trying," "concentrating," "picking up on cues," "tuned in," "making the best possible effort," and so forth. Rather than dismiss correlates of these quotes from clinicians as too subjective to study, we initiated research to explore their role in successful treatment.

Figure 5–5 is a representation of a two-parameter framework that attempts to subsume all elements relevant to intervention under two domains termed *capability* and *focus*. Degree and rate of *learning*, as measured by probes of trained and untrained targets, is viewed as requiring some minimum level of capability and focus. As shown in Figure 5–5, a child's capability is assessed by measures of linguistic status and is constrained by risk factors. The construct of focus, reflecting a child's need for extrinsic motivational events, is assessed using brief diagnostic therapy procedures that vary levels of contingent reinforcement. Focus is operationally defined as the amount of motivational support a child needs to persist at a difficult task (Kwiatkowski & Shriberg, 1996). Notice in Figure 5–5 that two processes associated with treatment outcomes, stimulability and self-monitoring, are viewed as reflecting both capability and focus.

Findings from retrospective (Kwiatkowski & Shriberg, 1993) and prospective (Kwiatkowski & Shriberg, 1996) studies support the potential contribution of the focus concept for prediction and treatment decisions. Pretreatment capability is the most significant predictor of normalization rate, but pretreatment measures of focus add statistically significant predictive variance. Specifically, lack of focus is associated with minimal rather than maximal progress in treatment—even in children with high capability scores. Records for children making minimal progress have included such clinician comments as "lack of motivation for speech change," "highly distractible," "fear of failure," "unwilling to risk being incorrect," "easily

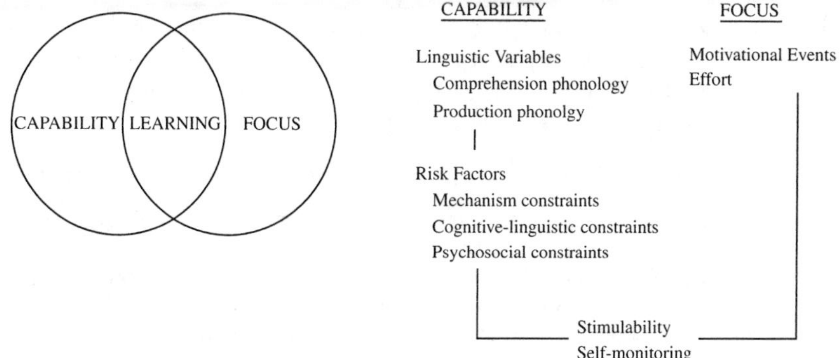

Figure 5–5 The Capability-Focus Framework for Intervention in Childhood Speech Disorders. *Source:* Reprinted with permission from J. Kwiatowski and L.D. Shriberg, *Language, Speech, and Hearing in the Schools*, Vol. 24, p. 11, © 1993, American Speech-Language-Hearing Association.

frustrated and discouraged if not immediately successful," and "unwilling to attempt difficult speech tasks." We use the construct of focus as the common denominator among these observations, reflecting attentional-motivational constraints on learning.

The two parameters of capability and focus seem to be interactive. Some threshold level of capability appears to be required for a child to be self-focused without the need for clinicians to manipulate teaching tasks and reinforcers to motivate focus. And for some children, lack of focus inhibits learning and generalization. These studies have suggested to us that no matter how well developed our linguistic analysis and treatment procedures, individual differences in children's motivation and effort play a central role in normalization outcomes.

CONCLUSION

I hope these few observations have captured the flavor of some challenging questions in past, present, and future research in childhood speech disorders. Emerging research worldwide promises a variety of new technologies to study etiology, prognosis, treatment, and ultimately approaches to the prevention of childhood speech disorders. Our own work will continue to emphasize etiology projects, including collaborative studies using techniques in molecular and behavioral genetics. We envision a day when computer-aided procedures will be used routinely to diagnose subtypes of involvement, provide accurate prognostic information to concerned caregivers, and suggest the most effective and efficient treatment regimens for each child. Indeed, throughout the chapters in this volume and in other contemporary texts, one can discern the progress that has been made toward such applied technologies. Clearly, for the talented generations of new students who will skillfully assess and successfully treat children with speech disorders, the best is yet to come.

I have had the good fortune of pursuing the questions presented in this chapter with many talented people, including my long-time friend and colleague Joan Kwiatkowski, several dozen speech-language pathologists in the Madison Metropolitan School District, collaborators at several research centers, former and current graduate students, and a long line of talented and congenial people who have worked with us in our laboratory facilities at the Department of Communicative Disorders and at the Waisman Center on Mental Retardation and Human Development.

Preparation of this chapter was supported by The National Institute on Deafness and Other Communication Disorders, National Institutes of Health, Grant Numbers 5 R01 DC00496-07, 5 R01 DC00528-07, and 1 P50 DC02746-01.

REFERENCES

Bernthal, J.E., & Bankson, N.W. (Eds.). (1994). *Child phonology: Characteristics, assessment, and intervention with special populations.* New York: Thieme.

Bishop, D.V.M., & Edmundson, A. (1987). Language-impaired 4-year-olds: Distinguishing transient from persistent impairment. *Journal of Speech and Hearing Disorders, 52*, 156–173.

Felsenfeld, S., McGue, M., & Broen, P.A. (1995). Family aggregation of phonological disorders: Results from a 28-year follow-up. *Journal of Speech and Hearing Research, 38*, 1091–1107.

Hall, P.K., Jordan, L.S., & Robin, D.A. (1993). *Developmental apraxia of speech: Theory and clinical practice.* Austin, TX: Pro-Ed.

Hodson, B.W. (1994). Helping individuals become intelligible, literate, and articulate: The role of phonology. *Topics in Language Disorders, 14*(2), 1–16.

Ingram, D. (1976). *Procedures for the phonological analysis of children's language.* Baltimore: University Park.

Kent, R.D. (1996). Hearing and believing: Some limits to the auditory-perceptual assessment of speech and voice disorders. *American Journal of Speech-Language Pathology, 5*, 7–23.

Kwiatkowski, J., & Shriberg, L.D. (1992). Intelligibility assessment in developmental phonological disorders: Accuracy of caregiver gloss. *Journal of Speech and Hearing Research, 35*, 1095–1104.

Kwiatkowski, J., & Shriberg, L.D. (1993). Speech normalization in developmental phonological disorders: A retrospective study of capability-focus theory. *Language, Speech, and Hearing Services in Schools, 24*, 10–18.

Kwiatkowski, J., & Shriberg, L.D. (1996). *The capability-focus framework for treatment of speech delay II: Predictive validity and clinical application.* Manuscript submitted for publication.

Lahey, M. (1990). Who shall be called language disordered? Some reflections and one perspective. *Journal of Speech and Hearing Disorders, 55*, 612–620.

Lahey, M., & Edwards, J. (1995). Specific language impairment: Preliminary investigation of factors associated with family history and with patterns of language performance. *Journal of Speech and Hearing Research, 38*, 643–657.

Locke, J.L. (1994). Gradual emergence of developmental language disorders. *Journal of Speech and Hearing Research, 37*, 608–616.

McSweeny, J.L., & Shriberg, L.D. (1995). *Segmental and suprasegmental transcription reliability* (Tech. Rep. No. 2). University of Wisconsin-Madison, Waisman Center on Mental Retardation and Human Development, Phonology Project.

Morrison, J.A., & Shriberg, L.D. (1992). Articulation testing versus conversational speech sampling. *Journal of Speech and Hearing Research, 35*, 259–273.

Morrison, J.A., & Shriberg, L.D. (1994). Response to Ingram letter. *Journal of Speech and Hearing Research, 37*, 936–937.

Odell, K.H., & Shriberg, L.D. (1996). *Inappropriate stress in adults with apraxia of speech and children with suspected developmental apraxia of speech.* Manuscript in preparation.

Oller, D.K., Eilers, R., Steffens, M.L., Lynch, M.P., & Urbano, R. (1994). Speech-like vocalizations in infancy: An evaluation of potential risk factors. *Journal of Child Language, 21*, 33–58.

Paul, R. (1993). Patterns of development in late talkers: Preschool years. *Journal of Childhood Communication Disorders, 15*(1), 7–14.

Shriberg, L.D. (1972). Articulation judgments: Some perceptual considerations. *Journal of Speech and Hearing Research, 15*, 876–882.

Shriberg, L.D. (1975a, November). *Preliminaries to a social learning theory view of deviant child phonology.* Paper presented at the annual meeting of the American Speech and Hearing Association, Washington, DC.

Shriberg, L.D. (1975b). A response evocation program for /ɝ/. *Journal of Speech and Hearing Disorders, 40*, 92–103.

Shriberg, L.D. (1980a). Developmental phonological disorders. In T.J. Hixon, L.D. Shriberg, & J.S. Saxman (Eds.), *Introduction to communicative disorders* (pp. 262–309). Englewood Cliffs, NJ: Prentice Hall.

Shriberg, L.D. (1980b). An intervention procedure for children with persistent /**r**/ errors. *Language, Speech, and Hearing Services in Schools, 11*, 102–110.

Shriberg, L.D. (1982a). Programming for the language component in developmental phonological disorders. *Seminars in Speech, Language, and Hearing, 3*(2), 115–126.

Shriberg, L.D. (1982b). Toward classification of developmental phonological disorders. In N.J. Lass (Ed.), *Speech and language: Advances in basic research and practice* (pp. 2–18). New York: Academic Press.

Shriberg, L.D. (1986). *PEPPER: Programs to Examine Phonetic and Phonologic Evaluation Records* [Computer software manual]. Hillsdale, NJ: Lawrence Erlbaum.

Shriberg, L.D. (1987). In search of the otitis media-speech connection. *Journal of the National Student Speech Language Hearing Association, 15*, 56–67.

Shriberg, L.D. (1991). Directions for research in developmental phonological disorders. In J. Miller (Ed.), *Research on child language disorders: A decade of progress* (pp. 267–276). Austin, TX: Pro-Ed.

Shriberg, L.D. (1993). Four new speech and prosody-voice measures for genetics research and other studies in developmental phonological disorders. *Journal of Speech and Hearing Research, 36*, 105–140.

Shriberg, L.D. (1994). Five subtypes of developmental phonological disorders. *Clinics in Communication Disorders, 41*, 38–45.

Shriberg, L.D., Aram, D.M., & Kwiatkowski, J. (in press). Developmental apraxia of speech: I. Descriptive and theoretical perspectives. *Journal of Speech and Hearing Research.*

Shriberg, L.D., Austin, D., Lewis, B.A., McSweeny, J.L., & Wilson, D.L. (in press a). The Percentage of Consonants Correct (PCC) metric: Extensions and reliability data. *Journal of Speech and Hearing Research.*

Shriberg, L.D., Austin, D., Lewis, B.A., McSweeny, J.L., & Wilson, D.L. (in press b). The Speech Disorders Classification System (SDCS): Extensions and lifespan reference data. *Journal of Speech and Hearing Research.*

Shriberg, L.D., & Flipsen, P., Jr. (1996, November). *Otitis media and speech delay: Relative risk and diagnostic markers.* Miniseminar presented at the annual meeting of the American Speech-Language-Hearing Association, Seattle.

Shriberg, L.D., Gruber, F.A., & Kwiatkowski, J. (1994). Developmental phonological disorders III: Long-term speech-sound normalization. *Journal of Speech and Hearing Research, 37*, 1151–1177.

Shriberg, L.D., Hinke, R., & Trost-Steffen, C. (1987). A procedure to select and train persons for narrow phonetic transcription by consensus. *Clinical Linguistics and Phonetics, 1*, 171–189.

Shriberg, L.D., & Kent, R.D. (1982). *Clinical phonetics*. New York: Macmillan.

Shriberg, L.D., & Kwiatkowski, J. (1978, November). *Natural process analyses for children with severely delayed speech.* Paper presented at the annual meeting of the American Speech and Hearing Association, San Francisco.

Shriberg, L.D., & Kwiatkowski, J. (1980). *Natural process analysis: A procedure for phonological analysis of continuous speech samples.* New York: Macmillan.

Shriberg, L.D., & Kwiatkowski, J. (1982). Phonological disorders III: A procedure for assessing severity of involvement. *Journal of Speech and Hearing Disorders, 47*, 256–270.

Shriberg, L.D., & Kwiatkowski, J. (1983). Computer-assisted natural process analysis (NPA): Recent issues and data. *Seminars in Speech and Language, 4*, 389–406.

Shriberg, L.D., & Kwiatkowski, J. (1985). Continuous speech sampling for phonologic analyses of speech-delayed children. *Journal of Speech and Hearing Disorders, 50*, 323–334.

Shriberg, L.D., & Kwiatkowski, J. (1988). A follow-up study of children with phonologic disorders of unknown origin. *Journal of Speech and Hearing Disorders, 53*, 144–155.

Shriberg, L.D., & Kwiatkowski, J. (1990). Self-monitoring and generalization in preschool speech-delayed children. *Language, Speech, and Hearing Services in Schools, 21*, 157–170.

Shriberg, L.D., & Kwiatkowski, J. (1994). Developmental phonological disorders I: A clinical profile. *Journal of Speech and Hearing Research, 37*, 1100–1126.

Shriberg, L.D., Kwiatkowski, J., Best, S., Hengst, J., & Terselic-Weber, B. (1986). Characteristics of children with phonologic disorders of unknown origin. *Journal of Speech and Hearing Disorders, 51*, 140–161.

Shriberg, L.D., Kwiatkowski, J., & Gruber, F.A. (1994). Developmental phonological disorders II: Short-term speech-sound normalization. *Journal of Speech and Hearing Research, 37*, 1127–1150.

Shriberg, L.D., Kwiatkowski, J., & Hoffmann, K.A. (1984). A procedure for phonetic transcription by consensus. *Journal of Speech and Hearing Research, 27*, 456–465.

Shriberg, L.D., Kwiatkowski, J., & Rasmussen, C. (1990). *The Prosody-Voice Screening Profile.* Tucson, AZ: Communication Skill Builders.

Shriberg, L.D., Kwiatkowski, J., Rasmussen, C., Lof, G.L., & Miller, J.F. (1992). *The Prosody-Voice Screening Profile (PVSP): Psychometric data and reference information for children* (Tech. Rep.

No. 1). Madison, WI: University of Wisconsin—Madison, Waisman Center on Mental Retardation and Human Development.

Shriberg, L.D., Kwiatkowski, J., & Snyder, T. (1989). Tabletop versus microcomputer-assisted speech management: Stabilization phase. *Journal of Speech and Hearing Disorders, 54*, 233–248.

Shriberg, L.D., Kwiatkowski, J., & Snyder, T. (1990). Tabletop versus microcomputer-assisted speech management: Response evocation phase. *Journal of Speech and Hearing Disorders, 55*, 635–655.

Shriberg, L.D., & Lof, G.L. (1991). Reliability studies in broad and narrow phonetic transcription. *Clinical Linguistics and Phonetics, 5*, 225–227.

Shriberg, L.D., & Olson, D. (1988). *PEPAGREE: A program to compute transcription reliability* [Computer software]. University of Wisconsin-Madison, Waisman Center Research Computing Facility.

Shriberg, L.D., & Widder, C.J. (1990). Speech and prosody characteristics of adults with mental retardation. *Journal of Speech and Hearing Research, 33*, 627–653.

Smit, A.B., Hand, L., Freilinger, J.J., Bernthal, J.E., & Bird, A. (1990). The Iowa Articulation Norms Project and its Nebraska replication. *Journal of Speech and Hearing Disorders, 55*, 779–798.

Stampe, D. (1979). *A dissertation on natural phonology.* New York: Garland. (Original dissertation completed 1973)

Thielke, H.M., & Shriberg, L.D. (1990). Effects of recurrent otitis media on language, speech, and educational achievement in Menominee Indian children. *Journal of Native American Education, 29*, 25–33.

U.S. Education Department, Office of Special Education Programs. (1992). *To assure a free appropriate education: Fourteenth annual report to Congress on the implementation of the Individuals with Disabilities Education Act.* Washington, DC: Author.

Velleman, S.L., & Shriberg, L.D. (1996). *Syllabic stress constraints as the proximal loci of a subtype of developmental apraxia of speech (DAS).* Manuscript in preparation.

Chapter 6

Child Phonology and Infant Vocalizations: Theory and Methodology

D. Kimbrough Oller

HOW MODERN RESEARCH IN CHILD PHONOLOGY BEGAN

For a quarter of a century, I have been engaged in research on language, speech, and developmental linguistics. In 1971, as a beginning faculty member at the University of Washington, I was introduced to child phonology through a guest lecture by David Stampe. Soon thereafter I obtained copies of Stampe's writings on natural phonology (in particular, Stampe, 1969) and Roman Jakobson's (1941) famous treatise on child language. These writings offered a starting point and a measure of inspiration to initiate a body of research in young child speech. Both Stampe and Jakobson provided reasons to believe that child phonology was rich in structure and full of implications regarding the biological underpinnings of speech capacity.

The contributions of Stampe and Jakobson were important because they showed that child speech errors were systematic rather than "random." When children produce phonological substitutions, deletions, and other kinds of modifications of target words, they do so in a way that is rule governed. Further, the characterization of the rules by which children modify target words can be deeply revealing regarding the structure of the emerging capacity for speech and the relationship between child speech and patterns of speech-sound occurrence in languages in general. It turns out that the kinds of errors children make result in the production of sounds that are common in the world's languages, whereas the sounds deleted and replaced tend to be uncommonly occurring sounds.

Inspired by reading these fundamental works of child phonology, I made arrangements to visit Stanford University, where a major effort in empirical research in child phonology was underway. There Charles Ferguson had established a program of graduate education and investigation where many of today's key figures in child phonology (including David Ingram, Mary Louise Edwards, Marlys Macken, Carol Farwell, Carol Stoel-Gammon, and Marilyn Vihman) were being educated. From that point forward, by choice of subject matter in research and partly under the influence of the Stanford group, I have been a child phonologist myself.

It was no idle choice, for the nature of the sounds of languages has always fascinated me. Still, throughout these 20-odd years, it has seemed that the field was on the verge of something new, that the whole framework of description and understanding through which we approached the elucidation of what John Locke (1993) called (by the title of his recent book) "the child's path to spoken language" has been ripe for a radical restructuring.

To have anticipated a major restructuring during the era of the early 1970s was somewhat iconoclastic, for it seemed in the early 1970s that prevailing approaches represented a revolutionary new way of approaching the study of speech in children. Investigators had abandoned purely segmental (phonemic) inventory descriptions in favor of rule-based, phonological-feature-manipulating, generative descriptions (see Edwards, 1978; Ingram, 1976). Both research and clinical practice were entertaining natural phonology and Jakobsonian assumptions that claimed to provide broadly integrative frames.

My own work in this area had focused on providing applications of generative phonological tools (Chomsky & Halle, 1968) to the description of disordered phonological systems. The primary finding of that research was that children with speech disorders were often no less systematic in their mistaken pronunciations of target words than were younger, normally developing infants and children. Rules of generative phonology could be formulated to characterize the errors and to illustrate the ways in which those errors resembled commonly occurring errors of normally developing children and, in some cases, ways in which the disordered phonological systems were distinct (Oller, 1973b). In some cases the generative descriptions provided surprising outcomes, showing that children who had been thought, on the basis of clinical evaluations, to produce wildly random errors were in fact abiding by a rather rigid system of rules. In the case of deaf children, the results were more mixed (Oller & Eilers, 1981; Oller, Jensen, & Lafayette, 1978), indicating that although deaf children often produced *systematic* substitutions and deletions that were typical of younger hearing children, there were also many special errors of deaf children (some of which were predictable on the basis of the important role of lipreading in cases of hearing impairment) and errors of "bidirectional" substitution (e.g., /m/ for /b/ in some cases and /b/ for /m/ in others), a pattern rarely if ever found in hearing children. Presumably, the bidirectional alternations were the result of inability to discriminate among the alternatives: /m/ and /b/, for example, look identical, and in cases of very profound deafness, amplification may not be able to transmit the distinction. In contrast, hearing children appear to be capable of perceiving the relevant distinctions of their language, and when they make substitution errors they routinely seem to favor one sound or the other (so /s/ becomes /t/, but /t/ does *not* become /s/).

The work in child phonology based on this generative approach was exciting and fruitful in producing a new understanding of the nature of the phonological systems children present. But there were important limits to how far these approaches could go. Very soon, both Jakobson's and Stampe's theoretical models failed to survive scrutiny from the standpoint of conformity with apparent facts of phonological development. For example, Jakobson had attempted to reverse an earlier trend that had emphasized "ease of articulation" as an important factor in the nature of child phonological errors. In so doing, he had claimed that children's errors were unassociated with articulatory factors and instead were purely the result of universal sound laws that were found to apply in child speech as well as in disorders such as aphasia. The problem with this reasoning was that it could not effectively dispense with the explanatory appeal of ease of articulation as a factor in accounting for why sound laws have the form that they do. Deletions of final consonants and cluster reductions, for example, do result in the production of CV syllables, which are the universally preferred types of syllables in languages, but the question of why children delete consonants to maximize CV syllable production is not entirely answered by an appeal to universal laws. The laws appear in part to be the result of a tendency to seek simple forms that involve a minimum of articulatory adjustments. By deleting consonants, much of the articulatory difficulty of complex sequences can be reduced. Jakobson's theoretical claims were thus weakened by the inherent attractiveness of ease of articulation in explaining why sound laws exist in the first place.

Stampe insisted on the idea that the prime units of child phonological function were "natural processes" specifying particular alternations (unidirectional substitutions) and deletions. The advantage of the approach was that it offered a quick and clean account for many commonly occurring errors in phonological development (and in phonological disorders), an account that has substantial clinical value in providing a structural model of systematic errors (Hodson & Paden, 1981; Shriberg & Kwiatkowski, 1980). This model was limited, however, by its focus on the level of rules specifying individual alternations and deletions. It became clear that such processes fit into groupings sometimes referred to as "conspiracies." Each grouping consisted of rules that had very different superficial form but accomplished a similar broad phonological goal. For example, one presumed goal might be the maximization of the production of CV syllables. A conspiracy of rules to accomplish that goal could consist of final-consonant deletions, consonant-cluster reductions, and sometimes even rules of insertion of vowels between consonants in clusters (e.g., such an insertion might result in "buhlue" for "blue") or insertion of brief "epenthetic" vowels at the end of CVC syllables, resulting in CVCV sequences. Because individual children with normally developing (Oller & Warren, 1976) or disordered phonologies (Oller et al., 1978) often show such conspiracies of rules, it became appealing to consider the possibility that the "processes" were organized by broader principles and that these broader principles were the guiding forces in development. In my own work, I came to think of processes as the product of application of the principles rather than the primes of child phonological theory. Similarly, the child was seen within this perspective as an active creator of rules rather than as a passive implementer of innate processes.

Generative phonology provided the framework of description in the 1970s revolution that sought to apply Jakobsonian and Stampian approaches. Although clearly an improvement over what had preceded it, it began to suffer from the lack of ability to see beyond its own structural confines. The need for a system of description with general phonological principles (rather than rules or processes) at the center and the need for more integration of the descriptive framework with information about the motivations lying behind phonological principles began to push the field toward new frameworks that would consider ease of perception, ease of production, and the organizational principles for lexical and phonological material in long-term storage (Ingram, 1976; Oller & Warren, 1976).

My own interests in broadening of the framework of child phonology were substantial. I believed that it should be possible to evaluate child phonology synchronically and thereby to see the essence of deeper phenomena. It was appealing to address the roots of communicative systems both in the individual child and in humanity as a species and to seek ways to capture the likely communicative futures of individual children through the evaluation of their current speech or speechlike actions.

Although many (including me) have attempted to contribute to a fundamental change in framework, it is clear that more is needed. This chapter represents an attempt both to address the need for more lasting solutions to our theoretical needs and to clarify certain methodological needs that will surely persist through the transition into whatever new theoretical postures may be adopted over the coming decades. The field's methodology in part reflects its theoretical assumptions and, in a variety of ways, limits the potential for revising theory. And certain characteristics of the methodologies may be fundamentally transferable even when a new theory is embraced.

A HISTORICAL PERSPECTIVE ON HOW SCIENTIFIC PROGRESS CAN BE LIMITED BY THEORY

Before addressing methodological and theoretical issues for the future, it may be useful to look in detail at a problem that is of constant concern in any scientific enterprise. Any theoretical model is a two-edged sword. It may offer new and richer interpretations, but it may also limit perspectives toward further growth. Ideally, a theory is a tool of interpretation rather than a yoke to hold its users in place. But in fact, in the history of science, theory has often been perspective limiting rather than perspective broadening.

Consider a classical example. From medieval times through most of the Renaissance, the stars and planets were assumed to revolve around the earth. This theory, attributable to Ptolemy, accounted for a wide variety of phenomena quite accurately. When Copernicus (1514/1978) provided an equally accurate account of movements of heavenly bodies, using a more elegant model in which the earth and planets were seen as revolving about the sun, there was fundamental resistance that persisted for decades. The resistance was imposed by prevailing theory and the authority that backed it. That resistance held off the Copernican revolution for many years, even though by adopting the newer model a whole series of phenomena would become accessible (e.g., the much greater distance from the earth of stars than of observable planets, the fundamental differences between stars and planets, and the remarkable possibility, as considered within the context of the 16th century, that the sun was only one of thousands of visible astral bodies).

One might imagine that such limitations of viewpoint occurred only in ancient times. Not so. The re-publication in 1968 in English of Jakobson's book (1941) provided impetus for the growth of some modern efforts in child phonology. But the book's ideas also imposed a disastrous restriction on the realms of inquiry that were later considered legitimate, and those limitations have prevailed until very recently. I have encountered both linguists and psychologists within the present decade who remain fundamentally influenced by Jakobsonian thinking regarding infant vocal development. A key narrowing of view imposed by Jakobson's theory was associated with his claim that a sharp discontinuity existed between prelinguistic vocalization and early speech. This view of early phonology fit within a general conception in which language was expected to emerge, as a biological entity, from the natural maturational process. Learning was deemphasized, and Jakobson seemed to be trying to analogize the emergence of phonological capabilities to other biological (not cultural or environmental) phenomena of development. Perhaps he had in mind metamorphosis. Here was a phenomenon that seemed to proceed according to lockstep principles of maturation, guided by the organism's heredity, largely ignoring environment, and involving changes that are dramatic and unmistakable.

Jakobson thought that in the first words of children he could see a behavioral phenomenon of dramatic, sudden change. His description of early speech focused on systematic tendencies of pronunciation in which certain sound types that had by then been designated as relatively universal in natural languages, the most frequently occurring sounds worldwide, were also the sounds that children tended first to use in the formation of words. It should be granted that on this point Jakobson was at least superficially correct: The early sounds of children do indeed resemble sounds primarily drawn from an inventory of elements that are universal or near-universal in natural languages. The primary error was on a different point. He claimed that the appearance of children's preference for universal sounds was sudden in development, corresponding precisely to the onset of speech. He asserted that in the prior periods of babbling, infants produced all the sounds of all the world's languages in a sort of random sound play. He even emphasized a "silent period" that was supposed to occur between babbling and speech.

In this view, speech begins with two simultaneous extraordinary events: systematic, sound-limited phonology and learned morphology based on associations between meanings and phonological sequences. Two such remarkable occurrences could not coincide by chance, he reasoned, and the sharp distinction between the child's language capabilities and prelinguistic actions could hardly be interpreted as anything other than a crisp, biologically based transition. He hammered home the point that in the transition the child was transformed from having a broad capability to produce any kind of speechlike sounds to having a narrow capability limited by universal tendencies of language.

It is now clear to those of us who study child phonology that the empirical claim Jakobson used to support the discontinuity theory was incorrect. The presumed metamorphic change appears to have been constructed from speculation rather than from empirical evidence. Late babbling is composed of sound productions that in very large measure resemble the types found in early speech and in phonological universals (see Cruttenden, 1970; Locke, 1983; Menyuk, 1968; Oller, Wieman, Doyle, & Ross, 1975). The similarity, to the present observer, appears to be overwhelming. The presumed "silent period" may happen in some child somewhere, but it most assuredly is not the typical pattern of speech acquisition. In fact, there is typically a long period of overlap in which babbling and speech commingle (Elbers, 1982; Vihman, Ferguson, & Elbert, 1986; Vihman & Miller, 1988), and for my own part, in many longitudinal studies involving scores of children, I have never observed a child to develop as Jakobson predicted (i.e., to stop babbling, stay silent for a period of days or weeks, and then begin speaking without further babbling).

Before dealing with how Jakobson could have been so wrong empirically, it is important to make clear that using a discontinuity model in child language is not necessarily a mistake in principle. There may indeed exist relatively discontinuous events in language development, events that may reveal important aspects of the maturational and biological nature of the language capacity. So to say that Jakobson was wrong in positing a particular kind of discontinuity is not to say that the idea of discontinuity might not have merit in a different formulation. Perhaps the reason that the empirically untenable view was cited so frequently in reviews on child development and child language was that it fit with other, more well-documented observations of discontinuity in human ontogeny.

Yet for Jakobson's claims of discontinuity and randomness in babbling and speech, there is no supportable evidence and no modern empirical source to cite. How could he have strayed so far from empirical fact? The approach seems to have been the product of bias and preformed expectation, the same sort of theoretical limitation that was imposed in the long era of Ptolemy's influence in astronomy. In whatever observations he made of infant babbling and in the various studies he reviewed, Jakobson must have focused on what he wished to find and ignored the rest. To obtain a more secure grasp of the way such theoretical expectations might have guided him and held in sway the many who were persuaded by his writings, let us consider certain more concrete claims that Jakobson made. In particular, he noted that infants often produce uvular and labial trills, sounds that are rare in natural languages. True enough, the sounds are rare, and true enough, they are produced by some individual infants at a certain point in development, but his interpretation of the occurrence of such sounds was blown out of proportion. He claimed that the infant produced "the most varied sounds with ease," leaving the implication that all sorts of other potential sounds of natural languages were also commonly present in infancy.

In fact, there are many other types of sounds that do occur in mature languages but that observational research in infancy has been scarcely able to document at all: implosives, ejectives, retroflex articulations, palatalized, coronal trills, and many more. Even uvular trills, on which Jakobson rests part of his claim that infants produce sounds of all the world's languages, are relatively rare in infancy. Uvular trills do occur occasionally during the early "primitive articulation" or "gooing" stage (prior to two months of age), and in some individuals that occurrence is fairly frequent. During the primitive articulation stage, however, velar or uvular friction sounds are much more common. Both these and uvular trills tend to subside with the onset of the following "expansion" or "vocal play" stage (see Oller, 1980; Roug, Landberg, & Lundberg, 1989; Stark, 1980; Zlatin, 1975; or Oller, 1995, for review of the stages). Labial trills, another focus of Jakobson's contention that infants have unlimited sound production capabilities, are among the common productions of this later stage, but they fit into a broader category referred to as "raspberries" that includes vibrants and fricativelike sounds as well as trills. One key point here is that only *some* children produce trills commonly, and then primarily only during a particular stage of development.

An even more important point is that neither uvular trills nor labial trills occur commonly in well-formed syllables in infancy during the canonical stage (when well-formed syllables come under the infant's control). Trills almost always occur either in isolation or in primitive syllablelike structures in which either the nucleus is ill formed (a "quasivowel," in the terminology of current vocal literature) or the transitions between the nucleus and the margins are ill formed (usually they are too slow, producing what are termed *marginal syllables*). I once spent most of an evening at a party observing a child who, well into the canonical stage, produced reduplicated babbling sequences in which the consonantlike margins of the syllables were indeed labial trills. The reason for the particular interest in this child was that he was the *only* child I have ever observed producing trills of any kind in reduplicated babbling. In the research in our laboratories at the University of Miami and earlier at the University of Washington over a 25-year period, no infant has been found to produce reduplicated syllables with trills during four major longitudinal studies involving more than 100 infants. Jakobson wanted to make much of the fact that babies sometimes produce trills, but he chose systematically to ignore that the vast majority of babies show little or no capability to produce such sounds within a phoneticlike context including vowel-like articulations and well-formed transitions.

Once children reach the canonical stage, it becomes relatively easy to focus attention on the well-formed syllables that are the hallmark of the stage and to assign these syllables to categories that bear reliable resemblance to those of natural languages. To put the matter another way, it is easy to transcribe well-formed syllables phonetically. When one conducts observational research based on transcription of canonical syllables in infants, one finds that trills of any kind are almost entirely absent—that in fact, the only consonantlike elements that occur frequently in babbling are those that are near-universal in languages and thus nearly a perfect match with the sounds that occur in early speech.

Jakobson's error was one of systematic, directed attention guided by a theoretical assumption. It was quite a different error from that of Ptolemy, although no less misleading. Ptolemy did not acquire faulty information about movements of celestial bodies, nor did he ignore the oddities (e.g., retrograde motion of planets) that made his geocentric model complicated. Copernicus, also well aware of the oddities, redesigned the model but left the data alone. It is worthwhile to consider the difference between Jakobson's error and Ptolemy's because it presents the opportunity to take stock of a particular vulnerability of work in phonology and of work in the natural sciences in general.

The data obtained through observing movements of planetary bodies in early astronomy involved very few variables: position in space (of stars and planets) and time. In contrast, the subject matter addressed in child phonology is amazingly complex. Events are categorized along a remarkable number of dimensions: nasality, frication, vocal quality, loudness, duration, timbre, pitch, to name a few. The complexity is so great that it is necessary to impose certain limitations of framing because to do otherwise would be to open a Pandora's box of descriptive confusion. For practical reasons, if not theoretical ones, it is necessary to look at certain aspects of infant babbling, of early speech, and systematically to ignore others. This limitation of observation leaves the enterprise wide open to fundamental errors of judgment. Theoretical biases can lead investigators to see exactly what they are looking for and to ignore the rest. Consequently, unless there is good reason to believe that the *right* choices have been made about what aspects of infant sounds to observe, it seems likely that the resulting model may be no less flawed than Jakobson's was.

IN SEARCH OF NEW FRAMEWORKS, OR AT LEAST NEW PROTECTIONS

The change in current views about babbling, moving away from the Jakobsonian perspective, has had one undeniable salutory effect. It has encouraged research on infant vocal development and its relationship with later speech, an endeavor that was treated as a waste of time by many scholars prior to the 1970s, purely under Jakobson's influence. The systematic look that is being taken nowadays at young children's speech has brought with it certain new tools of description, although nothing terribly fancy: tape recorders, the international phonetic alphabet, transcription training, sometimes some minimal acoustic analysis hardware, and at least the beginnings of tools of experimental design.

One thing that has *not* changed much in this new era of research is the *elemental basis* of the descriptions that can be performed. The problem concerns the very units in terms of which descriptions are patterned. For example, researchers still primarily characterize infant and young child sounds segmentally, even though there is increasingly good reason for suspecting that children have no segmental system at their disposal until at least the second and perhaps the third year of life (Ferguson & Farwell, 1975; MacNeilage & Davis, 1990). So even though traditional Jakobsonian contentions about infant vocal development have been left behind, there is little reason for confidence that in the current era, research is less vulnerable to errors of judgment that might resemble those of the prior traditions. When frameworks are limited in this way and methodologies are relatively primitive, there is reason for concern that research may produce data that are basically flawed.

The question is, are there ways to constrain the extent of impact of such investigatory dangers to make the engine of progress more efficient? If we evaluate the mechanisms that impose limits on understanding in child phonology, perhaps we can provide a basis for more graceful and productive growth in our conception of the ontogeny of the speech capacity.

Methodologies in linguistic research (and child phonology is merely the example of present focus) are by their very nature extremely blunt instruments. This is a problem all by itself, but when one combines unavoidable vulnerability of methods with unavoidable theoretical biases, one obtains an unfortunate mixture. To limit the potential damage to our investigatory enterprise, it is important to seek ways to neutralize the effects of both *bluntness* and *bias* to the extent that it is possible. In the remainder of this chapter, both issues are considered.

SUGGESTIONS ABOUT METHODOLOGICAL PROTECTIONS IN CHILD PHONOLOGY

Group Comparisons and Transcription

To limit the effects of inherent biases in empirical research, it is critical to acknowledge their existence and design research in ways that eliminate or at least constrain the potential effects of bias. Explanation and attempts to construct explanatory frameworks are inherently and inevitably constrained in validity by the effectiveness of the controls provided to ensure that results reported conform to the reality observed. In the field of child phonology, as in many others in which data are extremely complex, scientific controls are of paramount importance.

Child phonology is a relatively new science, drawing its approaches partly from linguistics, partly from speech science, and partly from experimental psychology. The mixture has not always been felicitous. This chapter considers just a few salient problems in the domain of design, problems that are particularly worrisome in terms of their potential for fostering the sorts of errors of observation noted above. The first of these concerns relates to the need for unbiased observations when comparing groups of subjects.

Consider a hypothetical example of two groups of children, one learning Spanish and the other learning English. We might wish to know at what point the two groups produce sounds that differ in accordance with the phonetic characteristics of the two languages. The example is not entirely hypothetical because research at the University of Miami has pursued such questions for some years (Eilers, Oller, & Benito-García, 1984; Thevenin, Eilers, Oller, & LaVoie, 1985). In the studies in question, it has been reported that children from both language backgrounds produce extremely similar sounds. Others have reported notable differences in sounds produced by infants growing up in differing language communities (e.g., de Boysson-Bardies, Sagart, & Durand, 1984). The study of such possible differences is important because it offers the opportunity to glimpse the early stages of experiential effects on speech (or speechlike) sound production.

Considering the case of infants in a Spanish- and/or English-speaking environment, it is worthwhile to note that the two groups of children are likely to produce very similar sound types during canonical babbling because both are likely to produce many sounds from the universal inventory discussed above and to resist pronunciation of language-specific elements that would not be universal. But perhaps there might nevertheless be subtle differences between the groups, and surely, by some point in development, such differences do occur. When? How can the point at which such differences occur be determined reliably?

Of course, in the abstract it would seem possible that such differences would occur (though subtly) from the very beginning of vocal development in the first year. So imagine a longitudinal study of two groups of children, one from English-speaking homes in the United States and one from Spanish-speaking homes in Spain. Further assume that the environments are fairly pure linguistically and very representative of competent monolingual environments for the languages in question. Imagine that vocalizations from the infants are tape recorded every month and that those recordings are subjected to transcriptional analysis. Suppose that after such transcriptions are performed and outcomes are quantitatively analyzed, the two groups appear to differ by 9 months of age in how often they produce dark l's (characteristic of English but not Spanish) and the vowel [e] produced without diphthongization, a pattern typical of Spanish but not (most varieties of) English. The differences found are statistically reliable and are as predicted: English-learning babies produce more of the dark l's, and Spanish-learning babies produce more of the [e] vowels. Prior to 9 months, no reliable differences are found. What can be made of this outcome?

To interpret appropriately, it is important to know a series of things about methodology. First, who did the transcriptions, and what did they know about the infants? Often in studies conducted to compare groups of children from differing language backgrounds, transcriptions are performed on site where the infants are, and consequently the transcribers of the two groups are different people. If the transcribers are different people, one set of transcribers for Spanish and another for English, one must immediately face a major interpretive problem. The differences obtained may be due to differences in the infants, but they may also be due to differences in the transcribers. The Spanish transcribers may simply have different tendencies from the English transcribers, and this could be so whether the transcribers in the two cases are monolingual speakers or bilingual speakers of either language.

Suppose that a portion of the data is transcribed by all the transcribers in both groups to attain a reliability estimate. Such information could help mitigate concerns about potential transcriber biases, but the interpretive problem does not go away so easily. Unless the reliability is perfect, some proportion of the apparent difference between groups could still be attributed to the differences among transcribers. Without special quantitative analysis to determine the potential role of transcriber effects on the group outcome, we cannot know that the obtained "significant" difference will still be significant after extracting the role of transcriber.

The point here is that there is no simple way out of this bind once the study design specifies the "yoking" of transcribers to groups of infants. A solution might be to break the yoking from the beginning of the study and to mail the tapes back and forth so that all transcribers could be assigned equally to the two language groups of infants, effectively spreading whatever transcriber effect might occur equally (or as equally as possible) across the infant groups.

Suppose that such a precaution is taken. Is it now safe to assume that the two groups, which differ in some phonetic dimension according to the transcriptions, really differ in pronunciation? Not necessarily. Consider another transcriber problem. Every individual transcriber listens to tapes of infants vocalizing, but under normal circumstances the tapes have the voices of parents, experimenters, or other persons in the background. These voices reveal the language background of the child. The transcriber may be affected in terms of expectation by knowing what language the child is hearing. The effect could be subtle, but it could produce differences in the way transcriptions are made: perhaps the dark /l/ heard in the background of the tape recordings of infants in English settings subtly influences the expectations of transcribers, who tend, not often, but once in a while, to transcribe an infant sound as dark /l/, even though they would not transcribe it in that way without the background context.

Experimental Blinding

One might think these to be unreasonable or obsessive concerns, but they are not. There is solid evidence that phonetic transcription—indeed, all of phonetic perception—is subject to a wide variety of context effects. Sounds that are excised from their original contexts and replaced by noise are sometimes heard as if still there when the full manipulated contexts are played back (Warren & Obusek, 1971). The expectation of the listener forces an illusion that is encouraged, and in some cases demanded, by context. If listeners are told that a particular unintelligible pronunciation has a particular meaning, the listeners are systematically biased to hear the utterances in ways that conform to the phonetic expectations associated with the particular meaning (Oller & Eilers, 1975). The listeners transcribe what they think the speaker is saying, but that transcription is systematically altered when they are given reason to believe the speaker is saying something else. The physical utterance does not change; the listener's interpretation does.

Now, if the background of a tape recording hints to the listener about the infant's language experience or simply provides the transcriber with a contagious language-specific model, there would seem to be the potential for vexing transcriber effects in the hypothetical study. Of course, the problem could be even worse because however honest one intends to be as a scientist, it is not possible to be sure that awareness of a child's background would not influence transcription: One might simply shift transcriptions subtly due to expectations about what *should* happen in different circumstances of language learning, on the basis of inherent biases that might be impossible to control.

So the differences between the groups of children are confounded with possible transcriber effects unless the potential effects are controlled through experimental blinding. This has been hard to accomplish in the past because it has required laborious dubbing of each individual infant utterance from tapes while exercising caution to prevent even small snatches of other vocalizations from getting through. Apparently it was the biasing effect of voices in the background of tape recordings that persuaded Weir (1966) that she could detect differences in the babbling among Chinese- and English-learning infants. After her death, when recordings were presented to listeners in a special arrangement in which background voices could not be heard, listeners detected no differences in the vocalizations of infants from differing backgrounds (Atkinson, MacWhinney, & Stoel, 1970). In work conducted at the University of Miami seeking to evaluate possible detection by adult listeners of language background differences in babbling (Thevenin et al., 1985) it was also found that listeners could not reliably differentiate between Spanish- and English-learning infants. But the study was small in scale (eight infant subjects per group, 10 utterances per subject) because the dubbing problem prevented use of a large data set. Perhaps with a larger corpus, subtle differences between the infant groups could have been discerned. Some recent studies have reported abilities of listeners to detect differences in vocalizations of infants from different backgrounds (de Boysson-Bardies et al., 1984), but given the inconsistency of outcomes and the tremendous difficulty of ensuring that biases are not present in this sort of research, it remains uncertain that babbling of infants from different language settings can be distinguished in the first year of life.

Modern instrumental methods are about to make the problem of dubbing infant utterances (and thus isolating them from background voices) enormously easier. Adaptations to computer-based transcription programs (see Masterson & Pagan, 1993; Oller, 1991) have been developed that allow a convenient mouse-interface selection of utterances using a real-time screen display of an oscillographic or spectrographic representation, followed by digitized storage of the utterance in a convenient location that will allow it (and all the other utterances selected and stored in this way) to be accessed randomly for transcription by an experimentally blind observer. In this new scheme, utterances can be presented in whatever order one pleases. For example, they can be presented in mixed fashion so that the listener hears utterances at random from different children at different ages in different language backgrounds. If the hypothetical study is conducted in this way, the problem of transcriber bias may be effectively eliminated.

The Role of Acoustic Analysis

Why use transcription at all? Why not just analyze the utterances acoustically? Wouldn't that solve the problem of potential bias? These questions are routinely presented when the inherent problems of transcription are posed. Unfortunately, it is naive to imagine that a pure acoustic analysis approach could provide a general solution to the problem of bias. There exists no general-purpose, acoustically based speech recognition system capable of identifying phonological units in speech of children or other nonstandard speakers. In addition, however, it is important to recognize the more fundamental fact that acoustic analyses of speech are now (and will be in the future) founded upon assumptions about what aspects of acoustic signals are relevant to the speech code. At each step of acoustic analysis, bias can be introduced in terms of choices made about what features are extracted instrumentally and how they are measured. There is no such thing as error-free analysis of complex signals: The complexity of the signals implies lack of uniqueness of possible interpretations. Whether any particular interpretation of an acoustic speech signal is judged correct is dependent upon the assumptions (biases, if you will) of the judge.

Consider, for example, the measurement of speech segment durations. Bias in duration judgment can be manifest at several levels. First of all, duration judgments must be made at some designated level of analysis. Suppose one chooses to measure syllable durations. One requirement will be to define (acoustically) the notion of the syllable, and another will be to face the fact that there are a variety of options, none of which will satisfy the whole speech science community. The choice of one of the various options will result in a bias in analysis owing to the particular definition of the syllable that is chosen. It is possible, of course, to choose an utterly different level of analysis—segments, for example, or phrases—but here again there would be a variety of options for definition among which potentially biasing choices would have to be made. In trying to avoid linguistically based biases, one could abandon the phonological realm altogether and decide to measure arbitrarily defined chunks of information: for example, at every 10-ms interval. The arbitrary choice would, however, solve nothing because it would provide a reference unrelated to the goals of the inquiry—which, of course, concern the nature of speech, not the nature of 10-ms chunks of anything.

Second, it will be necessary to choose an instrumental approach to extract information at a designated level. Different options (including whether to monitor time domain or spectral domain and how to establish gain settings, frequency ranges, time constants, bandwidths of analysis, dynamic range of display, etc.) all have an effect on resulting measurements. Further, the choice of instruments and settings has undeniable *theoretical* consequences because the nature of the resulting characterization of speech units is affected by the choices.

My early research (see Oller, 1973a) focused primarily on the relative durations of final and nonfinal syllables in English, durations now known to favor the final syllables in adult subjects speaking, for example, English, Swedish, or French (Delattre, 1966; Lindblom, 1968; Oller, 1973a) but known to show less clear advantages for final syllables in other languages such as Finnish, Estonian, or Spanish (Lehiste, 1970; Oller, 1979). Klatt (1976) and others have provided reasons to believe that final lengthening is one of the ways that some languages mark the boundaries of chunks of speech information (such as sentences or phrases). How and when children learn the appropriate pattern of syllable duration has become a topic of substantial interest because it offers a perspective on acquisition of suprasegmental factors that appear to influence listeners' abilities to chunk the complex stream of speech (see, e.g., Konopczynski, 1985; Lynch, Oller, Steffens, & Buder, 1995).

In such work, instrumental choices produce unavoidable biases in relative outcomes for a variety of reasons. One of those reasons is that final syllables are inherently less intense than nonfinal ones under declarative intonation (the most commonly occurring type of intonation). Consequently there is a differential effect of instrument settings (such as gain or dynamic range) on acoustically displayed final- and nonfinal-syllable durations: The difference favoring final syllables is found to be highest at high signal-to-noise ratios and to be reduced systematically at lower ratios. How to decide what instruments and instrument settings to use is not a purely acoustic matter, and the choices made are inherently theoretical.

Third, it is important to choose standards of measurement to be used upon the acoustic analysis that is obtained. What constitutes the beginning of a syllable, and what the end? Does high-frequency noise at the end of a syllable (resulting from gradual cessation of expiration) count as part of the syllable? If not, how should high-frequency noise produced by other mechanisms (such as frication) be treated? Choices such as these also have unavoidable theoretical consequences and may substantially affect outcomes. In the final- versus nonfinal-syllable studies, relative durations can be affected fundamentally by measurement criterion choices: If high-frequency noise is included, final syllables are deemed relatively longer. Again, whether one chooses to include such noise is a theoretical matter that cannot be resolved on purely acoustic grounds. External information about the nature of speech and speech perception is commonly invoked to help make the choices, but it must be remembered that once such information has been introduced into the process, the potential perspective is biased by the choice of what is considered relevant external information.

Acoustic analysis cannot, then, solve the problem of bias in transcription. Acoustic analysis has its own inherent biases. An important goal of research in acoustics of infant vocalizations should be the development of a standard of interpretation (which, of course, will constitute a kind of bias) based, at least in part, upon the auditory perceptions of normal mature listeners. This may sound like putting the cart before the horse, but it is an inevitable feature of appropriate studies in the sounds of speech.

The need for auditory referencing of acoustic data may best be illustrated by example. Consider a description of a series of vocalizations by an infant. Suppose that by spectrographic measurement it is determined that the infant produced 20 utterances, with average duration of 500 ms, resonance characteristics with a median peak at 1,500 Hz, and a mean F0 of 350 Hz. What does this description by itself tell about the extent to which the infant's vocalizations are or are not speechlike? What stage of development has the infant reached? Is the child normal or handicapped? One might gather large amounts of such data on normal and abnormal development at various stages and try to reference the outcomes to standards established in such normative work. Even the normative work, however, requires limiting assumptions about what features of sounds are important. How does one determine which features are most important? One suggestion worth considering is to make the determination by focusing on which features of the acoustic signal are used by the normal auditory system in judging the sounds. According to the suggestion, one starts with how the normal listener perceives speech and which features of the acoustic signal play the most critical roles, and from there one develops a theory on the acoustic nature of speech that is based on the listener's systematic perceptual strategies. Having once developed such a theory, one can attend to the infant sounds with a perspective that gives new meaning to each of the acoustic facts that may be discovered.

The perspective constitutes a sort of bias to be sure, but this is the kind of bias that should be sought because it is founded on the natural goals of the learner. It guides investigation toward the kinds of information in the acoustic signal that are relevant to the development of functional (i.e., understandable) speech. If we return to the hypothetical study, the median peak of acoustic energy at 1,500 Hz may be discarded as relatively unimportant, replaced by information about the range of values for two or three resonance peaks (or formants) that are known (through perceptual research) to be relevant to vowel perception. The durational information may be interpreted more thoroughly in the context of what is known about the duration of syllables and other rhythmic units in speech—information also gleaned from acoustic research on the perception of sounds. The F0 data may be referenced to what is known of intonation and stress, features of the signal that can be understood only in the context of perceptual research.

The point is that there is no perfectly objective standard of acoustic description. Every description requires assumptions. It is better to develop assumptions that appeal to appropriate goals of description and that seek external support from other sources of information relevant to those goals than to shoot in the dark. When Lynip (1951) tried to describe infant vocalizations with nothing but acoustic methods, he produced a body of data that created only a little ripple in the history of child phonology. His descriptions were unreferenced to the auditory standard of normal listeners and thus were largely uninterpreted. In retrospect, their potential usefulness appears to have been largely lost.

SUGGESTIONS ABOUT THEORETICAL GROWTH

Infrastructural Descriptions: The Development of Well-Formed Syllables

The consideration of the role of acoustics in the study of infant vocalizations and child phonology highlights the need for integrated descriptions that unite acoustic and perceptual information about the nature of speech within a single framework. Articulatory descriptions provide additional perspectives in the context of the framework. Much of my own work in infant vocalizations has focused on the development and elaboration of a framework that might provide deeper insights into infant sounds through integration of perceptual and acoustic/articulatory data in the context of a broadened perspective on the nature of the human sound-making capacity. The work is founded on the idea that only in the context of such a perspective can the relationship between sounds of infants and sounds of mature speech be characterized insightfully. It is advantageous to begin by knowing what speech is in a very general way. In a sense, this is the same problem as that mentioned above in the context of the discussion of acoustic analysis of speech. It is important to provide a set of acoustic (and/or articulatory) characterizations of the most fundamental properties of speech elements at every level of the rhythmic hierarchy of speech. The realm of study that seeks to accomplish such characterization has come to be called "infraphonology" (Oller & Lynch, 1992) to focus attention on the sense in which the enterprise specifies the foundational structures of potential phonological systems.

Theoretical infraphonological efforts began with characterizations of the minimal rhythmic unit of speech, the syllable. The prototypical or "canonical" syllable was defined in both acoustic and articulatory terms that made reference only to infrastructural properties of abstract units such as nuclei (prototypical vowels), margins (prototypical consonants), and transitions between them. The work scrupulously avoided reference to concrete, segmental phonetic units (e.g., [b], [β], [ɛ], [ɪ], [θ]) because these were seen in the infraphonological model as concrete and language-specific products of the more general infrastructural capability. The infraphonological model addresses only those properties of speech that are thoroughly universal.

There are a number of advantages of infraphonologically oriented descriptions of infant vocalizations. In such descriptions, one finds the ability to characterize infant sounds in terms of the extent to which they resemble speech. One can note that infants do or do not produce this or that feature of canonical syllables, for example. To the extent that they do command any of the designated features, they show a greater speech capacity than infants who do not. The infraphonological approach proves far superior to segmental description of infant sounds in the first half year of life because segmental phonetic transcription proves not only utterly unreliable but also deeply misleading for infants prior to entry to the canonical babbling stage. To transcribe phonetically when an infant is gooing, squealing, and growling does little more than confuse issues. On the other hand, infraphonological description provides useful descriptions of ways that such vocalizations manifest an emerging, if immature, capacity. In gooing, infants show that they are developing a capacity to differentiate nuclei and margins (because gooing involves supraglottal articulation during normal phonation), and squealing and growling show exploration of the capacity to use a full range of pitches.

Another advantage of an infraphonological approach is that it provides the basis for a stage model of infant vocal development, a model that is interpretable in terms of the external standards of what canonical, or well-formed, speech is in an entirely universal sense. There now exists an international consensus model of infant vocal development, based essentially on infraphonological principles (see review in Oller, 1995).

Perhaps the greatest appeal of the model has been in its ability to provide broadened empirical perspectives. For example, the stage model has provided a basis for differentiation of vocal development patterns in deaf and hearing infants. Deaf infants show extremely delayed onset of the canonical stage by comparison with normally developing infants, a pattern of differentiation that occurs almost without exception (Eilers & Oller, 1994; Kent, Osberger, Netsell, & Hustedde, 1987; Oller & Eilers, 1988; Stoel-Gammon & Otomo, 1986; Vinter, 1987).

Infrastructural Descriptions: The Development of Well-Formed Higher Order Rhythmic Units

Research on the development of well-formed syllables was not until recently paralleled by similar work on well-formed higher order units, such as phrases or rhythmic feet. But such work is now underway (Lynch et al., 1995), and the results are also encouraging. Infants as young as 2 months have been shown to structure the production of utterances into clusters that resemble mature phonological phrases in both duration and intonation. In fact, even at 2 months, there appear to be at least three levels in the hierarchy of vocal rhythm (syllables, multisyllabic utterances, and utterance clusters), and the durational dimensions of that hierarchy appear to be comparable to the dimensions found for syllables, rhythmic feet, and phonological phrases of adults in conversational speech. Even Down syndrome infants show the hierarchical pattern of rhythm, but they show it as if in slow motion: Every level of the hierarchy is slowed down by about one third.

The work in infraphonological development of higher order rhythmic units provides a glimpse of possibilities that may lie just over the horizon when traditional descriptive patterns (that are so heavily focused on segments) are replaced by broader descriptive schemes encompassing the understructure of speech systems at a variety of rhythmic levels. The infraphonological approach facilitates illumination of patterns that emerge early in life, patterns that may be of such importance that their failure to emerge as expected may reveal deep aberrations of development.

Nonlinear Approaches and the Need for Nonsegmental Descriptions

A number of recent efforts presage the development of new approaches to description in child phonology that emphasize nonsegmental tools. The efforts are founded in part in developments from linguistics proper (e.g., Goldsmith, 1976; Liberman & Prince, 1977), in which nonlinear phonological description has solved a number of vexing problems of analysis that proved treatable in traditional segmental systems only when the tools were contorted and twisted to accommodate phenomena that clearly do not operate at a segmental level. When notions such as "syllable" and "phrase" are incorporated into descriptions (as nonlinear models require), many such problems prove easily manageable.

In child phonology, nonlinear models have shown promise in dealing with similar problems. For example, natural accounts of phenomena such as assimilation and metathesis, in which changes occur across long stretches of segmental material, prove easier to achieve with nonlinear approaches (Bernhardt, 1992; Stemberger, 1992; Stoel-Gammon & Stemberger, 1994). It has been suggested that accounts of phonological disorders may be enhanced through nonlinear approaches as well and that intervention strategies may be improved.

Work in infant vocal development has also recently focused on nonsegmental levels of function. In particular, MacNeilage and Davis (1990) have presented data suggesting that infants use consonant-vowel combinations in highly limited fashion. Early in canonical babbling, front vowels tend to go with front (coronal) consonants, back vowels with back consonants, and low vowels with labials. The tendency suggests that infants producing reduplicated sequences merely adjust the jaw position in repetitive rhythmicity, producing the vowel that is most proximal or requires the least additional adjustment for each consonantal articulatory target. The pattern of production suggests that infants do not actually possess a distinction among different vowel and consonant types and that the level of function, at this stage of development, is the syllable. Two or three syllable types appear to occur, one with a labial, one with a coronal, and sometimes one with a velar onset, but the vowels that occur are predictable, given specification of the onset. The tendency of infants to produce syllables with no obvious segmental differentiation early in life provides further support for nonlinear descriptive tools in child phonology.

One difficulty in application of nonlinear approaches in child phonology is associated with uncertainty about the optimal form for coding of data. If infants possess no segments but only syllables, how can the syllables be characterized without implying the presence of segments? Transcription of a syllable as [ba] appears to imply a suborganization of consonant and vowel that infants may not possess. The problem is, of course, more general, because infants and children produce many variations of pronunciation that adults can both perceive and assign to adultlike categories, even though the differentiations may be irrelevant to the child. For example, in a sequence of syllables produced by an infant, one might hear [baβʌbawæ], and to the ears of sophisticated listeners, the sequence might indeed have had the phonetic characteristics implied by the transcription. But at the same time, the infant may not have *intended* the distinctions implied by the various vowels and consonants in the sequence. The infant may instead have intended to produce a sequence of four syllables, all with labial onset, and the vowel-like elements associated with each onset may have occurred without the child's having had a specific intention to differentiate among them. Even the consonantlike onsets may show differences that are incidental from the child's perspective. What sounds like a [b], a [β], and a [w] to adult ears may be all in the same realm to the child. How, then, can one best characterize (i.e., transcribe) such a sequence? It might be best to adopt syllabic symbols with superscript or subscript onset markers to help capture the investigator's necessary lack of certainty about whether the infant has control of segmental units. A syllable that sounds like [ba], [wa], or [βa], for example, might be characterized as [^{Labial}S], where the capital S is intended to represent an undifferentiated syllable and the onset is specified in a global way without implication regarding manner of articulation. [di], [θɩ], and [zm], on the other hand, might be characterized as [^{Coronal}S]. Such an approach would be consistent with the implications of the MacNeilage and Davis (1990) theoretical model and would conform in some ways to the global featural rules and "underspecifications" of nonlinear systems of phonology.

This sort of symbology may seem cumbersome, but it may be necessary to use new symbological alternatives to break out of the confines of segmentally based expectations. There is a persistent tendency to ask segmental questions about infant sounds. Did he produce more [h]s than she did? What proportion of [p]s did that child use? Do Down syndrome infants use more [m]s than normally developing infants? Such questions encourage "shoe-horning" of infant sounds into the segmental categories upon which the questions are based. The questions drive the enterprise into a hole and force the data into categories where they do not belong. Consequently it is increasingly appealing to consider proposals that abandon segmental characterizations explicitly in infancy and introduce them (presumably for infants of greater age) only as justified by observations that suggest that the infants or children really do possess segments. Even further, it may be justifiable to insist that narrow transcriptions of infant or child utterances be specially marked to indicate features that the transcriber has reason to believe are contrastive in the infant or child inventory, as opposed to those features that merely conform to categorizations that can be imposed by the listener.

The problem of transcribing or categorizing in a way that differentiates the perspective of the listener's ear and the speaker's intended contrasts will not disappear by virtue of theoretical innovations. There are reasons to consider both perspectives. Up to the present, research has almost exclusively considered the listener's perspective, a perspective that provides a view of the *potential* communicative abilities of the infant or child's pronunciations but can lead interpretations astray if there is interest in knowing about the child's mental organization.

CONCLUSION

It is encouraging that new ways of categorizing the sounds of infants and young children are being entertained. It seems clear that syllables and higher order rhythmic units will be the focus of much future attention in child phonology and that nonlinear and infrastructural descriptions will largely replace our earlier, purely segmental approaches. But many fundamental questions remain unresolved, and as we proceed to implement new models, it is critical that methodological tools be applied with special care. The primary intent of this chapter is to note the importance of implementing protections to thwart unintended biases and, perhaps most of all, to encourage a constant vigilance with regard to unavoidable effects of bias within research designs that do not effectively control for them. Theoretical structures and the possibility of obtaining reliable observations, whether segmental or nonlinear, are inherently blunt. In the context of the bluntness of the instruments of child phonology, it is important to impose extreme measures to prevent bias from yielding illusory, and ultimately misleading, outcomes.

The work reported here was supported by a grant from the National Institutes of Deafness and Other Communication Disorders (R01 DC00484) and by philanthropic support from Austin Weeks.

REFERENCES

Atkinson, K., MacWhinney, B., & Stoel, C. (1970). *An experiment in the recognition of babbling* (Papers and Reports on Child Language Development, No. 1). Stanford, CA: Stanford University Press.

Bernhardt, B. (1992). Developmental implications of nonlinear phonological theory. *Clinical Linguistics and Phonetics, 6*, 259–281.

Chomsky, N., & Halle, M. (1968). *The sound pattern of English*. New York: Harper & Row.

Copernicus, N. (1978). *On the revolutions* (E. Rosen, Trans. and Comm.; J. Dobrzycki, Ed.). Baltimore: Johns Hopkins Press. (Original work published 1514)

Cruttenden, A. (1970). A phonetic study of babbling. *British Journal of Disordered Communication, 5*, 110–118.

de Boysson-Bardies, B., Sagart, L., & Durand, C. (1984). Discernible differences in the babbling of infants according to target language. *Journal of Child Language, 11*, 1–15.

Delattre, P. (1966). A comparison of syllable length conditioning among languages. *International Review of Applied Linguistics, 4*, 183–198.

Edwards, M.L. (1978). *Patterns and processes in fricative acquisition: Longitudinal evidence from six English-learning children*. Unpublished doctoral dissertation, Stanford University.

Eilers, R.E., & Oller, D.K. (1994). Infant vocalizations and the early diagnosis of severe hearing impairment. *Journal of Pediatrics, 124*, 199–203.

Eilers, R.E., Oller, D.K., & Benito-García, C.R. (1984). The acquisition of voicing contrasts in Spanish and English learning infants and children: A longitudinal study. *Journal of Child Language, 11*, 313–336.

Elbers, L. (1982). Operating principles in repetitive babbling: A cognitive continuity approach. *Cognition, 12*, 45–63.

Ferguson, C.A., & Farwell, C.B. (1975). Words and sounds in early language acquisition: English initial consonants in the first fifty words. *Language, 51*, 419–439.

Goldsmith, J. (1976). An overview of autosegmental phonology. *Linguistic Analysis, 2*, 23–68.

Hodson, B.W., & Paden, E.P. (1981). Phonological processes which characterize unintelligible and intelligible speech in early childhood. *Journal of Speech and Hearing Disorders, 46*, 369–373.

Ingram, D. (1976). *Phonological disability in children.* New York: American Elsevier.

Jakobson, R. (1941). *Kindersprache, Aphasie, und allgemeine Lautgesetze*. Uppsala: Almqvist & Wiksell.

Kent, R., Osberger, M.J., Netsell, R., & Hustedde, C. (1987). Phonetic development in identical twins differing in auditory function. *Journal of Speech and Hearing Disorders, 52*, 64–75.

Klatt, D. (1976). Linguistic uses of segmental duration in English: Acoustic and perceptual evidence. *Journal of the Acoustical Society of America, 59*, 1208–1221.

Konopczynski, G. (1985). Acquisition du langage: La période charnière et sa structuration mélodique. *Bulletin d'Audiophonologie: Annales Scientifiques de l'Université de Franche-Comté, 11*, 63–92.

Lehiste, I. (1970). *Suprasegmentals.* Cambridge, MA: MIT Press.

Liberman, M., & Prince, A. (1977). On stress and linguistic rhythm. *Linguistic Inquiry, 8*, 249–336.

Lindblom, B. (1968). Temporal organization of syllable production. *STL-QPSR, 2*(3), 1–5.

Locke, J.L. (1983). *Phonological acquisition and change*. New York: Academic Press.

Locke, J.L. (1993). *The child's path to spoken language*. Cambridge, MA: Harvard University Press.

Lynch, M.P., Oller, D.K., Steffens, M.L., & Buder, E.H. (1995). Phrasing in prelinguistic vocalizations. *Developmental Psychobiology, 28*, 3–23.

Lynip, A. (1951). The use of magnetic devices in the collection and analysis of the preverbal utterances of an infant. *Genetic Psychology Monographs, 44*, 221–262.

MacNeilage, P.F., & Davis, B.L. (1990). Acquisition of speech production: The achievement of segmental independence. In W.J. Hardcastel & A. Marchal (Eds.), *Speech production and speech modelling.* Dordrecht, the Netherlands: Kluwer.

Masterson, J., & Pagan, F. (1993). *Macintosh interactive system for phonological analysis* [Computer software]. San Antonio, TX: Psychological Corporation.

Menyuk, P. (1968). The role of distinctive features in children's acquisition of phonology. *Journal of Speech and Hearing Research, 11*, 138–146.

Oller, D.K. (1973a). The effect of position-in-utterance on speech segment duration in English. *Journal of the Acoustical Society of America, 54*, 1235–1247.

Oller, D.K. (1973b). Regularities in abnormal child phonology. *Journal of Speech and Hearing Disorders, 38*, 36–47.

Oller, D.K. (1979). Syllable timing in English, Spanish and Finnish. *Current Issues in the Phonetic Sciences, 9*, 331–343.

Oller, D.K. (1980). The emergence of the sounds of speech in infancy. In G. Yeni-Komshian, J. Kavanagh, & C. Ferguson (Eds.), *Child phonology: Vol. 1. Production* (pp. 93–112). New York: Academic Press.

Oller, D.K. (1991). Computational approaches to transcription and analysis in child phonology. *Journal for Computer Users in Speech and Hearing, 7*, 44–59.

Oller, D.K. (1995). Development of vocalizations in infancy. In H. Winitz (Ed.), *Human communication and its disorders: A review* (Vol. 4, pp. 1–30). Timonium, MD: York.

Oller, D.K., & Eilers, R.E. (1975). Phonetic expectation and transcription validity. *Phonetica, 31*, 288–304.

Oller, D.K., & Eilers, R.E. (1981). A pragmatic approach to phonological systems of deaf speakers. In N. Lass (Ed.), *Speech and language: Advances in basic research and practice* (Vol. 6, pp. 103–141). New York: Academic Press.

Oller, D.K., & Eilers, R.E. (1988). The role of audition in infant babbling. *Child Development, 59*, 441–449.

Oller, D.K., Jensen, H., & Lafayette, R. (1978). The relatedness of phonological processes of a hearing impaired child. *Journal of Communication Disorders, 11*, 97–106.

Oller, D.K., & Lynch, M.P. (1992). Infant vocalizations and innovations in infraphonology: Toward a broader theory of development and disorders. In C. Ferguson, L. Menn, & C. Stoel-Gammon (Eds.), *Phonological development* (pp. 509–536). Parkton, MD: York.

Oller, D.K., & Warren, I. (1976). On the nature of the phonological capacity. *Lingua, 39*, 183–199.

Oller, D.K., Wieman, L., Doyle, W., & Ross, C. (1975). Infant babbling and speech. *Journal of Child Language, 3*, 1–11.

Roug, L., Landberg, I., & Lundberg, L.-J. (1989). Phonetic development in early infancy: A study of four Swedish children during the first eighteen months of life. *Journal of Child Language, 16*, 19–40.

Shriberg, L.D. & Kwiatkowski, J. (1980). *Natural process analysis: A procedure for phonological analysis of continuous speech samples.* New York: Macmillan.

Stampe, D. (1969). The acquisition of phonetic representation. In R.T. Binnick, A. Davison, G.M. Green, & J.L. Morgan (Eds.), *Papers from the fifth regional meeting of the Chicago Linguistic Society* (pp. 443–454). Chicago: Chicago Linguistic Society.

Stark, R.E. (1980). Stages of speech development in the first year of life. In G. Yeni-Komshian, J. Kavanagh, & C. Ferguson (Eds.), *Child phonology: Vol. 1. Production* (pp. 73–90). New York: Academic Press.

Stemberger, J.P. (1992). Vocalic underspecifiation in English language production. *Language, 68*, 492–524.

Stoel-Gammon, C., & Otomo, K. (1986). Babbling development of hearing impaired and normally hearing subjects. *Journal of Speech and Hearing Disorders, 51*, 33–41.

Stoel-Gammon, C., & Stemberger, J.P. (1994). Consonant harmony and phonological underspecification in child speech. In M. Yavas (Ed.), *First and second language phonology* (pp. 63–80). San Diego: Singular.

Thevenin, D., Eilers, R.E., Oller, D.K., & LaVoie, L. (1985). Where's the drift in babbling drift? A cross-linguistic study. *Applied Psycholinguistics, 6*, 3–15.

Vihman, M.M., Ferguson, C.A., & Elbert, M. (1986). Phonological development from babbling to speech: Common tendencies and individual differences. *Applied Psycholinguistics, 7*, 3–40.

Vihman, M.M., & Miller, R. (1988). Words and babble at the threshold of language. In M. Smith & J. Locke (Eds.), *The emergent lexicon* (pp. 151–183). New York: Academic Press.

Vinter, S. (1987). Contrôle de premières productions vocales du bébé sourd. *Bulletin d'Audiophonologie, 3*, 659–670.

Warren, R.M., & Obusek, C.J. (1971). Speech perception and phonemic restoration. *Perception and Psychophysics, 9*, 358–362.

Weir, R. (1966). Some questions on the child's learning of phonology. In F. Smith & G. Miller (Eds.), *The genesis of language* (pp. 153–168). Cambridge, MA: MIT Press.

Zlatin, M. (1975). *Preliminary descriptive model of infant vocalization during the first 24 weeks: Primitive syllabification and phonetic exploratory behavior* (Final Report, Project No 3-4014, NE-G-00-3-0077).

CHAPTER 7

Phonological Awareness: Connecting Speech and Literacy Problems

Joy Stackhouse

Phonological awareness refers to the ability to reflect on and manipulate the structure of an utterance (e.g., into words, syllables, or sounds) as distinct from its meaning. Children need to develop this awareness to make sense of an alphabetic script, such as English, when learning to read and to spell. For example, children have to learn that the sounds (phonemes) in a word can be represented by letters (graphemes). When spelling a new word, children have to be able to segment the word into its sounds before they can attach the appropriate letters, and when reading an unfamiliar word, they have to be able to decode the printed letters back to sounds. Environmental exposure to nursery rhymes, sound games, and the printed word helps them to distinguish form from meaning and facilitates the sound play and literacy development typical of normally developing children.

Children with expressive phonological impairments have particular difficulty with developing phonological awareness skills (Stackhouse, 1992a). Further, the severity of the phonological output impairment, when measured by speech intelligibility, may be a significant predictor of performance on phonological awareness tasks (Webster & Plante, 1992).

Over the last few years, I have been involved in investigating the relationship between spoken and written language difficulties in children. This chapter summarizes some of the findings from this research programme. It discusses why children with phonological impairments are particularly at risk for problems with phonological awareness and literacy development. Phonological awareness is defined, and the relationship between phonological awareness and literacy development is examined. Phonological awareness problems in children with reading impairments and literacy problems in children with phonological impairments are discussed with reference to stage models of speech and literacy development. Longitudinal case studies of children with severe expressive phonological impairments are presented to illustrate how phonological awareness skills can be assessed, as well as to demonstrate the unfolding effect of phonological awareness problems on literacy development.

WHAT IS PHONOLOGICAL AWARENESS?

Phonological awareness has been defined by Goswami and Bryant (1990) as awareness of "the ways in which words and syllables can be divided into smaller units" (p. 2). It refers to rhyme knowledge, syllable and sound segmentation, manipulation, and blending. Investigations of children's phonological awareness skills have incorporated a variety of tasks that differ in the knowledge and experience a child needs to complete them successfully. Lewkowicz (1980) noted that at least 10 different types of tasks were available. These included:

- recognition of rhyme (e.g., Do these words rhyme—*fish dish*?; Which is the odd one out—fish dish *ball*?)
- isolation of a beginning, medial, or final sound (e.g., What is the last sound in *fish*?)
- sound segmentation (e.g., What are the three sounds in *fish*?)
- identifying the number of syllables or sounds in a word (e.g., How many beats in *potato*; How many sounds in *fish*?)
- sound-to-word matching (e.g., Does *fish* start with /f/?)
- word-to-word matching (e.g., Does *fish* start with the same sound as *foot?*)
- syllable and sound blending (e.g., What does *po-ta-to* say? What does *f-i-sh* say?)
- sound deletion (e.g., Say *fish* without /f/; Say *fish* without the first sound)
- specifying which phoneme has been deleted (e.g., Say *meat*, now say *eat*—what sound was left out of the second word?)
- sound substitution (e.g., Say *meat*; now say it with /f/ instead of /m/)

This is by no means an exhaustive list. Two other popular phonological awareness tasks involve rhyme production (e.g., Tell me as many words as you can that rhyme with *fish*), and sound exchange (e.g., Give me a spoonerism on *big fish*—answer: *fig bish*).

Normally developing children not only learn how to perform these phonological awareness tasks but incorporate phonological awareness skills into their everyday lives: For example, rhyme games are very common in the play of young children (Chukovsky, 1963). This is in contrast to children with phonological impairments and reading impairments, who find such tasks extraordinarily difficult (Hulme &

Snowling, 1992; Snowling, Goulandris, & Stackhouse, 1994; Snowling, Hulme, Wells, & Goulandris, 1992).

THE RELATIONSHIP BETWEEN PHONOLOGICAL AWARENESS AND LITERACY DEVELOPMENT

Phonological Awareness as a Predictor of Literacy Development

Phonological awareness has been found to be a strong predictor of literacy development. Given the range of phonological awareness tasks above, however, it is clear that some tasks might be better predictors than others. In general, early phonological awareness skills such as syllable segmentation (Liberman, Shankweiler, Fischer, & Carter, 1974) and knowledge of nursery rhymes (Maclean, Bryant, & Bradley, 1987) are not such powerful predictors of literacy outcome as later developing phonological awareness skills, such as sound segmentation and manipulation (Adams, 1990). This does not mean that rhyme is not a useful skill. A longitudinal study by Bryant, Bradley, Maclean, and Crossland (1989) monitored the rhyme awareness and literacy progress of 65 children from the ages of 4:07 to 6:07. Their data suggested that sensitivity to rhyme is a prerequisite for sound segmentation, which in turn plays an important role in learning to read. The development of proficient rhyme skills may also be an indicator of children's abilities to read by analogy with similar words, by recognising the similarities in sound and appearance between groups of words (e.g., *cat, hat, sat, fat*; Goswami, 1990). In contrast, phoneme segmentation skills and letter knowledge may be more predictive of a child's ability to read unfamiliar words by a sounding-out strategy (e.g., *c-a-t* → *cat*; Muter, 1996).

Phonological Awareness: Prerequisite or Consequence of Literacy Development?

During the 1970s and 1980s, there was much debate about whether phonological awareness was a prerequisite or consequence of literacy development (e.g, Mann, 1986; Read, Yun-Fei, Hong-Yin, & Bao-Qing, 1986). It is now clear that the relationship is a reciprocal one, and that children's phonological awareness develops from a tacit to a more explicit level through increased orthographic experience. For example, Zhurova (1963) reports that when a young child called Igor was asked if his name was "Gor," he confidently replied that it was not, but he was unable to supply the missing initial sound. Instead, Igor responded by elongating the initial sound without segmenting it from the rest of the word: "*Eeeee*gor." This suggests that although Igor had developed some phonological awareness, he did not have the skills necessary to complete the task. To become really efficient at more advanced phonological awareness tasks, children are aided by their orthographic knowledge. Adolescents who were good spellers, for example, performed better on a spoonerism test than adolescents who were poor spellers (Perin, 1983). The good spellers were able to conjure up the orthographic forms of the words and use this to help them transpose the appropriate letters/sounds in order to produce a spoonerism on popular singers' names (e.g., Bob Dylan → Dob Bylan).

Not all phonological awareness tasks, however, are dependent on literacy skill. Liberman et al. (1974), for example, demonstrated that normally developing preschool children could perform syllable segmentation tasks. Young children can also identify initial sounds in words before they can read, often by reflecting on their speech sound production. Orthographic experience, however, sharpens children's phonological awareness skills and allows them to make finer distinctions, such as identifying sounds *within* words, or the components of clusters (e.g., spl, scr). For example, a normally developing prereader, aged 4:6, was able to say that *strawberries* began with "str," but could not identify what sounds were within the cluster *str.* She was therefore proficient at onset/rhyme segmentation, but not at segmentation within the onset. To segment within the cluster, children need to *see* the written form in order to help them identify the components and be able to spell it for themselves.

Exhibit 7–1 illustrates how a child's phonological awareness develops along a continuum of tacit to explicit awareness (see "level of awareness") and is the cumulative result of auditory, articulatory, and reading experience (see "feedback"). Popular phonological awareness tasks are presented in a developmental progression from left to right (see "level of analysis") and are related to children's increasing feedback experience. From left to right, the phonological awareness tasks become progressively more dependent on literacy experience. Orthographic experience *shows* the child how words are structured (e.g., word/syllable boundaries, vowels, clusters) and thus facilitates a more explicit level of phonological awareness. The effect of orthography on phonological awareness was demonstrated by Ehri and Wilce (1980). They presented 24 nine-year-old children with counters to mark the number of phonemes detected in a series of single words that they then had to spell. Half of the words contained hidden letters (e.g., pi*t*ch/rich, com*b*/home). The results indicated that those children who could spell the words also marked with a counter the hidden letters as additional *sounds* in their segmentation of the word.

Training Studies

Findings from training studies in particular have contributed to our understanding of the relationship between phonological awareness and literacy development. Bradley and Bryant (1983) studied 65 children who were nonreaders and below average on phonological awareness tasks when starting school. The group was divided into four subgroups:

Exhibit 7–1 Development of Phonological Awareness Skills

FEEDBACK	Auditory	Articulatory	Orthographic
		Lip reading	

LEVEL OF ANALYSIS

Syllable Segmentation

Rhyme

Blending

Sound Segmentation

Sound Manipulation

Cluster Segmentation

LEVEL OF AWARENESS Tacit ——→ Explicit

Source: Copyright © Joy Stackhouse.

- *Group 1 (experimental group):* trained in sound categorization tasks involving listening for shared sounds in words (e.g., *hen/hat; hen/man*) or odd-one-out tasks (e.g., cat, sat, *leg*, hat)
- *Group 2 (experimental group):* trained like Group 1, but the children were shown how each sound was represented in the alphabet by the presentation of plastic letters
- *Group 3 (control group):* trained in semantic categorization involving listening for words that were associated in meaning (e.g., *hen* and *pig* are both farm animals) or odd-one-out tasks (horse, cow, *lion*, sheep)
- *Group 4 (control group)*: received no training

Training took place in 40 individual sessions over 2 years. At the end of this time, Group 1, which had received sound categorization training, was no different from Group 3, the group that had received semantic categorization training. In contrast, the children in Group 2 were significantly better than controls on reading and spelling measures. The findings from this study suggest that phonological awareness training needs to be linked with explicit letter knowledge teaching for gains to be made in children's literacy development.

Similar results were obtained in a more recent training study targetting 7-year-old children who were reading around the 5:9 year level. Hatcher, Hulme, and Ellis (1994) divided 128 poor readers matched on IQ and reading age into three experimental groups—Group 1, trained in phonological awareness alone; Group 2, trained in reading alone; and Group 3, trained in phonological awareness plus reading—and a control group, Group 4, that received no training other than routine classroom experience. Each of the experimental groups received forty 30-minute sessions over a 20-week period. A range of reading, spelling, and phonological awareness measures were taken before and after the training period. The results showed that Group 3, which had received both phonological awareness training and reading instruction, was the only group to make significantly more progress than the controls on reading and spelling measures. Group 2—reading alone—was significantly better than the controls on one measure only: early word reading (a reading recognition task). Group 1—phonology alone—was no better than the controls on any of the reading and spelling measures. The results of this study support the earlier findings of Bradley and Bryant (1983) that phonological awareness training alone does not necessarily facilitate literacy development. Literacy development is dependent on children's ability to *link* their phonological awareness skills to letter knowledge and reading experience. Hatcher et al. (1994) termed this the *phonological linkage hypothesis.*

A STAGE MODEL OF LITERACY DEVELOPMENT

To understand how phonological awareness fits into literacy development, it is necessary to examine briefly the normal development of reading and spelling skills. In 1985, Uta Frith presented a three-stage model of literacy development in which the child moves from an initial *logographic* or visual whole-word-recognition stage of reading to an *alphabetic* stage using letter-sound correspondences and finally to an *orthographic* stage dependent on segmentation of larger units: morphemes.

In the first stage, children's reading is limited by the extent of their orthographic lexicon (their store of written words). They can recognise only words that they know and are not able to decode unfamiliar words. When spelling, children may have some automatic programmes for familiar words such as their own name, but in general, spelling is *nonphonetic* in this stage and does not show sound-letter correspondences. For example, a normally developing 5-year-old spelt *orange* as *oearasrie*. This was perfectly acceptable, in fact rather good, for her age. She had segmented the onset correctly and showed an awareness of letter forms and word length. This type of spelling soon diminishes in young, normally developing children (Stackhouse, 1989) but persists in children with a history of speech difficulties (Clarke-Klein & Hodson, 1995; Robinson, Beresford, & Dodd, 1982).

Breakthrough to the alphabetic stage occurs when the child can apply letter-sound rules to decode new words. When reading, the child may sound out letters in the word and then blend them together to produce the target (e.g., *f-i-sh* → *fish*). At the beginning of this stage, *semiphonetic* spelling occurs. Vowels are often not transcribed, and letter sounds may be used to represent syllables (e.g., *burglar* → *bgl*; sounded out as [bə gə lə] to represent the three syllables in the word). Gradually, the child learns how to fill in the gaps. Vowel names are helpful (e.g., *boat* → *bot*), and spelling becomes more logical or *phonetic*. Targets are recognisable even if the spelling is not conventionally correct (e.g., *orange* → *orinj*). Although this may appear a little odd, phonological awareness skills are developing normally. The child is segmenting the word successfully and applying letter knowledge but has not yet learned (or been taught) the conventions of English spelling.

In the final stage, the child is able to recognize larger chunks of words, such as prefixes and suffixes (e.g., addi*tion*), and to read more efficiently by analogy with known words. Once the child has the skills to perform at each stage, the most appropriate strategy for the task presented can be adopted.

Frith (1985) suggested that the failure to progress through these stages is characteristic of children with literacy problems. Children with delayed development may progress through these stages, though at a slower rate than their peer group. Children with *specific* literacy difficulties, however (i.e., surprising reading and spelling impairments given their cognitive abilities), may be unable to progress through the normal stages outlined above and need to develop compensatory strategies or ways around barriers to their literacy development. These children may be called *dyslexic.* Although sometimes a contentious term (see Stanovich, 1994), there is overwhelming evidence that such a condition exists, that it is often inherited, and that a key characteristic is phonological difficulties (Snowling, 1996).

A particularly severe form of dyslexia that occurs when a child's development is arrested at the logographic stage of literacy development is known as *phonological dyslexia.* This is characterized by a particular difficulty with applying phonological processing skills to literacy. Children with phonological dyslexia have poor phonological awareness skills, limited phonological short-term memory, and poor verbal repetition and naming skills. A consequence of these deficits is that they are unable to break through to the alphabetic stage of literacy development. They are unable to read new words because they cannot decode letters into sounds and blend them together to produce the word. Further, their spellings may be predominantly nonphonetic, particularly in longer and more complex words (Snowling, 1987).

A modified version of Frith's model is presented in Figure 7–1. A list of the skills necessary to progress from stage to stage has been added on the right-hand side of the figure. The majority of these skills involve spoken language. Although recent work has clarified how visual deficits may also affect reading performance, there

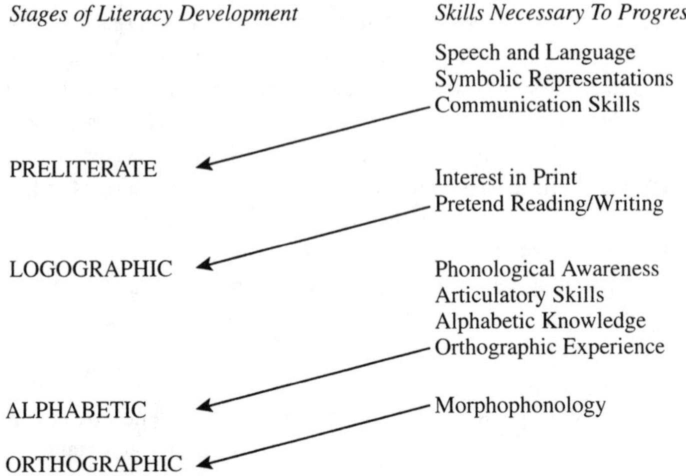

Figure 7–1 Prerequisite Skills for Each Stage of Frith's (1985) Model of Literacy Development. *Source*: Reprinted with permission from Promoting Reading and Spelling Skills through Speech Therapy, in *Specific Speech and Language Disorders in Children*, P. Fletcher and D. Hall, eds., p. 202, © 1992. AFASIC.

is an overwhelming consensus that verbal skills are the most influential in literacy development (Catts, Hu, Larrivee, & Swank, 1994).

Phonological awareness plays a major role in the child's progression from the logographic to alphabetic stage of literacy development. Children who fail to develop adequate phonological awareness skills cannot progress to the alphabetic stage of literacy development.

WHY MIGHT CHILDREN FAIL TO DEVELOP PHONOLOGICAL AWARENESS SKILLS?

Phonological awareness is dependent on an intact phonological processing system. This system is illustrated in its simplest form in Figure 7–2. A problem at any point within this system may interfere with phonological awareness development.

Without intact *input* (auditory processing) skills, children cannot discriminate and sequence what they hear. This auditory processing problem not only interferes with performance on phonological awareness tasks such as rhyme detection but also affects how words are stored in the lexicon. Inaccurate or incomplete phonological *representations* in the lexicon will be particularly problematic when the child wants to name or spell (Constable, Stackhouse, & Wells, 1994; Stackhouse, 1996) and will interfere with the child's performance on phonological

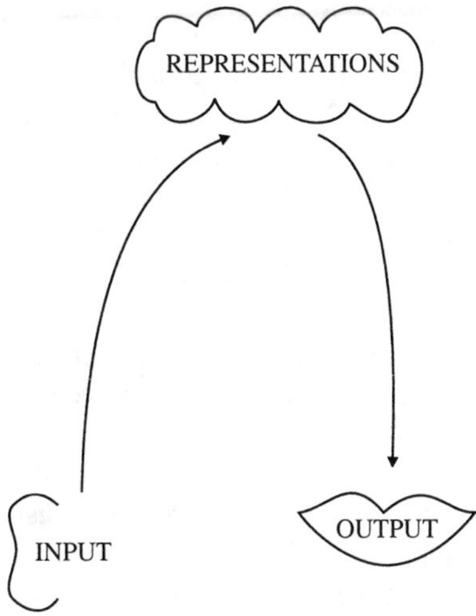

Figure 7–2 The Basic Structure of the Phonological Processing System. *Source*: Copyright © Joy Stackhouse.

awareness tasks involving pictures in which the child is dependent on his or her own representations to complete the task (e.g., when matching pictures that rhyme or that begin with the same onset; see Vance, 1996). *Output* skills are particularly important for rehearsing verbal material in memory and for reflecting on the structure of words in preparation for speech and spelling. Problems with spoken output affect not only the child's ability to imitate new words but also his or her ability to perform phonological awareness tasks such as rhyme production or sound blending (Stackhouse, 1993). Successful literacy development depends on coupling these phonological processing skills at the input, representation, and output levels with alphabetic (letter) knowledge gained through orthographic experience.

PHONOLOGICAL PROCESSING PROBLEMS IN CHILDREN WITH READING IMPAIRMENTS

The work of Vellutino (1979) in particular shifted the emphasis from visual to verbal processing deficits in children as an explanation of specific reading difficulties (dyslexia). Vellutino, Harding, Phillips, and Steger (1975) demonstrated that children with dyslexia could visually match and select abstract shapes as well as normal children in Grades 4 through 6. The children with dyslexia, however, did less well at associating abstract shapes with a verbal response and had difficulty transferring their verbal codes to new tasks. This became known as the *verbal deficit hypothesis* of dyslexia. More recently, the emphasis has been on the specific phonological processing deficits demonstrated by children with specific reading impairments: the *phonological deficit hypothesis* (Snowling & Hulme, 1994).

Before learning to read and spell, children have already established a phonological processing system to deal with spoken language. This system is also the foundation for their written language development (Pring & Snowling, 1986). To test the hypothesis that weaknesses in this foundation will be reflected in children's literacy performance, Snowling, Stackhouse, and Rack (1986) investigated the underlying phonological processing skills in seven cases of developmental phonological dyslexia (defined above), six of whom were in the age range from 8 to 13 years and the other of whom was an adult. The cases were selected on the basis of (a) normal IQ, (b) specific reading and spelling difficulties, and (c) poor nonword reading compared to real-word reading. None had serious speech difficulties at the time of testing, but three had received speech-language therapy in the past. Tests of reading, spelling, auditory processing, phoneme segmentation, and articulation were administered. The results, which were analysed quantitatively and qualitatively, indicated that all of the cases, regardless of their reading age (range 7:5 to 12:0), adopted a visual rather than a sound approach to reading. When spelling, those with low reading ages (range 6:11 to 7:5) performed less well than normal controls and made more nonphonetic errors than would be predicted by their reading age (e.g., *traffic* spelt as *tatin*, and *polish* as *phins*), indicating difficulties with sound segmentation skills. Indeed, although all could segment words at the syllable level, none was proficient at rhyme or sound segmentation tasks, suggesting difficulties at the alphabetic stage of literacy development.

The cases in this study were similar to each other in that they all had difficulties with phonological processing skills. Qualitative analysis, however, revealed individual differences in the *nature* of the phonological processing deficit and how this affected their spelling. One of the children, Tina, had input (auditory processing) problems. On tests of auditory discrimination (e.g., Wepman & Reynolds, 1987), she could not discriminate minimal pairs such as *map/nap* or *cope/coke*. When spelling, Tina failed to represent the initial phoneme on 18 out of 30 occasions. She often wrote the last sound of the target first, for example *lip* spelt as *persye*, and *tulip* as *peper*. Tina appeared to be relying on lipreading and therefore confused sounds made in the same place of articulation. When these two errors were combined, her spelling was difficult to decipher (e.g., *trap* → *mupter*). Sound/letter order seemed unimportant to her (e.g., *nest* → *teryes*, *bank* → *capuny*). On three-syllable spellings, Tina showed an awareness of increased word length but often substituted words that she knew for individual syllables (e.g., *catalogue* → *catofleg*, *refreshment* → *threesleling*).

In contrast, another child, Annie, had intact input skills but specific segmentation and memory problems. Her spellings were more accurate than Tina's; she was able to represent the initial phoneme of targets correctly and showed normal immaturities when spelling (e.g., short-vowel confusion, as in *pet* → *pat* and *lip* → *lap*, and deletion of the unstressed syllable as in *packet* → *pak* and *finger* → *fing*). Her segmentation difficulties, however, were apparent at the end of words in particular (e.g., *bump* → *bunt*, *nest* → *nent*) and were more serious as word length increased (e.g., *adventure* → *avatan*, *instructed* → *inshumdin*).

A third child, John, had output (i.e., expressive phonology) problems and had attended speech-language therapy when he was younger. Like Annie, John was able to transcribe the initial phoneme in words on most occasions, and errors revealed normal immaturities. Unlike both Tina and Annie, however, he had difficulties transcribing particular sounds, even though he could distinguish them perfectly well on an auditory discrimination test. The voice/voiceless contrast (e.g., b/p, g/k) was particularly difficult for him to produce and spell (e.g., *polish* → *bols*, *sack* → *sag*, and *cap* → *gab*). Of the three children, John experienced the most difficulty when spelling three-syllable words. These were unrecognizable (e.g., *membership* spelt as *meaofe*, and *adventure* as *afvoerl*). His output difficulty affected his ability to segment these longer words into smaller units (i.e., syllables and sounds).

The findings of this study suggested that the level at which phonological processing broke down influenced the nature of the reading and spelling difficulties in children with specific reading impairments. This raises the question of what happens to reading and spelling development in children with more obvious expressive phonological impairments whose underlying processing skills might be more impaired.

LITERACY DEVELOPMENT IN CHILDREN WITH PHONOLOGICAL IMPAIRMENTS

The Critical Age Hypothesis

Children with speech and language problems often have associated difficulties with phonological awareness and literacy. Group studies have shown that children with speech and language disorders do significantly less well than matched normally developing children on phonological awareness tasks (Bird & Bishop, 1992; Marion, Sussman, & Marquardt, 1993; Webster & Plante, 1992). Results of a study by Bird, Bishop, and Freeman (1995) confirm that children with *persisting* speech-sound difficulties have phonological awareness and literacy problems. They investigated a group of 31 boys in the age range of 5 to 7 years with phonological impairments to see if the severity of the speech problem and the presence of additional language impairments were significant prognostic factors for literacy development. The boys' performance on a range of phonological awareness tasks (e.g., rhyme and phoneme segmentation) and reading and spelling tasks (including nonword reading and spelling) was compared to that of a group of normally developing boys matched for chronological age and nonverbal ability. The boys with phonological impairments had particular difficulty with phonological awareness tasks, even when the tasks did not require a spoken response, and the majority had significant literacy problems when followed up at age 7:6. The presence of additional language impairments did not significantly affect the children's literacy development in this study, but the severity and persistence of the speech problem did. This supports the *critical age hypothesis* posited by Bishop and Adams (1990): Persisting phonological impairments beyond the age of 5:6 years may be a sign that a child is at risk for literacy problems.

Are *All* Children with Persisting Speech Difficulties at Risk for Literacy Problems?

In a study designed to examine literacy development in children with different types of speech difficulties, Stackhouse (1982) compared the reading and spelling skills of children in the age range of 7 to 11 years whose speech difficulties were the direct result of a cleft lip and palate with children who had expressive phonological impairments but no abnormality of their oral structure. The latter were described by their speech-language therapists as having developmental verbal dyspraxia (based on the Nuffield Centre Dyspraxia Assessment; Connery, 1992). The children with cleft lip and palate were not significantly different from age-matched normally developing children without speech difficulties on tests of reading and spelling. When errors were made, they followed sounding-out strategies (e.g., *sabre* was read as ['seɪ'bri] and *ceiling* as ['kɛ'lɪn]). In contrast, the children with verbal dyspraxia were significantly poorer than the normally developing children on reading and spelling tests, and their errors suggested guesswork rather than principled sound out strategies (e.g., *canary* was read as *competition*, and *dream* as *under*).

Spelling performance also distinguished the two groups of children with speech difficulties. Again, the children with cleft lip and palate performed similarly to the normally developing children. The errors made by the children with cleft lip and palate reflected intact sound segmentation skills but a lack of conventional spelling-rule knowledge: for example,

Target		*Spelling*
sooner	→	soona
boat	→	bot

These were in sharp contrast to the errors produced by the children with verbal dyspraxia, which appeared much less logical: for example,

Target		*Spelling*
year	→	andere
slippery	→	greid

It would seem that children whose speech difficulty is an isolated articulatory difficulty arising from a physical abnormality can develop segmentation skills perfectly well and may be no more likely to have specific reading impairment than the population with normally developing speech. This finding has been supported by investigations of children with speech problems arising from physical handicap. Bishop (1985) tested seven teenagers with dysarthric speech as a result of cerebral palsy, using tasks requiring word and nonword homophone judgement and word and nonword spelling. There was no difference in performance on these tasks between this group and a matched group of children with cerebral palsy but no speech difficulties. Nevertheless, it is important not to become complacent about such children's literacy development. Any child with hearing and health problems or with periods of hospitalization that lead to absenteeism from school may be at risk for delayed literacy development. It is the children with persisting speech difficulties with no obvious medical etiology (who are often described as having phonological impairments or developmental verbal dyspraxia), however, who are most at risk for related and specific literacy problems (Bishop & Robson, 1989; Stackhouse, 1982).

Speech and Spelling Errors

The next question to address is whether there is a direct relationship between how children pronounce a word and their spelling of that word. In 1983, Snowling and Stackhouse studied a small group of children, in the age range of 8 to 10 years, with severe expressive phonological impairment who were described by their speech-language therapist as having developmental verbal dyspraxia (based on the Nuffield Centre Dyspraxia Assessment; Connery, 1992). Each child was asked to imitate, read, spell, and copy a series of consonant-vowel-consonant (CVC) syllables that varied in degree of articulatory place change (e.g., *mop*, *bat*, *peg)*. The children with phonological impairments performed as well as normally developing children, matched on reading age, on reading and copying the written form of these words but significantly less well on imitating and spelling them. Overall, there were more spelling than imitation errors, and there was no obvious one-to-one correspondence between imitation and spelling responses; a child might imitate a word wrongly but spell it correctly, and vice versa.

During the study, however, it became apparent that the children with phonological impairments had great difficulty in segmenting the target prior to spelling it. For example, *Pam* was repeated correctly, segmented as [pə tə], and spelt as *potm*. *Nick* was also repeated correctly, segmented as [kə kə nə ɪ tə], and spelt as *cat*. These spellings were not the direct result of the children's speech-sound errors but were a manifestation of the inaccurate segmentation process, which was audible. The first example shows how an intrusive sound was transcribed in spelling, whereas the second example reveals how the order in which the sounds were segmented determined the triggering of an automatic spelling of a known word.

In summary, the spelling difficulties encountered by children with expressive phonological impairments are not always the direct result of their mispronunciations. Rather, their spelling problems also stem from limited phonological awareness and, in particular, sound segmentation difficulties.

CHILDREN WITH ARRESTED SPEECH AND LITERACY DEVELOPMENT

To investigate further the relationship between speech and literacy problems, the development of speech, phonological awareness, reading, and spelling in two children with severe expressive phonological impairment was studied over a 5-year period (Stackhouse, 1989). At the beginning of the study, Michael was aged 10:7 and Caroline was 11:0. They attended a secondary school, where they were mainstreamed but where they received daily remedial teaching and twice-weekly speech and language therapy within a language unit attached to the school. Both were of average intelligence. On the British Ability Scales (Elliot, Murray, & Pearson, 1983), Michael obtained an estimated IQ of 100 and Caroline an IQ of 111. Their speech had been unintelligible during the preschool years, and they had persisting and obvious speech output difficulties. In addition, they had serious literacy problems. Both children had a history of fluctuating hearing loss, but hearing was within normal limits at the time of the study.

Speech

Michael and Caroline's speech output had characteristics associated with developmental verbal dyspraxia (see Stackhouse, 1992b, for a review). These included imprecise articulations (e.g., *crab* → [kxə'wæb]), syllable reduction (*television* → [tɛ'vɪʒ‿ˌn]), and difficulties with articulatory place change (*buttercup* → ['kʌkəˌkʌʔ]). Caroline, in particular, struggled to produce target words, making repeated attempts to get it right (*treasure* → [s st 'stɛɾə 'stɛvə 'ʤɛvə 'stɛɪə 'ʤɛlɪʃ 'ʤɛdə]). Michael and Caroline's speech errors were compared with those from a group of younger normally developing children matched on articulation age (measured by the Edinburgh Articulation Test; Anthony, Bogle, Ingram, & McIsaac, 1971). The normally developing children were in the chronological age range of 3:3 to 5:6 and had an articulation age range of 3:0 to 5:6. The tasks presented included single-word naming and imitation, a connected speech condition, and a nonword imitation task. The target words increased in syllable length (e.g., *kite*, *rocket*, *caravan*, and *television)* and also included clusters (e.g., *nest*, *spider*, *stamp)*.

The normally developing children performed equally well across all the conditions. In contrast, Michael and Caroline's performance was much more variable, with particular difficulties evident on the connected-speech condition. Qualitative analysis revealed that although young normally developing children made dyspraxic-like speech errors, these were not as frequent or in such a severe form as those from the older children with speech difficulties. Therefore it was decided to compare the number of speech errors occurring in the target words spoken by the children with speech difficulties and the normal controls. To make this comparison, the number of errors occurring in each target word was calculated. For example, *treasure* realized as ['ʤɛdə] contains a total number of three errors:

1. affrication of the cluster	['trɛʒə] → ['ʧɛʒə]
2. prevocalic voicing	['ʧɛʒə] → ['ʤɛʒə]
3. stopping	['ʤɛʒə] → ['ʤɛdə]

This analysis revealed that Michael and Caroline could pronounce more words correctly than the younger children. Unlike the younger normally developing children, however, when they were unable to pronounce a word, they made multiple errors. Thus Michael and Caroline either *could* or *could not* produce a word, and when they could not produce a word, it contained several errors. In contrast, the younger normally developing children made only one or two errors per word but in a wider range of words (Stackhouse & Snowling, 1992b).

Reading and Spelling

A parallel finding emerged from an analysis of Michael and Caroline's reading and spelling errors. Michael and Caroline both met the criteria for *phonological dyslexia* (defined above): that is, their reading and spelling performance was typical of the logographic stage of literacy development (Frith, 1985). The children read words as visual wholes rather than breaking them up into their sound components. This meant that they were likely to make visual errors when reading (e.g., *pint* read as *paint*, and *organ* as *orange*) and were unable to tackle new words. They had particular difficulty when spelling. Michael's attempts to apply the phonics he had been taught were unsuccessful, as seen in the following spellings of three-syllable words:

Target	*Spelling*
cigarette	satersatarhaelerar
umbrella	rberherrelrarlsrllles

Although these appear bizarre spellings, they can be explained by a problem with phonological awareness: a failure to segment the word into syllables and sounds. These nonphonetic spellings occurred as Michael transcribed his repeated attempts at segmentation. For example, the following illustrates Michael's spellings when mapped onto the words' syllable structure:

Target	*Spelling*
ci/ga/rette	sa/ ter/ sa/ tar/ haelerar
1 2 3	1 3 1 3 2
um/bre/lla	r/ be/ rher/ re/ l/ ra/ r/ l/ sr/ lll/ es
1 2 3	2 2 2 2 3 2 2 3 ?2 3 ?

The first example shows how Michael has more success with the first and last syllables, which are the most acoustically salient. The second example reveals deletion of the first syllable, which is unstressed, particular difficulty segmenting the cluster [br], which he cannot pronounce, and some visual notion that the word contains more than one letter "l."

Caroline's spellings also revealed segmentation difficulties, but these were of a different kind. She had adopted a lexical strategy in which she selected words she knew to represent the syllables—for example:

Target	*Spelling*
adventure	andbackself
refreshment	withfirstmint

Unlike Michael, all of her spellings include the correct number of syllables, indicating that she is able to segment at the syllable level. Like Michael, however, she cannot segment sounds *within* the syllable for spelling purposes.

A qualitative developmental analysis revealed that neither of the children's spellings were typical of younger normally developing children (Stackhouse & Snowling, 1992a). Just as in the speech study above, in which they either could or could not pronounce words, Michael and Caroline either could or could not read and spell words. When they could not read or spell a word, they made complex errors because they did not have the phonological processing skills necessary to segment and blend the components of the target.

In both speech and literacy development, Michael and Caroline tackled each new word separately, rather than using phonological processing skills to identify similarities across phonologically related words. This lexical approach to acquiring new words is typical of very young children (Ingram, 1989) and parallels Frith's (1985) description of the logographic stage of literacy development. The indications are that Michael and Caroline are "arrested" in their speech and literacy development at a stage prior to the development of phonological awareness. If this is the case, then they should be unable to perform tasks tapping phonological awareness skills, such as rhyme.

Rhyme

First, a rhyme detection task was devised in which Michael and Caroline were to select the word that rhymed with a target (e.g., *cat*) from two alternatives (e.g., *cat*: *fish* or *hat*, *goat*: *boat* or *gate*). The nonrhyming target was either semantically related to the target (*fish*) or an alliteration of it (*gate*). To compare performance in the auditory and visual modalities, the stimuli were either spoken words or presented as pictures. Normally developing 7-year old children matched on reading age were at ceiling on these tasks (Stackhouse, 1989). Caroline at age 11:0 performed at ceiling in the visual modality and scored 85% correct in the auditory modality, indicating that she was making connections between rhyming words. In contrast, Michael at age 10:7 performed significantly less well: 70% correct in the visual modality and only 60% correct (i.e., at chance) in the auditory modality. He was also more likely to choose a semantically related distractor as his response.

Second, Michael and Caroline were tested on a rhyme production task. They were asked to produce rhyme strings to a series of simple words (e.g., *map*, *sun*, *key*). This task requires the child to segment the stimulus into onset and rhyme (e.g., m/ap), and then either to search the lexicon for words with the same rhyme and retrieve and produce such words, or search for different onsets while maintaining the rhyme and then reassemble new rhyming words. The first strategy results in only real words being produced, whereas the second explains why children often produce a mixture of real and nonwords when producing rhymes. On this task, both Michael and Caroline could only produce one correct rhyme response to each target.

Although their rhyme detection skills improved over time, their persisting difficulty with rhyme production was evident at follow-up when Michael's chronological age was 14:5 and Caroline's was 15:0 years. At this age, Michael was still more proficient at making semantic than phonological links in his lexicon. For example, for a rhyme with *wool*, he replied "sheep." It also became clear that the rhyming responses he made had been well taught and were not spontaneous. When asked what rhymes with *draw*, he responded rather anxiously "Miss V (his speech and language therapist) not tell me about draw!"

In contrast, Caroline's responses indicated that she had made phonological links in her lexicon and was attempting to produce rhyming words. Persisting expressive phonological difficulties, however, which were no longer so apparent in Michael's speech output, interfered with her rhyme production by taking her further away from the target (e.g., wool → ['wiʊ 'wiʊl 'luʊ 'wɪl 'dɪl 'bɪl]). A similar pattern of performance was evident on other phonological awareness tasks such as sound blending.

Sound Blending

When Michael was asked to blend the word *pr-a-ṁ*, he first attempted to blend the segments as follows: "prom, promp" but then gave up on this and responded "we call it a pushchair!"—again indicating strong semantic links. Caroline, however, had more intrusive articulations (e.g., [sæŋg] was blended as *sazng*), and sometimes her distorted response led to access of the wrong lexical item (e.g., [b ʌ sk] was blended as *bussst, basket*).

The results from the phonological awareness tasks suggested that Michael and Caroline were arrested in an early stage of speech and literacy development. Michael's lexicon was not organised along phonological lines. He had not progressed to a stage in which phonologically similar words (e.g., words with a shared rhyme) were closely connected (Waterson, 1987). The connections within Michael's lexicon were predominantly semantic, as evidenced in his rhyme and blending responses. In contrast, Caroline had made some progress with her phonological organisation skills, but her attempts to search her lexicon were undermined by her persisting expressive phonological difficulties. Further investigation of their lexical skills was carried out.

Lexical Decision

On the nonword repetition task reported earlier, Michael produced a real-word response more often than did either Caroline or the normally developing children. For example, he reproduced *slepper* as *slipper* and *dacks* as *ducks*. Out of a total of 30 nonwords, the normally developing children lexicalised on average only 1.6 of the targets (range 1–3). Caroline lexicalised on three items (i.e., at the top of the normal range), but Michael lexicalised significantly more—7.

Michael, in particular, also had difficulties with a nonword spelling test (see Campbell, 1983) in which a spoken list of words was presented within which were embedded a number of nonwords (e.g., *dish, night, coal*, [brəʊl], *lady, boil*, [wɔɪl]). The task was for the child to stop the examiner every time a nonword was heard and then to write it down. Michael accepted 81% of the nonwords as real words, and Caroline accepted 58% of them. Unlike Caroline, Michael was very confident that he had responded correctly and went on to define the nonwords (e.g., [jaɪt] → light, [tid] → tea).

To check whether this difficulty was specific to the auditory modality, Michael and Caroline were presented with a written and spoken lexical decision task (after Coltheart, 1980). They had to sort words into real word and nonword categories (e.g., real word, *black*; nonword, *brack*). In the visual modality, Michael and Caroline did not perform significantly differently from a group of 33 normally developing children matched on reading age. When the stimuli were presented auditorily, however, both children performed significantly less well than the controls. Michael, in particular, found this task difficult.

These results support the hypothesis that Michael may have more difficulty with input phonological processing than Caroline. Both children, however, were more willing than reading-age-matched controls to accept similar sounding nonwords as real words. This indicated that their lexical representations were less precise than those of the younger normally developing children. This lexical disorder was particularly apparent in Michael's case and put him at a disadvantage when learning new words that might be misrepresented or falsely categorized as known words.

One hypothesis regarding the cause of Michael and Caroline's less precise lexical representations was that they had deficits in auditory discrimination, resulting in a failure to identify fine phonetic distinctions. This affected their ability to construct accurate phonological representations for new lexical items. Auditory discrimination tasks were administered to test this hypothesis.

Auditory Discrimination

Initial testing on detecting similarities and differences between simple minimal-pair words (Wepman & Reynolds, 1987) did not support the hypothesis. Michael and Caroline were able to detect perfectly well when two words were the same or different (e.g., *pin* vs. *bin*, *pin* vs. *pin*). A more stringent test was therefore designed. This consisted of a series of complex nonwords which differed in

1. place of articulation e.g., [spəʊb] vs. [spəʊd]
2. voicing e.g., [beɪt] vs. [peɪt]
3. cluster sequence e.g., [wɛsp] vs. [wɛps]
4. phoneme sequence e.g., ['bɪkʌt] vs. ['bɪtʌk]

The test was administered to Michael and Caroline and to 42 normally developing children in the age range of 3:3 to 8:11. On this test, both Michael and Caroline performed less well than the controls. Although able to detect same nonword pairs 100% of the time, they were able to detect different nonword pairs at only a 69% accuracy level. In comparison, the controls scored 88% correct on the detection of different nonword pairs.

These results indicated that although Michael and Caroline did not have an auditory discrimination problem on a simple auditory discrimination test made up of CVC words, they did have difficulties discriminating words that differed in the *sequence* of sounds, particularly if these words were new to them. This auditory discrimination task may itself be dependent on articulatory and phonological awareness skills because when children are asked to make a same/different judgement on a pair of complex and unfamiliar words, a common strategy is to repeat the words while reflecting on their structure. Michael and Caroline's variable speech production and poor segmentation skills prevented successful use of this strategy. An alternative support strategy of visualising the written form of the word was also problematic for them; neither Michael nor Caroline could read or spell simple nonwords and therefore were not able to use such a strategy on this task.

A study by Bridgeman and Snowling (1988) supports this finding. A group of children in the age range of 7:2 to 11:0 years with expressive phonological impairments (described as having developmental verbal dyspraxia) performed less well than reading-age-matched normally developing children on a test of nonword auditory discrimination in which the pairs of words presented differed in cluster sequence (e.g., *vots/vost)*. There was no difference, however, between the two groups of children when discriminating real word pairs with and without clusters (e.g., *lots/lost, loss/lot)*, and simple nonwords without clusters (e.g., *vos/vot*). These two studies together suggest that children with persisting phonological impairments have sound segmentation difficulties when processing sound sequences within novel words and thus are more likely to form inaccurate phonological representations.

This longitudinal study of Michael and Caroline, two children with severe expressive phonological impairment, revealed the pervasiveness of their underlying phonological processing difficulties. The difficulties with input, representation, and output processing resulted in poor performance on phonological awareness tasks and was directly related to their literacy problems. One of the most important findings from this study was the discovery of a similar pattern of development in both their speech and literacy skills; phonological skills were not developed sufficiently enough to tackle the next phase of development in either speech or literacy. Frith's (1985) model of literacy development explains this arrested development as a failure to pass from the logographic to alphabetic phase. Stackhouse and Wells (in press) have posited a similar stage model of speech development in order to explain how speech difficulties develop and can lead to problems with phonological awareness.

A STAGE MODEL OF SPEECH DEVELOPMENT

Stackhouse and Wells (1996) have stressed the importance of keeping a developmental perspective when investigating children's speech and literacy difficulties. One way of doing this is to think of children's speech difficulties as arising at different stages in development—at points at which a child encounters specific difficulties. This mirrors the approach taken by Frith (1985) to literacy development, discussed above. Children with normally developing speech move smoothly through the stages of speech development as a result of developing phonological and articulatory skills, whereas the child with phonological impairments will have arrested or troublesome development through these stages of development. Stackhouse and Wells (in press) have suggested the following stages of speech development (the ages assigned to each stage will overlap and are for guidelines only):

1. Prelexical (1st year)
2. Gestalt parametric (2nd year)
3. Systematic simplification (3rd year)
4. Assembly (4th year)
5. Metaphonological (5th year)

Prelexical Stage

The neonate is able to respond to sound and even detect phonetic differences between syllables (e.g., [bɑ] vs. [dɑ]; Eimas, Siqueland, Juszcyk, & Vigorito, 1971). Motor execution skills exist for feeding and crying, but the kinds of sounds produced do not resemble speech. In the 6- to 9-month period, the infant begins to form phonological and semantic representations of familiar words as perceptual gestalts (e.g., *teddy*, *mummy*). There is no evidence of any kind of segmentation analysis at this stage. On the output side, babble strings are programmed and produced by the articulators. Around the age of 9 months, babble sequences become more like the language of the environment (see Vihman, 1996).

Even at this early stage of speech development, a number of warning signs indicate the presence of a future speech disorder (Oller, Eilers, Steffens, Lynch, & Urbano, 1994). Children with learning difficulties may be slow to move through this stage. In contrast, children with hearing loss may begin to babble but then stop (Eilers & Oller, 1994). Children with verbal dyspraxia are reported not to babble or readily engage in sound play at this stage (Milloy & Morgan-Barry, 1990).

Gestalt Parametric Stage

Usually around 12 months of age, the first spoken words begin to emerge. The first 50 words or so appear to be learned and stored as wholes or *gestalts* (Ingram, 1989). It is hypothesized that each phonological representation is unsegmented and consists of the most acoustically salient features, which allow it to be differentiated from other words (Juszcyk, 1992; Waterson, 1987). Similarly, the motor program or scheme for each word consists of a gestalt of gestures. This stage is analogous to Frith's logographic stage of literacy development because the whole word is the key structural unit.

As vocabulary size increases throughout the second year, there is a corresponding increase in the variability of how words are produced (Ferguson & Farwell, 1975). This variability occurs as the child attempts to reproduce the phonetic features of the word. Phonetic *parameters* rather than linear order of segments dominate their productions. For example, Laura at the age of 18 months produced *Muffin* (a cat's name) as [ˈβ^{n} ˌβ^{n}].

The speech of normally developing 1-year-olds therefore has many of the signs associated with developmental verbal dyspraxia, such as inconsistent and variable output, programming problems, and phonetic distortion (Stackhouse, 1992b). Michael and Caroline, described above, were arrested in the logographic stage of literacy development and in the gestalt parametric stage of speech development. Michael and Caroline's failure to move on to the next stage in both speech and literacy development was attributed to a pervasive phonological processing deficit affecting both input and output processing as well as lexical storage. Phonological awareness tasks, which, by definition, require segmentation skills, were extremely problematic for them because only in the next stage of speech development do children have sufficient skills to identify and produce smaller units—a prerequisite for breaking through to the alphabetic stage of literacy development.

Systematic Simplification Stage

This is the stage of speech development characterized by simplifying processes such as fronting, stopping, cluster reduction, and phonological mapping rules (Grunwell, 1982; Ingram, 1989). Children become more systematic and consistent in their speech output at this stage. As yet, *explicit* phonological awareness has not developed (see Exhibit 7–1), but many children will begin to remember and sing nursery rhymes and enjoy sound games around 3 years of age.

Children delayed in their speech development may reach this stage after 3 years of age and are often referred for help because the persisting use of simplifying processes renders their speech unintelligible beyond the accepted age. If they have moved through the previous stages smoothly, their problems may resolve following appropriate intervention or through maturation. Other children may reach this stage but continue to use simplifying processes for longer than expected. Children who are still in this stage at the point they begin school (at around 5 years of age) are likely to have phonological awareness problems and associated literacy difficulties (Bird et al., 1995; Bishop & Adams, 1990).

Assembly Stage

Having successfully passed through the previous stages focussing on single-word intelligibility, the child is faced with what happens to words when they are joined together. For example, compare the different pronunciations of the final [t] in *great* in the following: *great elephant*, *great tiger*, *great cat*. Morphological issues need to be tackled: for example, learning that "a pear" is appropriate but "a apple" is not. Junction between words is a complex business. Children who have had the diagnosis of verbal dyspraxia or phonological disorder may have particular difficulties at this stage and have persisting speech problems around the junction between words in connected speech (Wells, 1994).

There are also still some tricky pronunciations to sort out, such as the acoustically close f/th, r/w distinction and the articulation of words with complex clusters (e.g., *scrape*, *splatter)* and increasing syllable length (e.g., *hippopotamus*). Children with specific reading impairment (dyslexia) often have persisting difficulties with this stage of speech development (Stackhouse, 1996; Stackhouse & Wells, 1991).

This stage of understanding how words are joined together in connected speech has received less attention in clinical practice than the previous two stages, which are related to more traditional articulatory and phonological intervention programmes. Assessment in particular has been limited because of the lack of research into the normal development of how children deal with junctions between words in connected speech (Wells, 1994).

Metaphonological Stage

Children enter the metaphonological stage when they can apply their phonological processing skills, developed in the earlier stages for storing and producing speech, to phonological awareness tasks such as rhyme and syllable or sound segmentation. Metaphonological development is facilitated by environmental experience of sound awareness games, nursery rhymes, letters, alphabet books, and friezes. Normally developing children have reached this stage by around 5 years of age, at a point when they can take advantage of reading instruction offered at school. In turn, literacy instruction accelerates metaphonological awareness, which becomes more explicit as the child's orthographic experience increases (see Exhibit 7–1). The corollary of this is that children who do not reach this stage at the appropriate time are disadvantaged when exposed to literacy instruction and may experience failure early on in their literacy development. If this disadvantage is not recognized and appropriate intervention is not taken, the disadvantage can persist throughout the school years (Hatcher et al., 1994).

Inevitably, these stages overlap and are not as clear-cut as presented here. Examining children's speech difficulties within a stage model is an alternative but not necessarily incompatible approach to the one of subgrouping speech disorders on the basis of group studies (Dodd, 1995; and see Shriberg, Chapter 5 of this volume). An advantage of the developmental perspective on children's speech disorders is that it allows the unfolding nature of speech problems to be charted. Further, for the purposes of the present chapter, the stage model makes explicit how phonological awareness is related to normal speech development. The following case study illustrates the consequences of atypical speech development for the development of phonological awareness.

ZOE: A LONGITUDINAL CASE STUDY OF PHONOLOGICAL AWARENESS DEVELOPMENT

Zoe was referred for speech-language therapy when she was 2:2. It was reported that she had babbled normally and that her first word had appeared at 11 months. Her mother became concerned, however, about Zoe's speech development at 16 months. There were no medical problems at Zoe's birth, and her health was good. Zoe's general motor coordination was age appropriate, and she had no chewing or feeding problems. There was no family history of speech-language problems, but her younger brother was subsequently referred for speech-language therapy.

Zoe's verbal comprehension was age appropriate when tested on the Reynell Developmental Language Scales (Reynell & Huntley, 1985) at chronological age 2:10 (standard score: 0.4; age equivalent: 2:11). Expressive language was well behind her receptive skills, however. At this time, all her spontaneous utterances were reduplicated single words (e.g., *dog* → "wowo," *car* → "gaga"). There were atypical oral movements before vocalization, and sound production was described as inconsistent. The speech-language therapist at that time concluded that Zoe showed signs of developmental verbal dyspraxia (based on the Nuffield Centre Dyspraxia Assessment; Connery, 1992), and regular speech-language therapy sessions were offered from the age of 2:10.

Zoe at 3:9

Zoe presented as a neat and quiet girl at age 3:9. Tests of hearing and vision had been passed at 3:7, and her visuomotor and visuoperceptual skills were age appropriate on colour-matching and copying tasks. Her limited expressive vocabulary was used solely for object labelling and was mostly unintelligible. Zoe had good eye contact but very rarely initiated communication. She seemed able to understand others and communicated her needs using simple gesture.

Speech

The Nuffield Centre Dyspraxia Assessment (Connery, 1992) revealed that although Zoe had normal oral structure and function, she had a specific problem with sound production. For example, on imitation tasks, she distorted fricatives, affricates, and some vowels and found it difficult to maintain a sound sequence (e.g., t-t-t-t), particularly when this involved articulatory place change (e.g., p-t-p-t-p-t; p-t-k-p-t-k-p-t-k). In addition, her voice was low in pitch and had a quiet volume. In general, intonation was flat, and there was a disjointed, irregular rhythm during the sequencing tasks.

Language

On the British Picture Vocabulary Scales (Dunn, Dunn, Whetton, & Pintillie, 1982), Zoe scored at the 42nd centile (age equivalent: 3:05, confidence band of 3:0 to 3:10). Thus, receptive vocabulary was not a particular cause for concern, and she was able to understand sentences containing three information-carrying words (e.g., "Put teddy on the chair").

Auditory Discrimination

Zoe was presented with simple minimal-pair words and asked if each pair of words spoken was the same or different (e.g., *cart/tart, dig/dog, bib/big, cart/cart*). She scored 33 out of 38 correct, which indicated some possible auditory processing difficulty. Three of her errors involved the voice/voiceless contrast (*lock/log*, *tear/deer*, *robe/rope*), which she heard as being the same.

In summary, at age 3:9, there was no apparent physical cause for Zoe's expressive phonological impairment. The range of single words she produced indicated that she had passed through the prelexical stage of speech development. Some of her word productions, however, were inconsistent and characteristic of the gestalt parametric stage of speech development. She often had the correct phonetic ingredients in a production but not necessarily in the correct order (e.g., she produced target onset fricatives in coda position: *saw* → [ɔ:s]). Other aspects of her speech production were consistent and indicated some breakthrough into the systematic simplification stage. It was therefore proposed that Zoe was at a transitional point between these two stages of speech development (Stackhouse & Wells, in press).

Zoe's age-appropriate linguistic comprehension and her receptive vocabulary suggested that input difficulties were not as pervasive as her output difficulties. Nevertheless, there was some indication that in spite of normal hearing, Zoe had specific problems with auditory discrimination of the voice/voiceless contrast. Although phonological awareness skills were not tested explicitly at this age, this atypical profile did not bode well for developing phonological awareness abilities in time for starting school.

Zoe at 5:11

From the age of 5 years, Zoe attended a local language unit attached to a mainstream school, at which she received regular speech-language therapy. An educational psychologist's report 11 months earlier suggested that Zoe was a child with academic potential within the average range.

Speech

Zoe's single-word production, though not age appropriate, was adequate in signalling many of the necessary phonological contrasts. She did, however, have persisting speech difficulties with the voice/voiceless contrast and with clusters. Speech errors were more noticeable in connected utterances (see Stackhouse & Wells, 1993, and Wells, 1994, for detailed descriptions of her speech data at this age).

Language

Zoe's receptive vocabulary score on the British Picture Vocabulary Scales (Dunn et al., 1982) and grammar score on the Test of Reception of Grammar (Bishop, 1983) were at the lower end of the normal range. This was in contrast to her expressive grammar on the Renfrew Action Picture Test (Renfrew, 1989) and the

Language Assessment Remediation and Screening Procedure (LARSP; Crystal, Fletcher, & Garman, 1989), which was delayed by as much as 2 or 3 years.

Auditory Discrimination

Zoe's auditory discrimination was followed up by administering the Auditory Discrimination and Attention Test (Morgan-Barry, 1988). This test includes simple minimal pairs targetting various consonantal oppositions (e.g., place, manner, voicing). The child chooses a picture from a pair of minimally contrasting pictures (e.g., *log/lock*, *key/tea*, *mat/bat*, *crown/clown*) on hearing one of the two words spoken by the examiner over a number of trials. Zoe's errors on this test occurred on the voicing contrast items: She failed consistently on all four pairs. The only other contrasts that were confused more than twice were /r/ ~ /w/ and /m/ ~ /b/.

Rhyme

Because of Zoe's persisting phonological impairment, it was predicted that she would have specific difficulty with her phonological awareness development. Zoe's rhyme ability was therefore investigated. First, her ability to detect rhyme was tested at age 5:11 by using a picture-pointing task, which did not require any verbal output from her. After some practice and explanation of the concept of rhyme, Zoe was presented with a series of three picture stimuli and asked, "Which of these two pictures rhymes with the target picture?" (from Stackhouse, 1989). Neither the stimulus nor the target word was pronounced by the examiner, so Zoe had to draw on her own phonological representations of the targets to make a decision about the rhyming and nonrhyming words. In each item, the nonrhyming word is either a semantic or an alliterative distractor:

Rhyme target:	*cat*	*goat*
Choice:	*fish* or *mat*	*boat* or *gate*

Zoe scored 6/10 correct on this test, which was not significantly better than chance. Three of her errors were alliterative (e.g., she selected *gate* as a rhyme with *goat*, *pig* to rhyme with *peg*, and *cow* with *key)*. Only one of her errors was semantic: Zoe chose *spoon* to rhyme with *knife*.

Second, to test her rhyme output skills, Zoe was asked to produce as many words as she could that rhymed with a target word spoken by the examiner (e.g., *log*, *key*). Zoe was unable to produce rhyming words for 6 targets presented orally. Three of her responses were semantically related and two of these were also alliterations:

Target	*Response*
key	key, lock
hat	hair
four	five

Zoe also produced isolated sounds as part of her response. For example, in *key* above, she went on to produce [g] [j] [w] after her lexical search had failed, and for *log* she produced [l] [w].

Reading

At the age of 5:11, Zoe was approaching the end of her first year of formal schooling. It was now relevant to investigate her emerging reading and spelling skills as a baseline for measuring performance in later years. The Schonell Graded Word Reading Test (Newton & Thomson, 1982), which involves the child reading a list of single words, was administered. Zoe recognized the word *little* but no others. She made a number of visual errors (e.g., *milk* → *mum*, *sit* → *sun*). Her performance on this test put her below the 6-year level. This in itself does not constitute a problem, given her age. It was noted, however, that she did not know all of the letter names and sounds and that this restricted her ability to read novel material. Zoe presented as a typical beginning reader, functioning mainly in the logographic stage of literacy development. The question was, however, whether she would be able to move on from this stage, given her phonological difficulties.

Spelling

On the Schonell Graded Word Spelling Test (Newton & Thomson, 1982), Zoe achieved a spelling age of 5:1. She was able to spell one word correctly: *in*. For the other words, she tended to transcribe the initial and final consonants, though not always correctly. The voice/voiceless problem detected on the tests of speech and auditory discrimination was also evident in her spellings:

Target	*Spelling*
pet	bt
cap	cb
bank	bt

Given the wide variation in performance in beginner reader/spellers, these results alone would not be cause for concern. Her persisting speech and auditory discrimination difficulties, however, plus her poor rhyme performance suggested that she might find transition to the alphabetic stage of literacy development problematic.

In summary, compared to her performance at 3:9, there was a less pronounced deficit at age 5:11 in the production of real words. New deficits were emerging, however, notably those tapping metaphonological skills and also connected speech (Wells, 1994). This suggested that she was not passing smoothly through the normal assembly and metaphonological stages of speech development at a level expected for her age. To test the hypothesis that Zoe's difficulties would interfere with the normal course of reading and spelling development, she was reassessed at the age of 9:8.

Zoe at 9:8

Speech

Zoe was now intelligible and able to hold a conversation. She had made considerable progress with her speech, but residual speech errors were still apparent, and her speech sounded immature and disjointed. There were minimal segmental errors in one- and two-syllable words. Some immaturities remained, however (e.g., /r/ as in *reading* → ['ʋidɪn]). The voicing contrast had improved, but occasionally her earlier difficulty manifested itself through inappropriate aspiration (e.g., *polish* → ['p=ɒlɪʃ]). More complex articulations were still problematic for her (e.g., clusters such as /kw/ in *queen* → ['kjwɔin], and multisyllabic words such as *refreshment* → [ʋɪ'fʰʋɛʃmʰənt], and *instructed* → [ˌɪnˌdɪs'dʌkˌtɪd]). Zoe used glottal stops at the end of words (e.g., *bus* → [bʌʔ]) and would sometimes insert a glottal stop before the final sound, which broke up the syllable structure (e.g., *fish* → ['fɪʔəʃ]). This also occurred at syllable boundaries (e.g., *hockey* → ['hɒʔˌki]). In contrast, on other occasions, she ran words together (e.g., *but sometimes* → [ˌbʌ's:ʌmˌtaɪms]). This resulted in problems with speech intelligibility.

In addition, specific lexical items were consistently produced wrongly (e.g., the character name *Kipper* in her book was consistently pronounced as ['kjupə]). This suggested that she still had features of the gestalt parametric stage in her speech productions. Although she had moved on from this, she had not completed the transition from the systematic simplification stage to the assembly stage necessary for continuous speech. On the premise that breakthrough and functioning at the metaphonological stage is dependent on skills accumulated at these earlier stages of speech development, it was predicted that Zoe would have persisting problems with phonological awareness tasks such as rhyme.

Rhyme

Zoe was presented with four rhyme tests (three input and one output), for which normal control data had been collected on 100 children (Vance, Stackhouse, & Wells, 1994). The same or matched linguistic stimuli were used throughout so that comparisons could be made across tasks. Input tasks were presented both visually (via pictures) and auditorily, and nonword rhyme detection was included.

Zoe had little difficulty with the input tests in terms of accuracy of response. She was able to choose which of two words rhymed with a target (e.g., *sock*: *clock* or *dress*) and performed equally well when the items were nonwords (e.g., *poat*: *dath* or *hoat*). She therefore understood the concept of rhyme and could deal with novel as well as familiar words. On the picture-pointing rhyme test, however, for which she had to choose one out of two pictures that rhymed with a target, she routinely used verbal rehearsal to perform this visual task. In this respect, she resembled much younger children.

Zoe had specific difficulties when asked to produce as many rhyming words as she could think of in 20 seconds for a given target (e.g., *coat*). Although able to produce at least one rhyme response to 12 out of the 15 targets, her responses were very limited. Overall, she produced a total of 26 rhyme responses to 15 targets, which was less than a quarter of the total responses she gave. Compared to normally developing controls, this put her at around the 6-year level (total rhyme response = 29.7).

One of her best responses was to the item *ring*. She started off well, but was not able to maintain the rhyme strategy for the full 20 seconds:

Ring:	ring	ping	ting	ling
	ring	ping	[fə'lɛ]	boo
	ring	ping	['tɪli]	boo

This example also shows how she needed to repeat the target at regular intervals. Although this is a strategy typical of young children, only 15% of 7-year-old controls were still using it.

On a number of occasions, Zoe tried a frame strategy (particularly "silly old ——") to help her rhyme. Although to some extent this strategy was successful, it limited the number of correct rhyming words produced:

purse:	purse	the	worse	the	silly	old	turse
	purse	the	['lɜs	ə	'lɜsi	'gæ]	
sock:	sock	pock	silly	old	tock		
	sock	tock	peck	too			
	sock	['lju	'guli	'gu]			

Although her rhyme production skill had improved since age 5:11, this was not typical of normally developing children. Only one 6-year-old out of 100 normally developing children studied adopted a similar strategy:

sock:	sock the wock the pit pat pock
two:	two the woo the pit pat poo

The results suggested that Zoe's difficulty with rhyme production originated on the output side rather than with input or representations. More specifically, her output deficit appeared to be at the stage or stages in output processing in which she had to select an onset from her store of potential syllable onsets and attach it to the rhyme that had already been segmented from the stimulus word. Although Zoe no longer had the obvious expressive phonological impairments evident in earlier years, the investigation of her rhyme skills demonstrated that hidden deficits in phonological output processing remained (Wells, Stackhouse, & Vance, 1996).

Motor Programming

To investigate if her difficulties were at the level of motor programming, Zoe's performance on repetition of complex but familiar words was compared with her repetition of matched nonwords (i.e., unfamiliar words for which she did not have an existing motor programme). Zoe scored 17 out of 24 correct when repeating real words (e.g., *helicopter, supermarket)*, but only 8 out of 24 correctly on the nonword condition (e.g., ['grælɪˌdɛd]; stimuli from Ryder, 1991). This suggested that although she was able to produce familiar words quite well, she still had difficulty assembling motor programmes for new words. Further evidence for this came from her inconsistent responses when asked to produce a new word three times in succession (e.g., ['bɒˌbɪ'klæˌdɪd] → ['bɒˌbɪ' glæˌ dɪd] ['bɒˌbɪ' glæˌdɪd] [bɑ'b'bɑdi'blæˌgɪd]).

Auditory Discrimination

Two tests were administered to establish whether the earlier auditory discrimination problem had finally resolved. The first consisted of pairs of complex nonwords (e.g., *besket/bekset, ibikus/ikibus)*. Zoe was asked to say if each pair was the same or different. She performed at ceiling on this test but did make one error on a voicing contrast item (*baskoits/paskoits*).

In the second test, Zoe had to identify if a word spoken by the examiner (e.g., *fis*) was the correct name for the picture presented (e.g., *fish*; after Locke, 1980). This auditory/picture task allows examination of the link between auditory discrimination skills and phonological representations (see Vance, 1996). Ten three- and four-syllable words were presented. Zoe only made three errors on this test. Two of the errors (out of a possible 13), however, were on the voicing contrast (*caravan*/['kærəˌfæn] and *helicopter*/['hɛlɪˌgɒptə]). The other error (one out of a possible four) was on the w/r distinction (*parachute*/['pæwəˌʃut]), which was also one of Zoe's residual speech errors. Thus, compared to her performance at age 5:11, the same error types were still occurring, though more disguised. Zoe still had imprecise phonological representations of some lexical items. Given these subtle auditory lexical difficulties and her persisting speech output problems, it was not surprising to find that teachers and parents were concerned about her literacy skills.

Reading

On the Wechsler Objective Reading Dimensions (WORD) Basic Reading subtest (Wechsler, 1993), Zoe attained an age-equivalent score of 7:6 and a standard score of 81, which is at the ninth percentile for children of her age. Her errors indicated that she was attempting to identify words in a gestalt (i.e., whole-word) way and that she therefore sometimes confused visually similar words (e.g., she read *ruin* as *rain*). Zoe had considerable difficulty when words were unfamiliar and performed poorly on a nonword reading test (Snowling, Stothard, & McLean, in press). Overall, her reading performance suggested that she was still dependent on logographic skills for reading.

Spelling

When asked to spell words of increasing syllable length, Zoe managed to spell 4 out of 10 one-syllable words correctly but had particular difficulties transcribing the vowel (e.g., *tent* → *tant*). Voicing errors were still apparent (e.g., *sink* → *sing*, *desk* → *disg)*. Her spellings of longer words showed serious sound segmentation problems (e.g., *kitten* → *clke*, *envelope* → *ehfet*), which were compounded by the persisting speech output problems (e.g., *puppy* → *bopue*, *pyjamas* → *beg*).

In summary, by 9:8, Zoe could discriminate between minimal pair words and nonwords but still had some underspecified phonological representations. Her output phonology, however, was a more serious problem. Although she no longer had any obvious difficulty with nonverbal oral skills or the production of familiar words, she did have problems with assembling utterances in connected speech and with pronouncing longer, more complex words. This resulted in intermittent unintelligibility. Zoe's persisting speech difficulties were most apparent when she was asked to produce new words or to perform output phonological awareness tasks (e.g., rhyme production). This suggested that Zoe had a specific difficulty with motor programming skills because these are necessary for the production of new words as well as for the manipulation and production of phonological units on rhyme production tasks (Wells et al., 1996).

Implications for Zoe's Intervention Programme

Intervention with Zoe had two main aims: (a) to improve her speech intelligibility and (b) to promote her phonological awareness skills so that she could take full advantage of literacy instruction at school. To achieve these aims, the intervention programme involved addressing not only the surface patterns of simplification processes and error but also the *source* of the individual types of speech error. One of the most important findings of this study was that different aspects of Zoe's speech difficulties could be attributed to different loci of deficit (Stackhouse & Wells, 1993). The voice/voiceless difficulty present in her speech and spelling arose from *input (auditory processing) difficulties*. Zoe could not discriminate the difference between voice/voiceless sounds and had weak phonological representations of onsets involving this contrast. Her problem with producing unfamiliar words was attributed to a difficulty with *motor programming*, which resulted in errors characteristic of the gestalt parametric stage of speech development. Problems with connected speech occurred at the *motor planning* level of speech production resulting in errors typical of the assembly stage of speech development. Zoe's difficulties with some clusters and individual segments were best explained by a lower level *articulatory problem*. The overall effect of these speech difficulties was that Zoe was unable to move smoothly through the metaphonological stage—hence the literacy problems.

On the basis of this psycholinguistic profile, Zoe's intervention programme at the age of 5:11 included:

1. auditory tasks targetted specifically at the voicing opposition
2. self-monitoring work targetted at phonological retrieval errors
3. articulatory activities targetted at the postalveolar fricatives and affricates
4. games involving segmentation of the syllable into phonological constituents, including rhyme, to strengthen metaphonological awareness and thereby to provide the basis for reading and spelling development
5. games involving segmentation of words into syllables, to help Zoe with the acquisition of new vocabulary, particularly polysyllabic words
6. motor-programming drill games

These auditory, articulatory, programming, and phonological awareness strands were present throughout her intervention programme. Over time, the intervention focus shifted from single words to connected speech. Junction between words was targetted, and traditional voice production exercises were used to improve Zoe's rhythm and airflow control in her phrasing of connected speech.

Zoe's case illustrates that it is not appropriate to treat a speech problem as a single entity. Rather, a number of possible sources of difficulty may need to be tackled simultaneously in a child's intervention programme. The task for the clinician is, therefore, not only to *describe* a child's speech difficulties from a linguistic perspective but also to discover why they are occurring. This involves *explaining* the child's underlying phonological processing difficulties with reference to a model based on the simple diagram in Figure 7–2 (Stackhouse & Wells, 1993, in press).

CONCLUSION

Over the last 30 years, there has been overwhelming evidence that children with reading impairments have phonological impairments, and vice versa (see Snowling, 1987; Snowling & Stackhouse, 1996a; Vellutino, 1979). Successful speech and literacy development are both dependent on an intact underlying phonological processing system. Thus, children with phonological processing difficulties may have arrested, slow, or troublesome passage through the stages of speech and literacy development. The same pattern of developmental difficulty occurs in both spoken and written language problems: applying phonological processing skills to the segmentation of spoken and written material (i.e., phonological awareness).

Tests of phonological awareness (e.g., rhyme, segmentation, and blending) tap the integrity of the phonological processing system. Figure 7–3 illustrates how phonological awareness connects speech and literacy development. All three stem from the phonological processing system of input, output, and representations (illustrated in its simplest form in Figure 7–2). Through needing to develop the phonological processing system for the purposes of spoken communication, children develop awareness of the sounds and structure of their language. Once in the metaphonological stage, children are ready to match spoken output with the written form (e.g., through letter knowledge). There is then a much more reciprocal relationship between spoken and written language, mediated by phonological awareness skills. Failure or delay in reaching this metaphonological stage puts a child's literacy development at risk. In turn, lack of literacy experience can have negative consequences for a child's language development (e.g., vocabulary), and a downward spiral of disadvantage follows.

Intervention linking phonological awareness with both spoken and written language skills, however, can help the child to break out of this spiral (Hatcher, 1996). Targetting both spoken and written language skills in intervention programmes can begin before formal reading and spelling instruction takes place. Programmes promoting phonological awareness in preschool children at risk for literacy problems may help to prevent the full impact of a phonological impairment on later literacy development (Bradley & Bryant, 1983; Layton & Deeney, 1996).

Promoting literacy skills through speech and language therapy does not require clinicians to learn new techniques. Traditional therapy activities can be adapted easily to work on both spoken and written production (Gillon & Dodd, 1995; Hodson, 1994; Stackhouse, 1992c). Full advantage can be taken of well-established intervention programmes to promote phonological awareness (e.g., Hodson &

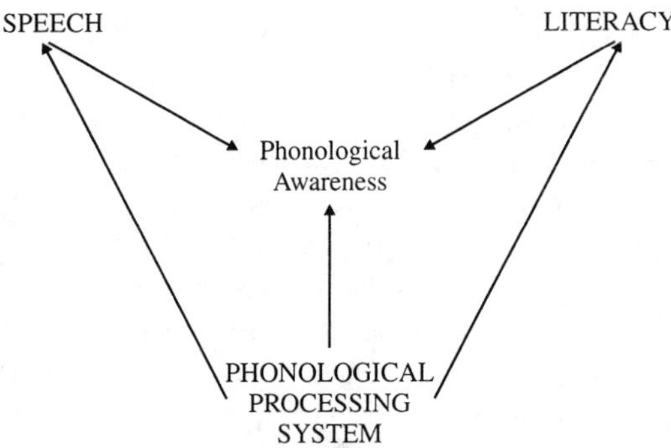

Figure 7–3 The Connection between Speech and Literacy Development. *Source*: Copyright © Joy Stackhouse.

Paden, 1991; Lindamood & Lindamood, 1975). Specific articulatory cueing through visual symbols (e.g., the Nuffield Centre Dyspraxia Programme; Connery, 1992) or gestures (e.g., Cued Articulation and Cued Vowels; Passy, 1993a, 1993b) are particularly helpful and can supplement more obvious phonological awareness training programmes (e.g., Catts & Vartiainen, 1993; Hatcher, 1994; Howell & Dean, 1994).

It is now expected that the work of speech-language therapists will promote and support literacy skills as an integral part of speech-language intervention programmes. This has led to a redefining of the role of speech-language therapists in the 1990s: "The role of the speech and language therapist does not include *teaching* reading and spelling which is traditionally and rightly the teacher's domain. Rather, the role is one of identification and promoting the underlying skills that contribute to literacy development" (Snowling & Stackhouse, 1996b, p. 240). Phonological awareness is not only the link here between spoken and written language for the children but also the meeting point for the professionals involved. Clarification of professional roles and the setting of common goals in phonological awareness programmes have resulted in closer collaboration between teachers and therapists (Popple & Wellington, 1996).

FUTURE DIRECTIONS

Although it has become accepted that tests of phonological awareness should be included routinely in the assessment of children with phonological impairments, further work needs to be done on designing appropriate phonological awareness assessment materials. In particular, more data need to be collected from normally developing children across a wide age range. Without these data for comparison purposes, it is not possible to identify who is delayed in phonological awareness development and when to intervene.

Comparing the phonological awareness and literacy development of children with phonological impairments over time will help us to understand the unfolding nature of phonological impairments and, in particular, how an expressive phonological impairment may interfere with phonological awareness and literacy development. One such longitudinal study is being carried out in the Department of Human Communication Science at University College London (Stackhouse, Goulandris, Nathan, & Snowling, in preparation). The study has been designed to profile the phonological processing skills of 50 children with expressive phonological impairments from the age of around 4:6 over a 4-year period. At the end of this period, their literacy skills will be measured. Each child is matched to a normally developing child on the basis of gender, IQ, and educational experience, making a total of 100 children in all. A main aim of this study is to identify, on the basis of the children's phonological processing profiles over the 4 years, which children go on to have literacy problems and why. As a result of group case studies like this, we should be able to identify children at risk for literacy problems earlier and to intervene in a more cost-effective manner.

An important aspect of these longitudinal studies is to follow the changing nature of expressive phonological impairments in children with reading impairments. Often speech problems are thought to have resolved if segmental difficulties are no longer obvious. Children with persisting reading impairments, however, may have persisting difficulties with specific lexical items, connected utterances, and junctions between words (Stackhouse, 1996). How these might be addressed in assessment procedures and intervention programmes needs further exploration (Wells, 1994).

The recent upsurge in availability of phonological awareness training materials reveals that clinicians and teachers recognise the importance of including phonological awareness activities in their intervention programmes. What is needed now is a better understanding of what works well, with whom, and why. Clearly, evaluation of the efficacy of different intervention programmes is high on the agenda. Research into phonological awareness training and literacy development in children with phonological impairments should benefit from the coming together of hitherto parallel research programmes. One such development would be to apply the rigorous research methodology from cognitive neuropsychology developed to evaluate treatment of *adults* with *acquired* speech and language disorders (Edmundson & McIntosh, 1995) to children with phonological impairments. This has already begun with children with phonological awareness and reading impairments (e.g., Broom & Doctor, 1995).

The increased availability of instrumentation should allow more objective measurement of progress made as a result of treatment. In particular, the use of electropalatography (Dent, Gibbon, & Hardcastle, 1995) coupled with acoustic measures (Tyler, 1995) will deepen our understanding of the nature of speech disorders in children, as well as providing techniques for remediating "intractable" speech problems. Interpreting the results from instrumentation studies within a psycholinguistic framework is helping to clarify the role of phonological output skills in phonological awareness and word-finding difficulties (Dent & Clarke, 1996).

Children with phonological impairments will continue to challenge our thinking about the role of phonological awareness in literacy development. Further research is needed on how and when to deliver an appropriate intervention programme to children with spoken and written language difficulties. More than ever, there will be a need for multidisciplinary approaches to research and practice to combine the skills from the range of methodologies now available.

The research programme on which this chapter is based has developed through collaboration with a number of colleagues. In particular, I thank Professor Maggie Snowling and Dr. Bill Wells for being a constant source of inspiration and support, and Professor Pamela Grunwell for her excellent teaching and encouragement.

REFERENCES

Adams, M.J. (1990). *Beginning to read: Learning and thinking about print.* Cambridge, MA: MIT Press.

Anthony, A., Bogle, D., Ingram, D., & McIsaac, M.W. (1971). *The Edinburgh Articulation Test.* New York: Churchill Livingstone.

Bird, J., & Bishop, D.V.M. (1992). Perception and awareness of phonemes in phonologically impaired children. *European Journal of Disorders of Communication, 27*, 289–311.

Bird, J., Bishop, D.V.M., & Freeman, N.H. (1995). Phonological awareness and literacy development in children with expressive phonological impairments. *Journal of Speech and Hearing Research, 38*, 446–462.

Bishop, D.V.M. (1983). *Test for Reception of Grammar* (2nd ed.). Manchester, UK: University of Manchester, Department of Psychology.

Bishop, D.V.M. (1985). Spelling ability in congenital dysarthria: Evidence against articulatory coding in translating between phonemes and graphemes. *Cognitive Neuropsychology, 2*, 229–251.

Bishop, D.V.M., & Adams, C. (1990). A prospective study of the relationship between specific language impairment, phonological disorders and reading retardation. *Journal of Child Psychology and Psychiatry, 31*, 1027–1050.

Bishop, D.V.M., & Robson, J. (1989). Unimpaired short-term memory and rhyme judgement in congenitally speechless individuals: Implications for the notion of articulatory coding. *Quarterly Journal of Experimental Psychology, 41A*, 123–140.

Bradley, L., & Bryant, P. (1983). Categorising sounds and learning to read: A causal connection. *Nature, 301*, 419.

Bridgeman, E., & Snowling, M. (1988). The perception of phoneme sequence: A comparison of dyspraxic and normal children. *British Journal of Disorders of Communication, 23*, 245–252.

Broom, Y.M., & Doctor, E.A. (1995). Developmental phonological dyslexia: A case study of the efficacy of a remediation programme. *Cognitive Neuropsychology, 12,* 725–766.

Bryant, P.E., Bradley, L., Maclean, M., & Crossland, J. (1989). Nursery rhymes, phonological skills and reading. *Journal of Child Language, 16*, 407–428.

Campbell, R. (1983). Writing nonwords to dictation. *Brain and Language, 19,* 153–179.

Catts, H.W., Hu, C-F., Larrivee, L., & Swank, L. (1994). Early identification of reading disabilities. In R.V. Watkins & M. Rice (Eds.), *Specific language impairments in children* (pp. 145–160). London: Paul H. Brookes.

Catts, H., & Vartiainen. (1993). *Sounds abound.* East Moline, IL: LinguiSystems.

Chukovsky, K. (1963). *From two to five.* Berkeley: University of California Press.

Clarke-Klein, S., & Hodson, B. (1995). A phonologically based analysis of misspellings by third graders with disordered-phonology histories. *Journal of Speech and Hearing Research, 38*, 839–849.

Coltheart, M. (1980). Analysing acquired disorders of reading. *Unpublished clinical tests.* London: Birkbeck College.

Connery, V. (1992). *Nuffield Centre Dyspraxia Programme.* (Available from the Nuffield Hearing and Speech Centre, Royal National Throat, Nose and Ear Hospital, Gray's Inn Road, London, WC1 8DA)

Constable, A., Stackhouse, J., & Wells, B. (1994). The case of the missing handcuffs: Phonological processing and word finding in a boy with language impairment. *Work in Progress, 4*, 1–27.

Crystal, D., Fletcher, P., & Garman, M. (1989). *Language Assessment Remediation and Screening Procedure (LARSP).* London: Whurr.

Dent, H., & Clarke, R. (1996). A two-pronged approach to assessment: Combining psycholinguistic and instrumental procedures in the investigation of a developmental speech and language disorder. *Work in Progress, 6*, 44–54.

Dent, H., Gibbon, F., & Hardcastle, B. (1995). The application of electropalatography (EPG) to the remediation of speech disorders in school-aged children and young adults. *European Journal of Disorders of Communication, 30,* 264–277.

Dodd, B. (1995). *Differential diagnosis and treatment of children with speech disorder.* London: Whurr.

Dunn, L.M., Dunn, L., Whetton, C., & Pintillie, D. (1982). *British Picture Vocabulary Scales.* Windsor, UK: NFER-Nelson.

Edmundson, A., & McIntosh, J. (1995). Cognitive neuropsychology and aphasia therapy: Putting theory into practice. In C. Code and D.J. Muller (Eds.), *Treatment of aphasia* (pp. 137–163). London: Whurr.

Ehri, L., & Wilce. (1980). The influence of orthography on readers' conceptualisation of the phonemic structure of words. *Applied Psycholinguistics, 1*, 371–386.

Eilers, R.E., & Oller, D.K. (1994). Infant vocalizations and the early diagnosis of severe hearing impairment. *Journal of Pediatrics, 124,* 199–203.

Eimas, P., Siqueland, E., Juszcyk, P., & Vigorito, J. (1971). Speech perception in infants. *Science, 171*, 303–306.

Elliot, C.D., Murray, D.J., & Pearson, L.S. (1983). *British Ability Scales.* Windsor, UK: NFER-Nelson.

Ferguson, C.A., & Farwell, C.B. (1975). Words and sounds in early language acquisition. *Language, 51*, 419–439.

Frith, U. (1985). Beneath the surface of developmental dyslexia. In K.E. Patterson, J.C. Marshall, & M. Coltheart (Eds.), *Surface dyslexia* (pp. 301–330). London: Routledge & Kegan-Paul.

Gillon, G., & Dodd, B.J. (1995). The effects of training phonological, semantic and syntactic processing skills in spoken language on reading ability. *Language, Speech, and Hearing Services in Schools, 26,* 58–68.

Goswami, U. (1990). A special link between rhyming skills and the use of orthographic analogies by beginning readers. *Journal of Child Psychology and Psychiatry, 31*, 301–311.

Goswami, U., & Bryant, P.E. (1990). *Phonological skills and learning to read.* Hillsdale, NJ: Lawrence Erlbaum.

Grunwell, P. (1982). *Clinical phonology.* London: Croom Helm.

Hatcher, P.J. (1994). *Sound linkage: An integrated programme for overcoming reading difficulties.* London: Whurr.

Hatcher, P.J. (1996). Practising sound links in reading intervention with the school-age child. In M. Snowling & J. Stackhouse (Eds.), *Dyslexia, speech and language: A practitioner's handbook* (pp. 146–170). London: Whurr.

Hatcher, P.J., Hulme, C., & Ellis, A.W. (1994). Ameliorating early reading failure by integrating the teaching of reading and phonological skills: The phonological linkage hypothesis. *Child Development, 65*, 41–57.

Hodson, B. (1994). Helping individuals become intelligible, literate, and articulate: The role of phonology. *Topics in Language Disorders, 14*(2), 1–16.

Hodson, B., & Paden, E. (1991). *Targeting intelligible speech: A phonological approach to remediation* (2nd ed.). Austin, TX: Pro-Ed.

Howell, J., & Dean, E. (1994). *Treating phonological disorders in children: Metaphon—theory to practice* (2nd ed.). London: Whurr.

Hulme, C., & Snowling, M. (1992). Deficits in output phonology: An explanation of reading failure? *Cognitive Neuropsychology, 9*, 47–72.

Ingram, D. (1989). *First language acquisition: Method, description and explanation.* Cambridge, UK: Cambridge University Press.

Juszcyk, P.W. (1992). Developing phonological categories from the speech signal. In C.A. Ferguson, L. Menn, & C. Stoel-Gammon (Eds.), *Phonological development: Models, research, implications* (pp. 17–64). Timonium, MD: York.

Layton, L., & Deeney, K. (1996). Promoting phonological awareness in preschool children. In M. Snowling & J. Stackhouse (Eds.), *Dyslexia, speech and language: A practitioner's handbook* (pp. 129–145). London: Whurr.

Lewkowicz, N.K. (1980). Phonemic awareness training: What to teach and how to teach it. *Journal of Educational Psychology, 72*, 686–700.

Liberman, I.Y., Shankweiler, D., Fischer, F.W., & Carter, B. (1974). Reading and the awareness of linguistic segments. *Journal of Experimental Child Psychology, 18*, 201–212.

Lindamood, C., & Lindamood, P. (1975). *Auditory discrimination in depth.* New York: Macmillan.

Locke, J. (1980). The inference of speech perception in the phonologically disordered child, Part II: Some clinically novel procedures, their use, some findings. *Journal of Speech and Hearing Disorders, 45*, 445–468.

Maclean, M., Bryant, P.E., & Bradley, L. (1987). Rhymes, nursery rhymes and reading in early childhood. *Merrill-Palmer Quarterly, 33*, 255–281.

Mann, V.A. (1986). Phonological awareness: The role of reading experience. *Cognition, 24*, 65–92.

Marion, M.J., Sussman, H.M., & Marquardt, T.P. (1993). The perception and production of rhyme in normal and developmentally apraxic children. *Journal of Communication Disorders, 26*, 129–160.

Milloy, N., & Morgan-Barry, R. (1990). Developmental neurological disorders. In P. Grunwell (Ed.), *Developmental speech disorders* (pp. 109–132). New York: Churchill Livingstone.

Morgan-Barry, R. (1988). *The Auditory Discrimination and Attention Test.* Windsor, UK: NFER-Nelson.

Muter, V. (1996). Predicting children's reading and spelling difficulties. In M. Snowling & J. Stackhouse (Eds.), *Dyslexia, speech and language: A practitioner's handbook* (pp. 31–44). London: Whurr.

Newton, M., & Thomson, M. (1982). *Aston Index*. Wisbech, UK: Learning Development Aids.

Oller, D.K., Eilers, R.E., Steffens, M.L., Lynch, M.P., & Urbano, R. (1994). Speech-like vocalizations in infancy: An evaluation of potential risk factors. *Journal of Child Language, 21*, 33–58.

Passy, J. (1993a). *Cued articulation*. Northumberland, UK: STASS.

Passy, J. (1993b). *Cued vowels.* Northumberland, UK: STASS.

Perin, D. (1983). Phonemic segmentation and spelling. *British Journal of Psychology, 74*, 129–144.

Popple, J., & Wellington, W. (1996). Collaborative working within a psycholinguistic framework. *Child Language Teaching and Therapy, 12*, 60–70.

Pring, L., & Snowling, M. (1986). Developmental changes in word recognition: An information processing account. *Journal of Experimental Psychology, 38A*, 395–418.

Read, C., Yun-Fei, Z., Hong-Yin, N., & Bao-Qing, D. (1986). The ability to manipulate speech sounds depends on knowing alphabetic writing. *Cognition, 24*, 31–44.

Renfrew, C. (1989). *Renfrew Action Picture Test.* London: Winslow.

Reynell, J., & Huntley, M. (1985). *Reynell Developmental Language Scales* (Rev. ed.). Windsor, UK: NFER-Nelson.

Robinson, P., Beresford, R., & Dodd, B. (1982). Spelling errors made by phonologically disordered children. *Spelling Progress Bulletin, 22,* 19–20.

Ryder, R. (1991). *Word and non-word repetition in normally developing children.* Unpublished MSc dissertation, University of London.

Snowling, M.J. (1987). *Dyslexia: A cognitive developmental perspective.* Oxford, UK: Basil Blackwell.

Snowling, M. (1996). Developmental dyslexia: An introduction and theoretical overview. In M. Snowling & J. Stackhouse (Eds.), *Dyslexia, speech and language: A practitioner's handbook* (pp. 1–11). London: Whurr.

Snowling, M., Goulandris, N., & Stackhouse, J. (1994). Phonological constraints on learning to read: Evidence from single case studies of reading difficulty. In C. Hulme & M. Snowling (Eds.), *Reading development and dyslexia* (pp. 86–104). London: Whurr.

Snowling, M., & Hulme, C. (1994). The development of phonological skills. *Transactions of the Royal Society B, 346,* 21–28.

Snowling, M., Hulme, C., Wells, B., & Goulandris, N. (1992). Continuities between speech and spelling in a case of developmental dyslexia. *Reading and Writing, 4,* 19–31.

Snowling, M., & Stackhouse, J. (1983). Spelling performance of children with developmental verbal dyspraxia. *Developmental Medicine and Child Neurology, 25,* 430–437.

Snowling, M., & Stackhouse, J. (Eds.). (1996a). *Dyslexia, speech and language: A practitioner's handbook.* London: Whurr.

Snowling, M., & Stackhouse, J. (1996b). Epilogue: Current themes and future directions. In M. Snowling & J. Stackhouse (Eds.), *Dyslexia, speech and language: A practitioner's handbook* (pp. 234–242). London: Whurr.

Snowling, M.J., Stackhouse, J., & Rack, J.P. (1986). Phonological dyslexia and dysgraphia: A developmental analysis. *Cognitive Neuropsychology, 3,* 309–339.

Snowling, M., Stothard, S.E., & McLean, J. (in press). *The Graded Nonword Reading Test.* Bury St. Edmunds: Thames Valley Test Publishers.

Stackhouse, J. (1982). An investigation of reading and spelling performance in speech disordered children. *British Journal of Disorders of Communication, 17,* 53–60.

Stackhouse, J. (1989). *Phonological dyslexia in children with developmental verbal dyspraxia.* PhD thesis, University College London.

Stackhouse, J. (1992a). Developmental verbal dyspraxia: A longitudinal case study. In R. Campbell, (Ed.), *Mental lives: Case studies in cognition* (pp. 84–98). Oxford, UK: Basil Blackwell.

Stackhouse, J. (1992b). Developmental verbal dyspraxia I: A review and critique. *European Journal of Disorders of Communication, 27,* 19–34.

Stackhouse, J. (1992c). Promoting reading and spelling skills through speech therapy. In P. Fletcher & D. Hall (Eds.), *Specific speech and language disorders in children* (pp. 194–203). London: Whurr.

Stackhouse, J. (1993). Phonological disorder and lexical development: Two case studies. *Child Language Teaching and Therapy, 9,* 230–241.

Stackhouse, J. (1996). Speech, spelling and reading: Who is at risk and why? In M. Snowling & J. Stackhouse (Eds.), *Dyslexia, speech and language: A practitioner's handbook* (pp. 12–30). London: Whurr.

Stackhouse, J., Goulandris, N., Nathan, L., & Snowling, M. (in preparation). *The relationship between speech disorders and literacy problems: Identification of the at risk child.* Department of Human Communication Science, University College London.

Stackhouse, J., & Snowling, M. (1992a). Barriers to literacy development in two children with developmental dyspraxia. *Cognitive Neuropsychology, 9*, 273–299.

Stackhouse, J., & Snowling, M. (1992b). Developmental verbal dyspraxia II: A developmental perspective on two case studies. *European Journal of Disorders of Communication, 27*, 35–54.

Stackhouse, J., & Wells, B. (1991). The obvious and hidden speech difficulty. In M. Snowling & M. Thomson (Eds.), *Dyslexia: Integrating theory and practice* (pp. 185–194). London: Whurr.

Stackhouse, J., & Wells, B. (1993). Psycholinguistic assessment of developmental speech disorders. *European Journal of Disorders of Communication, 28*, 331–348.

Stackhouse, J., & Wells, B. (1996). Developing models. *Bulletin of the Royal College of Speech and Language Therapists, 527*, 9–10.

Stackhouse, J., & Wells, B. (in press). *Psycholinguistic investigation of children with speech and literacy difficulties.* London: Whurr.

Stanovich, K.E. (1994). Does dyslexia exist? *Journal of Child Psychology and Psychiatry, 35*, 579–596.

Tyler, A.A. (1995). Durational analysis of stridency errors in children with phonological impairment. *Clinical Linguistics and Phonetics, 9*, 211–228.

Vance, M. (1996). Assessing speech processing skills in children: A task analysis. In M. Snowling & J. Stackhouse (Eds.), *Dyslexia, speech and language: A practitioner's handbook* (pp. 45–61). London: Whurr.

Vance, M., Stackhouse, J., & Wells, B. (1994). "Sock the wock the pit pat pock": Children's responses to measures of rhyming ability, 3–7 years. *Work in Progress, 4*, 171–185.

Vellutino, F. (1979). *Dyslexia: Theory and research.* Cambridge, MA: MIT Press.

Vellutino, F.R., Harding, C.J., Phillips, F., & Steger, J.A. (1975). Differential transfer in poor and normal readers. *Journal of Genetic Psychology, 126*, 3–18.

Vihman, M.M. (1996). *Phonological development: The origins of language in the child.* Oxford, UK: Basil Blackwell.

Waterson, N. (1987). *Prosodic phonology: The theory and its application to language acquisition and speech processing.* Newcastle upon Tyne, UK: Grevatt & Grevatt.

Webster, P.E., & Plante, A.S. (1992). Effects of phonological impairment on word, syllable, and phoneme segmentation and reading. *Language, Speech, and Hearing Services in Schools, 23*, 176–182.

Wechsler, D. (1993). *Wechsler Objective Reading Dimensions (WORD).* New York: Psychological Corporation.

Wells, B. (1994). Junction in developmental speech disorder: A case study. *Clinical Linguistics and Phonetics, 8*, 1–25.

Wells, B., Stackhouse, J., & Vance, M. (1996). A specific deficit in onset-rhyme assembly in a 9-year-old child with speech and literacy difficulties. In T. W. Powell (Ed.), *Pathology of speech and language: Contributions of clinical phonetics and linguistics.* New Orleans: International Clinical Phonetics and Linguistics Association.

Wepman, J.M., & Reynolds, W.M. (1987). *Wepman's Auditory Discrimination Test* (2nd ed.). Los Angeles: Western Psychological Services.

Zhurova, L.E. (1963). The development of analysis of words into their sounds by preschool children. *Soviet Psychology and Psychiatry, 2*, 17–27.

CHAPTER 8

Disordered Phonologies: What Have We Learned about Assessment and Treatment?

Barbara Williams Hodson

CLINICAL PHONOLOGY: THE EARLY YEARS

When I began my doctoral studies in 1972, not much seemed to be happening in the area of clinical phonology. Some attention was being given to theoretical phonology publications of the late 1960s (Chomsky & Halle, 1968; Stampe, 1969), as well as to Jakobson's (1941/1968) seminal writings. Applications for language (especially syntax) were "exploding" in our profession, but assessment and treatment procedures for children with speech-sound difficulties remained virtually the same as during preceding decades.

For the most part, clinicians were using standardized "articulation" tests (e.g., Goldman & Fristoe, 1969), which involve filling in blanks and do not require phonetic transcriptions of whole words. Scoring for these instruments is "all or none." Types of errors are not differentiated (i.e., distortions and substitutions are weighted the same as omissions in the final tally). In treatment, individual phonemes were taught one at a time (Van Riper, 1939) to perfection in initial, then final, positions of words (and sometimes in medial position and in clusters), then in phrases and sentences (for each word position), and finally in conversation.

As behaviorism principles and practices became popular, perfecting phonemes one by one to a criterion (e.g., 95%) was emphasized even more, and commercial programs for counting and charting specific phonemes with strict schedules of reinforcement (e.g., Baker & Ryan, 1971) proliferated. One behavioristic program (McCabe & Bradley, 1975) involved treating all phonemes simultaneously, but again the emphasis was on individual phonemes rather than patterns of deviations. Moreover, training all deficient phonemes simultaneously is rather overwhelming for the most unintelligible children.

Several studies in the early 1970s (Compton, 1970; Edwards & Bernhardt, 1973; Grunwell, 1975; Ingram, 1974; Oller, 1973; Smith, 1973) provided new directions for looking beyond singleton phonemes to patterns. As well, distinctive feature analysis (e.g., McReynolds & Engmann, 1975) provided a framework for analyzing patterns of substitutions and for planning treatment to teach distinctive features that would generalize across phonemes, but the emphasis in treatment still involved behavioristic training for each phoneme. It is generally acknowledged that all treatment methods (as well as maturation) yield gains (Ingram, 1983). Moreover, children with mild/moderate speech-sound impairments progress nicely in phoneme-oriented articulation programs.

Highly unintelligible children with extensive omissions and limited repertoires of sounds, however, typically require 5 or 6 years (or more) to become intelligible via phoneme-oriented programs. As we have become increasingly aware of possible long-term effects of highly unintelligible speech on the development of literacy (Bird, Bishop, & Freeman, 1995; Clarke-Klein & Hodson, 1995; Hodson, 1994a; Hodson, Nonomura, & Zappia, 1989; Stackhouse, Chapter 7 of this volume; Stackhouse & Snowling, 1992), we are more and more concerned about helping children become intelligible prior to entering school.

The most significant contribution in the 1970s for practitioners interested in expediting intelligibility gains was David Ingram's (1976) *Phonological Disability in Children.* Ingram's book served as a bridge to David Stampe's (1969) natural phonology theory and paved the way for clinicians to identify patterns of deviations, referred to as *phonological processes.*

DEVELOPMENTS IN EVALUATION OF CHILDREN'S PHONOLOGIES

Assessment Instruments/Procedures

During the 10 years following the publication of Ingram's (1976) landmark book, there was considerable assessment instrument publication activity (Compton & Hutton, 1978; Grunwell, 1985; Hodson, 1980, 1986a, 1986b; Ingram, 1981; Khan & Lewis, 1986; Lowe, 1986; Shriberg & Kwiatkowski, 1980; Weiner, 1979), and this activity continues into the 1990s (e.g., Bankson & Bernthal, 1990). As well, several additional clinical research procedures (e.g., generative phonology, Elbert & Gierut, 1986; nonlinear phonology, Bernhardt & Stoel-Gammon, 1994; Process Density Index, Edwards, 1994) are available in the literature. For the most part, these phonologically based procedures have the goal of identifying broad patterns of deviations.

Assessment/Analysis Methods: Alterations Resulting from University Phonology Clinic Research Findings

In 1975, we initiated a phonological intervention research clinic at the University of Illinois that accepted only highly unintelligible children (Hodson, 1978, 1982). Student clinicians who had completed the applied phonology graduate seminar were each assigned a highly unintelligible client. The basic goal of this clinic was to develop and test hypotheses involving innovative procedures for assessing disordered phonologies (Hodson, 1980, 1986a) and for expediting intelligibility gains (Hodson & Paden, 1983, 1991).

Similar clinics were initiated at San Diego State University in 1981 and at Wichita State University in 1989. The San Diego clinic also incorporated assessment and treatment for Spanish-speaking clients (Cabello, Contreras, & Hodson, 1987; Hodson, 1986b; Hodson, Becker, Diamond, & Meza, 1984), and the Wichita clinic added metaphonological components (Domnick, Hodson, Coffman, & Wynne, 1993; Hodson, 1994b; Hodson, Buckendorf, Conrad, & Swanson, 1994; Johnson, 1996). Findings from these three university clinics provided an impetus for a number of changes in our assessment/analysis procedures.

The initial focus in the Illinois clinic was on assessing and targeting distinctive features. It soon became apparent that distinctive feature analysis had a critical limitation. Syllable structure deficiencies (e.g., omission of final consonants, reduction of consonant clusters) were not adequately accounted for by distinctive feature procedures, and thus assessment results did not identify syllable structure deficiencies as treatment target patterns.

As our graduate student clinicians began incorporating phonological process analysis, a larger picture began to emerge. It soon became apparent, however, that phonological process analysis also had some limitations. Although one could identify constituent phonological processes (Edwards, 1992) affecting words (e.g., *die* for *sky* represents the syllable structure process of cluster reduction and the feature substitution processes of fronting and prevocalic voicing), such specifications did not always identify exactly what needed to be targeted. For example, a focus on fronting (or stopping) alone could be misleading. As a highly unintelligible child progresses along the continuum toward intelligibility, fronting occurrences often increase in number as the child replaces omissions of velars (e.g., *book* → /bʊ/) with substitutions (e.g., *book* → /bʊt/). Scoring fronting occurrences without considering phoneme class deficiencies (e.g., velars) as well as syllable structure omissions would not be likely to highlight all of the optimal target patterns and could yield potentially misleading results. Something was needed in addition to phonological processes.

We began identifying phoneme classes that were most often deficient in children's utterances (e.g., stridents, velars) in a manner similar to current nonlinear analysis procedures (see Bernhardt & Stoel-Gammon, 1994). These phoneme classes were analyzed by scoring omissions, as well as substitutions from other phoneme classes, as deficiencies (i.e., the phoneme class was lacking in the child's production). If an analysis procedure does not adequately differentiate omissions, phoneme class deficiencies, and substitutions in the scoring process (e.g., Khan & Lewis, 1986), a client may obtain a poorer score on the assessment instrument following treatment (Stokes, 1992), even when improvement in the child's phonological system and overall intelligibility has been observed.

Two major findings from the research with Spanish-speaking clients at the San Diego clinic were that (a) essentially the same major deviation patterns differentiated unintelligible Spanish-speaking and English-speaking children from their phonologically normal peers, and (b) consonant sequence reduction was a more appropriate category for analysis than cluster reduction. All of the highly unintelligible Spanish-speaking children, as well as their English-speaking counterparts, evidenced the greatest problems with consonant sequences, stridents, and (r), in contrast to their intelligible peers (Hodson et al., 1984). Moreover, normally developing Spanish-speaking (as well as English-speaking) 4-year-olds evidenced very few phonological deviations (see Mann & Hodson, 1994).

The second finding from the Spanish research projects was that it is more appropriate to score all omissions of consonants in sequences, including those that cross syllable boundaries, than to restrict the scoring of reductions to consonant clusters, which by definition must be in the same syllable. This became apparent because of the nature of Spanish consonant sequences that include /s/. Highly unintelligible children deleted /s/ in sequences (e.g., *espejo* → /ɛ pexo/) in a manner similar to their English-speaking counterparts. Because of the findings from Spanish, we changed the scoring for reductions of contiguous English consonants to include those that cross syllable boundaries (Hodson, 1986a). For example, if a child says "*too_b_ush*" for *toothbrush*, two consonant sequence omissions are scored (instead of only one, as would be the case for cluster reduction).

Research in the area of metaphonology at the Wichita State University Clinic led us to assess phonological awareness skills (Hodson, 1994b) of prereaders and emergent readers and to incorporate some metaphonological instruction (e.g., rhyming, syllable segmentation) in our treatment sessions. Children with severely disordered expressive phonologies typically perform below expectations on phonological awareness tasks (Apel, Shields, & Perrin, 1992; Domnick et al., 1993; Green & Edwards, 1992; Smith, Kneil, Hodson, Bernstorf, & Gladhart, 1993; Webster & Plante, 1992). Moreover, they lag behind their phonologically normal peers in later years on tasks measuring reading and spelling (Bird et al., 1995; Clarke-Klein & Hodson, 1995).

Clearly, a number of changes have occurred in our evaluation and treatment procedures because of findings from ongoing clinical research. We now realize that assessment of highly unintelligible utterances must include a means to differentiate and score (a) syllable structure deficiencies (including scoring omissions of all contiguous consonants in sequences as reductions even if syllable boundaries are crossed), (b) phoneme class deficiencies (whether by omission or by substitution from another phoneme class), and (c) substitution (e.g., *shoe* → /tu/, stopping and depalatalization) and assimilation (e.g., *smoke* → /fmoʊk/) strategies.

At a minimum, productions of whole words must be transcribed. As well, all phonemes should be assessed at least once, and representative consonant clusters/sequences must be included in the sample. We also believe that assessment instrument results should (a) indicate not only whether the phonology of the child is disordered but also the degree of severity (moderate, severe, profound), (b) provide a direction for intervention (i.e., identify optimal targets), and (c) yield scores that measure treatment outcomes accurately.

Identification of Disordered Phonologies

Phonological Acquisition: Differentiating Normal and Disordered Phonologies

To discern whether a child's phonological system is indeed disordered, we have to be able to compare the child's performance with that of phonologically normal children of the same age. Figure 8–1 provides guidelines that we use in our clinic when evaluating whether a child's phonology is developing normally. Assignments for these "steps" were derived by compiling phonological acquisition data from a number of studies (e.g., Dyson & Paden, 1983; Grunwell, 1981; Haelsig & Madison, 1986; Hodson & Paden, 1981; Lowe, Knutson, & Monson, 1985; Oller, 1980; Porter, 1989; Preisser, Hodson, & Paden, 1988; Smit, Hand, Freilinger, Bernthal, & Bird, 1990; Smith, 1973; Stoel-Gammon, 1987; Templin, 1957).

When children's phonologies are below what would be expected for their particular chronological ages, there is room for concern. The greater the discrepancy between the child's current performance and the expected performance for that child's age, the greater the concern. If, for example, a 4-year-old evidenced consistent omissions (e.g., consonant sequence reduction, final-consonant deletion), treatment most likely would be indicated in light of the fact that omissions are extremely rare in utterances of phonologically normal 4-year-olds.

If a 3-year-old evidenced a restricted repertoire of consonants (e.g., stops, nasals, and/or glides) and only consonant-vowel (CV) monosyllabic utterances (e.g., "ba," "da"), intervention also would be indicated. If, however, a child's phonology appeared to be only slightly delayed, and there were examples of emergence of appropriate patterns (i.e., inconsistent use), monitoring the child's phonological development via a reevaluation a few months later would be the recommendation. Needless to say, a complete diagnostic evaluation would be required to consider all possible etiological factors that might be operating and to make necessary referrals.

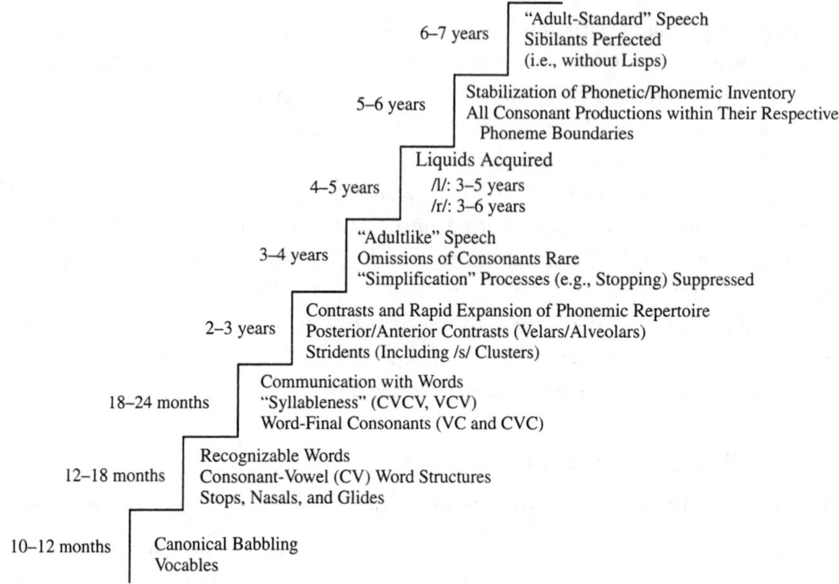

Figure 8–1 Phonological Acquisition Steps. *Source:* Copyright © Barbara Williams Hodson.

Severity Continuum

After deciding that a child's phonology is disordered, we must determine how severe the disorder is. Table 8–1 provides a summary of typical phonologies of children (age 3 years or older) for various levels of severity, as well as "accepted" deviations (including linguistic/cultural differences). Children with extensive omissions are considered to be profoundly involved. Because of the number of omissions, these children have fewer substitutions than children in less severe categories. Children in the profound or severe categories are candidates for intervention in our university phonology clinic.

In summary, substantial changes in evaluation procedures have occurred during the last 20 years. Now we need to review current treatment practices. Have advances in treatment methodology been commensurate with changes in evaluation procedures?

TREATMENT PRACTICES IN THE 1990s

Figure 8–2 provides an overview of treatment methods that currently are used most often by clinicians working with highly unintelligible children. For the most part, practitioners have individual preferences for initiating treatment with an emphasis on one of the following: (a) oral-motor exercises, (b) language, or (c) production of speech sounds.

Table 8–1 Speech Deviations Continuum for Children

Profound	*Severe*	*Moderate*	*Mild*	*Accepted Variations*
Extensive omissions Some substitutions Restricted repertoire of consonants	Extensive substitutions Some omissions	Some deviations from mild and some from severe categories Few omissions (if any)	Sibilant distortions Minimal shifts in place/manner Omissions rare	Utterance-final devoicing Regional/cultural/dialectal variations

Source: Copyright © Barbara Williams Hodson and Elaine Pagel Paden.

Oral-Motor Exercises

Clinicians who are prone to giving highly unintelligible children labels such as *dyspraxia* or *sensory integration deficit* commonly spend months having clients participate in "prespeech" activities. Children practice nonmeaningful exercises to "strengthen" their articulators and/or to increase sensory integration. For example, recommended activities include "stretching, stroking, icing" of the lips and "midline grooving" of the tongue (Marshalla, 1996). When sound productions are incorporated, they usually are nonmeaningful.

Clearly, children with severe neurological involvements (e.g., cerebral palsy) need comprehensive neurodevelopmental treatment. Some concern has been expressed, however, about excessive use of the labels *dyspraxia, developmental apraxia*, and *oral* or *sensorimotor impairment* for highly unintelligible children without definitive differential diagnostic criteria (see Guyette & Diedrich, 1981). Moreover, research data supporting efficacy of oral-motor exercises for unintelligible children as a whole are lacking.

Language Enhancement

Several approaches emphasize language (e.g., Backus & Beasley, 1951; Hoffman, Norris, & Monjure, 1990; Low, Crerar, & Lassers, 1959) and deemphasize production of speech sounds. The philosophy underlying these approaches is that treatment should occur in natural and meaningful contexts and that production practice at the word level is to be avoided. Will children who have difficulty producing certain sounds automatically begin producing such sounds in a language-rich environment? Fey (1992) questioned the efficacy of such approaches for

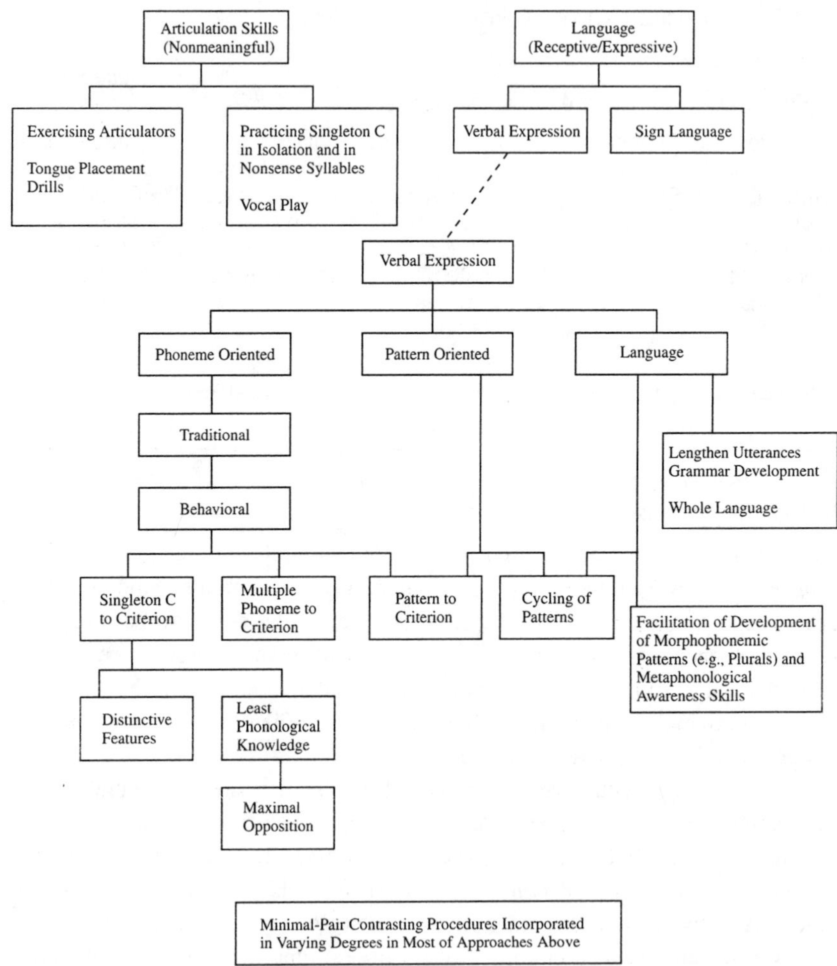

Figure 8–2 Prevalent Intervention Approaches/Options. *Source:* Reprinted with permission from Determining Phonological Intervention Priorities, p. 72, in *Children's Phonology Disorders*, 2nd ed., © ASHA.

---

children "who have severe limitations on the sounds their phonological systems can generate" (p. 605).

In American schools, a rather common practice is to place highly unintelligible children (with or without receptive language impairments) in self-contained early-childhood special education classrooms that emphasize language but devote little or no time to enhancing phonological development. Does language facilitation automatically enhance phonologies of highly unintelligible children? Results of several recent studies (Bopp, Bernhardt, & Johnson, 1996; Fey, Cleave, Ravida, Long, Dejmal, & Easton, 1994; Tyler & Watterson, 1991) indicated that phonological treatment results in improvement in language as well as phonology. The reverse, however, was not found to be true. Gains in phonology following language treatment alone were negligible.

Another language-oriented method employed by many clinicians for highly unintelligible children is sign language. Certainly, profoundly involved, nonverbal children need augmentative systems to communicate. If a child has the potential to communicate verbally, however, should time be spent teaching sign language? Clearly, a complete diagnostic evaluation (including prognosis for verbal communication) must be completed before determining the most efficacious method for each client.

Speech Production

Phoneme-Oriented Treatment

Even since practitioners began using phonological assessment instruments, most treatment methods for speech sounds have remained phoneme oriented (Fey, 1992; Hodson, 1992a). For example, /f/ (which usually is one of the first targets for highly unintelligible clients in phoneme-oriented programs and, in fact, often serves as an indicator that a child has been receiving phoneme-oriented treatment) is targeted in the initial position in words, phrases, sentences, and conversation to a criterion (e.g., 90%), then the process is repeated for word-final /f/, and so on.

Moreover, some phonologically based treatment programs (e.g., generative phonology; Elbert, 1983; Elbert & Gierut, 1986) also incorporate phoneme-oriented methods and behavioristic principles, even though they select quite different target phonemes. Elbert and her colleagues advocated teaching first those phonemes that the child experiences the most difficulty with, which they refer to as "least phonological knowledge." Their rationale, based on *implicational* principles, is that "learning the most difficult or complex distinction would enhance the learning of the less difficult or less complex sounds" (Elbert, 1992, p. 243).

Pattern-Oriented Treatment

Phonological analysis results have helped clinicians identify broad patterns of deviations (e.g., deletion of all final obstruents) that can be treated more holistically. For example, when the goal is "closing syllables," children are given opportunities to practice word endings involving several consonants. Even when targeting broad patterns, many clinicians still target each pattern to mastery (e.g., criterion of 95%) before targeting another pattern. As well, such clinicians commonly employ behavioristic counting and charting practices.

The approach that we have found to be most effective in expediting intelligibility gains for several hundred children in our university clinics is the cycles phonological remediation approach (Hodson & Paden, 1983, 1991). Deficient phonological patterns are targeted sequentially and recycled (i.e., re-presented) as often as needed until the pattern emerges in conversational speech (typically three to five cycles). Major components of the cycles approach are described briefly in the next section (see also Ingram, 1986).

CYCLES PHONOLOGICAL REMEDIATION APPROACH

A cycle is the period of time (varying in duration from 6 to 18 hours) when optimal phonological *patterns* are targeted (2 to 6 hours each). Phonemes, which are targeted approximately 60 minutes each per cycle, are used as a means to an end to help children learn to produce patterns needed for intelligibility. For example, when a child is targeting final consonants, common targets are final /p/ for an hour followed by final /t/ (or final /k/ if the child already produces velars) for an hour. A third final consonant may be targeted during the third hour, or, in most instances, final consonants are set aside after 2 hours of treatment. Then the next stimulable pattern is targeted (e. g., velars if the child is a "fronter" or alveolars if the child is a "backer") for at least 2 hours (depending on the number of readily stimulable phonemes in the pattern). Reassessment results at the end of each cycle, as well as conversational speech samples, indicate which patterns need to be recycled and which are already carrying over into spontaneous utterances.

Phonological Targets

Figure 8–3 provides a summary of patterns that have been targeted in the cycles approach (see also Hodson & Paden, 1991, for specific information about targets). The *primary* potential target patterns for beginning cycles for highly unintelligible children include (a) early developing patterns, (b) anterior/posterior contrasts, (c) /s/ clusters, and (d) liquids.

Early-developing patterns include "syllableness" and singleton consonants (prevocalic stops, nasals, and glides; postvocalic nasals and obstruents). Anterior/posterior contrasts refers to using velars and alveolars contrastively. /s/ clusters, which encompass stridency and consonant sequences, are targeted before singleton stridents (e.g., /f,s/) for two reasons: (a) overall effects on intelligibility, and (b) /s/ clusters are easier initially because highly unintelligible children retain the stop consonant anyway during initial attempts at producing singleton stridents (e.g., *see* → /sti/).

The initial goal for targeting /r/ is to suppress the gliding process. We do not expect adultlike productions of /r/ at this time. Rather, the child is to produce carefully selected production-practice words without an insertion of /w/. When modeling the practice word, the clinician emphasizes the vowel rather than the /r/.

For example, the clinician models /ɚɑ:k/. During initial cycles, the child's response of /ʊɑk/ would be accepted, but /ʊwɑk/ would be unacceptable.

All consistently deficient primary patterns that are stimulable are cycled and recycled until they begin to emerge in conversation, except liquid /r/. For /r/, which often lags behind the other patterns, the expectation is that the child is able to suppress gliding (i.e., not insert /w/) while naming the practice words. (The process of determining optimal targets for individual children is explained later in this chapter under the "Client Examples" section.)

Secondary patterns are then targeted as needed, along with further targeting of /r/. Even though a number of secondary patterns often are deficient during the initial phonological assessment session, many will no longer be problematic. For example, although many clients initially collapse voiced and voiceless prevocalic obstruents and/or *neutralize* vowels, considerable progress usually occurs for these two patterns while the child is targeting the primary beginning-cycles patterns, and thus vowels and voicing rarely need to be targeted. The secondary patterns that most often need to be targeted include other consonant sequences and palatals.

Advanced patterns often need to be targeted by children in upper elementary grades (i.e., around 9 years of age) who have problems being understood in conversation. Typically these children do not appear to have problems when naming articulation test pictures. Difficulties arise when saying certain complex multisyllablic words (e.g., *apostrophe, aluminum*). Children who "break down" on such words need to learn how to segment syllables and phonemes in complex multisyllabic words and then to blend them back together.

Remediation Basics

The seven underlying concepts listed in Exhibit 8–1 "drive" the cycles approach. The primary reason that we focus on a pattern for a short period of time and then sequentially target other deficient primary patterns is that acquisition is *gradual* (Ingram, 1976). Phonologically normal children do not master one sound before they begin to learn the next sound. Rather there is a considerable amount of vacillation (Dyson, 1988) as normally developing children explore and experiment in the process of learning the phonology of their linguistic community.

We also incorporate a short period of *auditory stimulation* (see Van Riper, 1939) with slight amplification at the beginning and end of each session because normally developing children typically learn to talk by *listening*. The child listens to (but must not repeat) 15 to 20 words containing the session's target pattern. We have found that our clients generally have poor listening skills. This phenomenon may be partially related to the fact that the majority of the unintelligible children we have worked with have histories of otitis media with effusion, accompanied by fluctuating levels of hearing. They appear to rely wholly on inaccurate kinesthetic images rather than to listen to their own utterances.

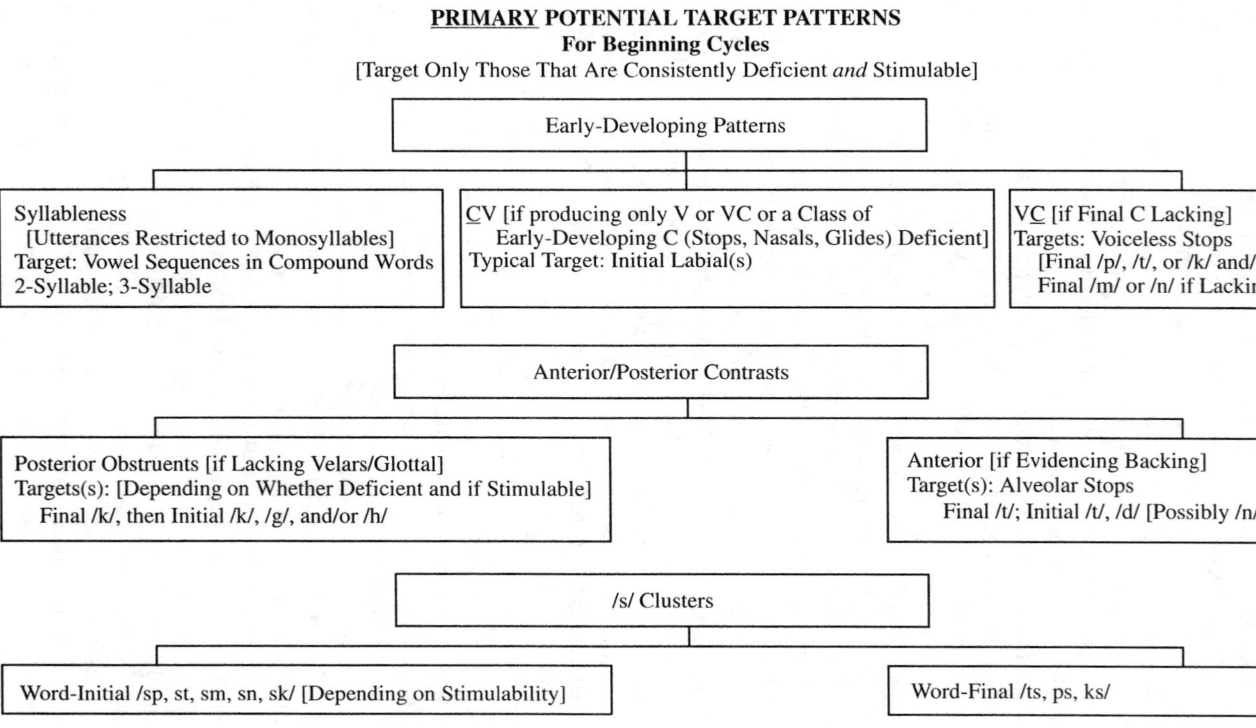
PRIMARY POTENTIAL TARGET PATTERNS
For Beginning Cycles
[Target Only Those That Are Consistently Deficient and Stimulable]
Early-Developing Patterns
Syllableness
[Utterances Restricted to Monosyllables]
Target: Vowel Sequences in Compound Words
2-Syllable; 3-Syllable
CV [if producing only V or VC or a Class of Early-Developing C (Stops, Nasals, Glides) Deficient]
Typical Target: Initial Labial(s)
VC [if Final C Lacking]
Targets: Voiceless Stops
[Final /p/, /t/, or /k/ and/or Final /m/ or /n/ if Lacking]
Anterior/Posterior Contrasts
Posterior Obstruents [if Lacking Velars/Glottal]
Targets(s): [Depending on Whether Deficient and if Stimulable]
Final /k/, then Initial /k/, /g/, and/or /h/
Anterior [if Evidencing Backing]
Target(s): Alveolar Stops
Final /t/; Initial /t/, /d/ [Possibly /n/]
/s/ Clusters
Word-Initial /sp, st, sm, sn, sk/ [Depending on Stimulability]
Word-Final /ts, ps, ks/

continues

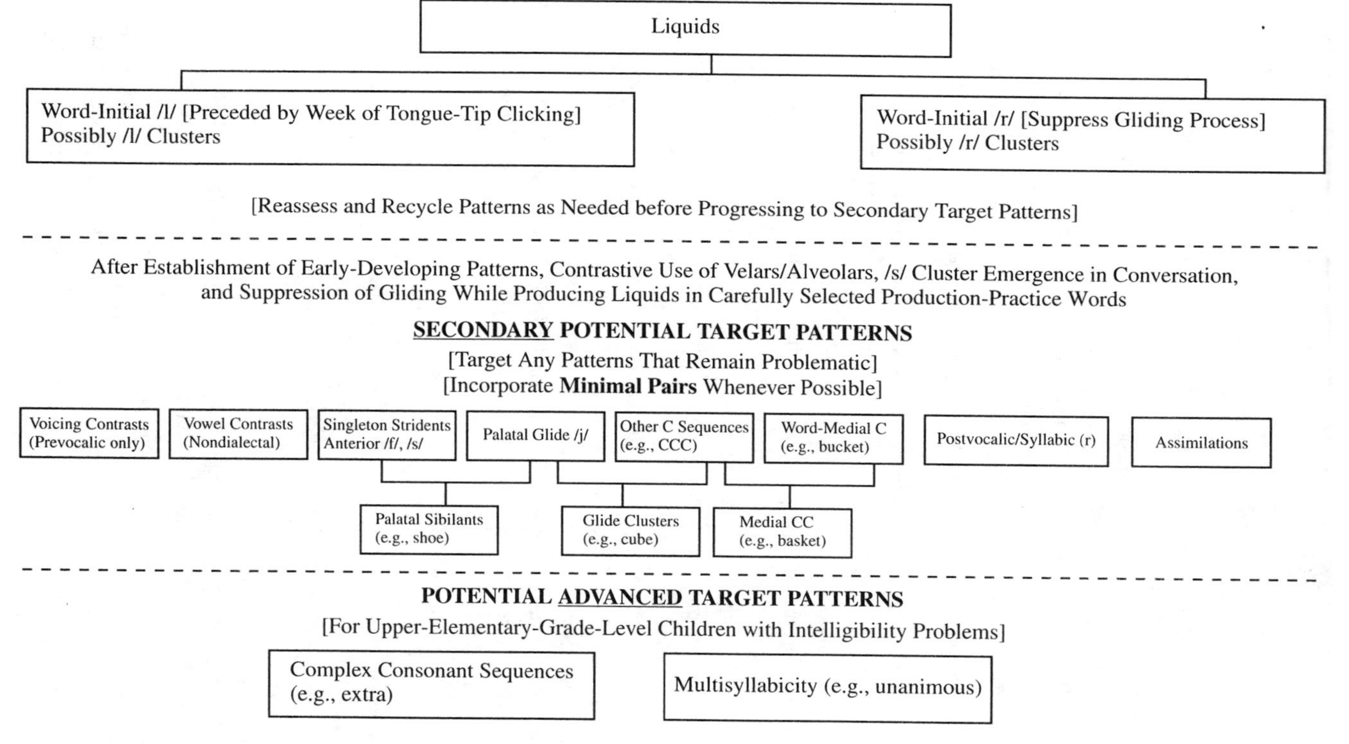

Figure 8–3 Potential Target Patterns. *Source:* Copyright © Barbara Williams Hodson.

Exhibit 8–1 Underlying Concepts for Cycles Phonological Remediation Approach

1. Phonological acquisition is a gradual process.
2. Children with normal hearing typically acquire the adult sound system primarily by listening.
3. Children associate kinesthetic and auditory sensations as they acquire new patterns, enabling later self-monitoring.
4. Phonetic environment can facilitate (or inhibit) correct sound production.
5. Children are actively involved in their phonological acquisition.
6. Children tend to generalize new speech production skills to other targets.
7. An optimal "match" facilitates a child's learning.

Source: Copyright © Barbara Williams Hodson and Elaine Pagel Paden.

Our goal for production practice is to help children develop new accurate *kinesthetic images* for the target phonological patterns. A small set of production-practice words with facilitative phonetic environments (Kent, 1982) are used for practice in a drill-play (Shriberg & Kwiatkowski, 1982a) format. Tactile cues and models are provided as needed to help the child consistently produce the target pattern correctly. Counting and charting, therefore, are not employed. Allowing the child to practice the error pattern while charting would be counterproductive. As children internalize kinesthetic and auditory sensations (Fairbanks, 1954), they develop their *self-monitoring* skills and *generalize* (McReynolds & Bennett, 1972) to other words and to conversational utterances (Elbert, Dinnsen, Swartzlander, & Chin, 1990).

Phonological analysis results provide a means for identifying the child's optimal "*match*." Hunt (1961), who discussed the "problem of the match," posited that optimal learning occurs when an individual is appropriately challenged yet successful. By identifying a child's current phonological level, treatment can be initiated one step higher, allowing clients to learn new patterns that they are ready to produce with success.

The session structure, although developed in a university clinic, has been adapted and used in public schools and other types of clinics. Each session begins with a review of the prior session's targets. This review is followed by amplified auditory stimulation. While still wearing the earphones, the child practices saying into the microphone a couple of new potential target words for the current session.

Pictures of four or five carefully selected target words (e.g., Buteau & Hodson, 1989) that the client is able to produce appropriately are drawn (or colored) on large 5 × 8 inch index cards. The word is then printed on the card for two reasons: (a) to make it possible for adults to know what the picture is and (b) to increase awareness of written words for overall development of literacy skills.

The child then participates in drill-play activities in as naturalistic an environment as possible. Each activity lasts approximately 7 or 8 minutes and can be used repeatedly during ensuing sessions. *Active participation* (mentally and physically) on the part of the child is fostered. At the end of the session, the clinician probes to determine the target for the next session. Auditory bombardment with amplification is then repeated prior to the child's departure.

A 2-minutes-per-day home program is recommended. The caregiver is to read the auditory bombardment listening list to the child once a day, and the child is to name the week's production-practice word cards.

CLIENT EXAMPLES

To exemplify our phonologically based assessment and treatment applications, case studies of four highly unintelligible clients (between 3:6 and 5:11) are summarized and compared. Their individual case studies have been presented in detail in other publications (Gordon-Brannan, Hodson, & Wynne, 1992; Hodson, 1994a; Hodson, Chin, Redmond, & Simpson, 1983; Hodson & Paden, 1983).

Background Information

All four of the clients had mild hearing losses or histories of fluctuating hearing related to recurrent episodes of otitis media with effusion. Receptive language measures yielded average or above-average scores for their respective ages. Expressive language samples could not be evaluated initially, nor could connected-speech samples be analyzed phonologically because of their low levels of intelligibility. Percentages of consonants correct (Shriberg & Kwiatkowski, 1982b) ranged from 8% to 29% at the time of initial phonological assessment. Phonetic transcriptions of 10 of the clients' word productions at that time are provided in Table 8–2.

Alan (Hodson & Paden, 1983) entered our university phonology clinic at the age of 5:11. He had been diagnosed at a major clinic in Minnesota as having "severe developmental dyspraxia." Alan had experienced seizures and was receiving phenobarbital and dilantin. In addition, he had a mild hearing loss. Alan had received 2 years of phoneme-oriented treatment and oral-motor practice in a special education preschool classroom. He was referred to our university phonology clinic by his public school clinician because progress had been limited.

Tim (Hodson et al., 1983) was 5:0 when he was referred. He had a repaired cleft palate and a history of recurrent otitis media. Pressure-equalizing tubes had been inserted nine times. His speech mechanism was judged to be adequate for speech purposes by his cleft palate team. Tim had received 2 years of phoneme-oriented treatment in an itinerant speech program in his local school district. Tim also was

Table 8–2 Phonetic Transcriptions of Word Productions: Samples from Four Clients

Stimulus	*Alan*	*Tim*	*Luke*	*Michael*
basket	bæwɛ	bædɛʔ	pɑtɛt	b̪ɑ
candle	næwo	ændʊ	tɑndə	gɛ
crayons	nɑ	eɪənʔ	tɑnə	g̊ʊᵊ
fork	bʌ	oɪʔ	poʊk	gi
glove	bʌ	dʌb̥	tʌp	g̊ɛ
jumprope	dɪʔoʊ	^{n}dʌmʔwoʊp	tɑmpwoʊp	gɛ
leaf	i	nip	jitə	dɪ
nose	moʊ	noʊd̥	noʊdə	n̊ʌ̃
shoe	tu	u	tʲu	ʃʊ
zipper	dɪpʊ	^{n}dɪbʊ	tɪpə	gɛ^{I}

referred to our clinic by his school clinician, who was concerned about Tim's lack of progress.

Luke (Gordon-Brannan et al., 1992) was 4:6 when he began phonological treatment. He had participated in a "modified multiple phoneme" program for four terms that targeted three phonemes simultaneously each term and emphasized high response rates. Luke had begun to evidence dysfluencies (see Edwards, Chapter 1 of this volume) during this time. He also had an unusual hearing loss—a mild conductive loss in the low frequencies, hearing within normal limits in the middle frequencies, and a moderate sensorineural loss in the high frequencies. Luke was referred to the phonology clinic by his clinical supervisor.

Michael (Hodson, 1994a) was 3:6 when he entered the university phonology clinic. He had experienced repeated episodes of otitis media and fluctuating hearing. In addition, his sequencing and oral-motor abilities appeared to be compromised. According to reports, Michael had been "blue" at birth and had remained in the hospital 1 week for a "jaundiced" condition. He had received 3 months of phoneme-oriented treatment and sign language instruction while attending an early childhood special education class in his local school district. Michael was referred to the phonology clinic by an audiologist who had tested his hearing.

Phonological Assessment Results

Phonological deviation percentage-of-occurrence scores during their initial evaluation sessions at our university clinic are listed in Table 8–3. Results for Luke and Michael are from the Assessment of Phonological Processes-Revised (APP-R;

Table 8–3 Phonological Deviation Percentage-of-Occurrence Scores for Four Clients

	APP		*APP-R*	
Deviation	*Alan*	*Tim*	*Luke*	*Michael*
Omissions				
Syllables	10	5	11	100
Clusters/sequences	106*	131*	90	125*
Prevocalic singletons	8	42	2	32
Postvocalic singletons	97	37	3	100
Class deficiencies				
Stridents	100	100	100	98
Velars	100	100	73	55
Liquid /l/	92	92	91	100
Liquid /r/	100	100	100	100
Nasals	53	5	0	79
Glides	60	50	50	70
Phonological deviation average	74	66	52	86
Severity interval	Profound	Profound	Severe	Profound

**Note*: Consonant sequence percentages over 100% reflect some "deletions" of total consonant clusters/sequences (in contrast to "reductions" with at least one consonant remaining).

Hodson, 1986a); scores for Alan and Tim are from the original version (APP; Hodson, 1980). Although some differences exist in stimuli and in category scoring, the percentages can be compared across children.

Phonological deviations that were evidenced most by all four boys were class deficiencies involving stridents (98%–100%, mean = 99.5%) and liquids (/r/ 100%; /l/ 92%–100%, mean = 94%), as well as reductions of consonant clusters/sequences (90%–131%, mean = 113%). These deviations have been prevalent in all speech samples of highly unintelligible children we have tested in our phonology clinics. It is interesting to note, however, that in spite of some commonalities across these four clients, as well as homonymy within individuals (e.g., Alan's productions of /bʌ/ for *fork* and *glove*), none of their productions in Table 8–2 are the same across any of the 10 words.

The next most commonly occurring deviation was velar deficiency (55%–100%, mean = 82.5%). Alan and Tim completely lacked velars; Alan was not even stimulable for velars at the onset of phonological treatment. Luke produced some word-final velars but completely lacked word-initial velars. Michael produced word-initial velars (in fact, /g/ was his preferred phoneme), but he omitted postvocalic velars along with all final consonants. Alan also omitted word-final consonants, except for a final nasal in his production for *spoon*.

Tim produced some final consonants. At times, however, he marked word endings by substituting a glottal stop, which is not uncommon for children with craniofacial anomalies. Luke, by contrast, "overproduced" final consonants, often adding a schwa. This phenomenon may have been related to the fact that he had targeted final obstruents the preceding term while involved in phoneme-oriented drill.

None of the children needed to target prevocalic consonants except Tim. He omitted voiceless word-initial consonants, a deviation pattern that has been observed in other children with repaired cleft palates.

All four boys produced some exemplars of sounds from each of the early-developing phoneme classes (i.e., stops, nasals, and glides). Each produced at least one example of both glides /w, j/ and also the anterior nasals /m, n/. Productions of stops were more scattered. Alan and Luke produced anterior stops /p, b, t, d/ prevocalically but no prevocalic velars, as stated above. Luke did evidence some final /k/ productions. Because Tim lacked prevocalic voiceless obstruents and velars, his prevocalic stops were limited to /b, d/. He did produce their voiceless cognates /p, t/ postvocalically. Michael's preferred production was /gɛ/. He also produced allophones of /b, d/. Michael dentalized bilabial consonants (i.e., labiodental placement for /p, b, m, w/), which may have resulted from having targeted /f/ the preceding term in phoneme-oriented sessions.

Sound productions other than stops, nasals, and glides were extremely limited in utterances of these four clients. Liquid /l/ was produced once each by Alan, Luke, and Tim. Luke and Michael also produced /h/, and Luke evidenced /ŋ/ as well. Stridents were lacking across the four boys (also see Churchill, Hodson, Jones, & Novak, 1988), except for a *phonological idiom* (Ferguson & Farwell, 1975) when Michael said *shoe* adequately.

Alan evidenced two additional interesting deviations. He substituted a glide to initiate final syllables (e.g., *basket* → /bæwɛ/). In addition, there were several examples of nasal assimilation (e.g., *candle* → /næwo/) and labial assimilation (e.g., *nose* → /mo/) in Alan's sample.

Tim inserted the alveolar nasal before producing the voiced alveolar stop and also substituted the alveolar nasal for the alveolar liquid in *leaf*. This may have been related to a lack of mastery of timing for velopharyngeal approximation.

For the most part, vowel productions were adequate for Alan and Tim. Luke substituted /ɑ/ for /æ/ rather consistently. Michael evidenced a number of mismatches for vowels. His preferred vowel was /ɛ/, which was often diphthongized, but he also produced /i,ɪ,ʊ,ʌ/ occasionally (but not necessarily appropriately).

Two of the boys also evidenced voicing/devoicing preferences for word-initial obstruents. Whereas most of Michael's prevocalic consonants were voiced, Luke devoiced most prevocalic (e.g., *boats* → /poʊt/), as well as postvocalic obstruents. Postvocalic obstruent devoicing is expected in light of the fact that phonologically normal children also devoice word-final obstruents (see Higgs & Hodson, 1978).

What did these boys need to target during beginning cycles? The factors that were considered when selecting optimal primary targets included (a) consideration of each client's phonological deviation percentage-of-occurrence scores, (b) a review of potential target patterns for beginning cycles, (c) further inspection of phonetic transcriptions of actual productions on the phonological assessment recording forms, and (d) stimulability (see Elbert, Chapter 3 of this volume). Table 8–4 provides a list of the phonological patterns that each boy targeted during the beginning cycles.

Beginning-Cycles Target Patterns

When selecting beginning-cycles target patterns for highly unintelligible children, we match each child's phonological deviations against the primary potential target patterns shown in Figure 8–3. Early-developing patterns include "syllableness" and singleton consonants. For word-initial singletons, the child needs to produce at least one exemplar for each of the early-developing phoneme classes (i.e., stops, nasals, glides). For word-final singletons, some postvocalic obstruents

Table 8–4 Beginning-Cycles Target Patterns for Four Clients

Alan (5:11)	*Tim (5:0)*	*Luke (4:6)*	*Michael (3:6)*
			Syllableness
Postvocalic singletons	Prevocalic voiceless singletons		Postvocalic singletons
Posterior obstruents (velars and glottal)	Velars (prevocalic and postvocalic)	Velars (prevocalic)	Velars (postvocalic)
/s/ clusters	/s/ clusters	/s/ clusters	/s/ clusters
Liquids	Liquids	Liquids	Liquids

as well as nasals must be evidenced. Only one of these four clients did not need to start with an early-developing pattern. Luke already produced singleton consonants and evidenced syllableness.

Michael was the only child who needed to target syllableness. He occasionally duplicated syllables but clearly did not sequence varied syllables. Therefore *syllableness* was Michael's first target pattern in Cycle 1.

All four boys produced some prevocalic stops, nasals, and glides. Tim, however, omitted word-initial voiceless obstruents (including stops). His postvocalic consonants were emerging, although in some instances he substituted glottal stops. The first Cycle 1 target for Tim was *voiceless prevocalic obstruents*.

The third early-developing pattern under consideration was postvocalic singletons. Alan and Michael both lacked word endings. *Voiceless final stops* became the first Cycle 1 target pattern for Alan and the second for Michael (after syllableness).

The next major pattern under consideration involved posterior/anterior contrasts. All four boys produced some anterior consonants (e.g., alveolars), but all evidenced some problems with posterior obstruents. Luke produced some word-final velars but no prevocalic velars. Michael produced word-initial velars (his preferred /g/). Neither Alan nor Tim produced any velars in any position. Alan also lacked the posterior glottal fricative /h/.

Alan and Tim needed to target both postvocalic and prevocalic velars. Word-final /k/, which is easier to elicit in most instances, was targeted before word-initial /k/. Alan was not stimulable for prevocalic /k/ until the third cycle. He was stimulable for /h/, however, which was added as a posterior obstruent target.

Michael needed to learn to produce postvocalic velars along with all final consonants. Final /k/ was one of his more stimulable postvocalic singletons, perhaps because of his demonstrated preference for velars prevocalically. Luke, on the other hand, already produced final /k/ but lacked velars prevocalically. Prevocalic velars became his first Cycle 1 target. (Recall that Luke did not need to target any early-developing patterns.)

The next major beginning-cycles target pattern to be considered involves /s/ clusters, which encompass consonant sequences as well as stridency. All four boys needed to target word-initial (e.g., /st, sk/) and word-final /s/ clusters (e.g., /ts, ps/). Each boy's current phonological system dictated the selection of specific /s/ clusters to be targeted. For example, /sm, sn/ were most successful for Tim (with a repaired cleft palate). Michael, who demonstrated a preference for velars, experienced success with /sk/, but Alan, who was not stimulable for /k/ initially, could not target /sk/ until several cycles later.

The last target pattern considered for each beginning cycle involves liquids. All four boys needed to target both /l/ and /r/. Alan, Tim, and Luke each produced one prevocalic /l/ during the initial phonological assessment session, but clearly they still needed additional practice. Michael and Luke, who were clients in more recent clinics, targeted liquids at the end of the first cycle. Because Alan and Tim attended our earlier phonology clinics (late 1970s), they did not target liquids at the end of Cycle 1. We were not yet aware at that time of the importance of facilitating liquid productions alongside the primary target patterns. Alan began targeting liquids at the end of his second cycle and Tim at the end of his third cycle. We have found that /l/ emerges rapidly and that /r/ productions improve with each cycle. Even though /r/ lags behind the other patterns, the earlier stimulation lays the foundation for successful /r/ productions at an earlier age in the future.

After an average of 35 weekly treatment sessions for Alan, Tim, and Luke and 43 for Michael, all of the above target patterns except liquid /r/ were emerging in conversation. Moreover, each boy's speech was considered to be essentially intelligible but certainly not perfect. *Secondary* target patterns were then reviewed to ascertain which were still problematic. None of the boys evidenced problems with vowel deviations or prevocalic voicing/devoicing at this time, even though Michael and Luke had substantial problems with vowels and prevocalic voicing/devoicing during their initial phonological assessment sessions.

Most of the remaining time was spent targeting other consonant clusters, including (a) postvocalic/intervocalic /s/ plus stop (e.g., *toast, toaster*), (b) glide clusters (e.g., *cube, queen*), (c) liquid clusters (e.g., *cloud, cry*), (d) CCC (e.g., *straw*), and (e) palatals (including /j/ for Michael, who had replaced /j/ with /l/ after he learned to produce /l/) and palatal sibilants as well as the palatal liquid /r/. (For actual targets for each cycle for each boy, see their detailed published case studies referenced earlier.)

Enhancing Metaphonological Skills

After we became aware of possible problems that might evolve in the area of emergent literacy for children whose expressive phonologies had been severely impaired, we began incorporating metaphonological skill enhancement activities (e.g., rhyming, syllable segmentation) for a few minutes during each session. Michael, who was one of our more recent clients, also participated in three short-term metaphonological treatment projects.

The first, which occurred the spring before he entered kindergarten, provided 11 individual half-hour instructional sessions (Domnick et al., 1993). The second involved six 2-hour group sessions the following year with four other kindergarten clients (Hodson et al., 1994). Components of *Animated Literacy* (Stone, 1992) were incorporated along with activities involving segmentation and blending of syllables, onset and rime, and finally phonemes.

Because Michael was experiencing considerable difficulty with spelling in the second grade, he returned to the university clinic during the summer before he entered third grade for six more 2-hour group sessions with three other former clients (Shields, 1996). During this last metaphonological project, vowels were emphasized. Stories and songs from Stone's *Animated Literacy* (1992) for vowels were presented. The large gestures, along with the names of the *Animated Literacy* characters in the stories and songs, were matched to the phonemes. Spelling and blending activities focusing on vowels also were incorporated.

In light of the fact that Michael did not talk intelligibly until he was almost 5 years of age, he appears to have some "catching up" to do. It might be that while phonologically normal children were developing their preliterate phonological awareness skills (e.g., rhyming), Michael was using his energies to develop intelligible speech. He has learned metaphonological aspects quickly, and teachers report gains following each project. It is possible that children like Michael may need periodic "boosts" to enhance their metaphonological skills to help them keep up with their peers as they advance in school.

Clearly, phonological awareness is an area that we must not neglect (Catts, 1991). After our clients with severely disordered expressive phonologies become intelligible, many experience problems developing literacy skills. In Chapter 7 of this volume, Stackhouse provides excellent information about relationships between speech impairments and literacy.

CLINICAL PHONOLOGY: THE NEXT 25 YEARS

Where do we go from here? Although clinical phonology is gaining in popularity, it still is not being used by most practitioners in the 1990s (Fey, 1992; Hodson, 1992a). Moreover, treatment applications have not kept up with gains in assessment/analysis. Clearly, a great deal more clinical research is needed in the area of phonology.

There is a growing recognition in our profession of the need for rigorously controlled treatment outcomes/efficacy research. We need to investigate all possible variables that might influence outcomes (see Shriberg, Chapter 5 of this volume). More detailed case studies (see Grunwell, Chapter 4 of this volume) of clients over time, including infants (see Oller, Chapter 6 of this volume) are needed, as well as studies with large numbers of clients in different types of treatment.

A great deal more information about phonologies of children with special needs (e.g., craniofacial anomalies, Down syndrome) and co-occurring communication impairments (e.g., stuttering, language) is needed. Some phonologists/practitioners have restricted phonological applications to children who are developing normally in all areas except intelligibility. A major distinction has often been made between "phonological disorders" and impairments related to some type of "organicity" (e.g., dyspraxia). We have found that a phonological approach can be used to expedite intelligibility gains in children with many different etiological factors. More needs to be known, however, about adaptations needed for assessment and treatment. The major question is how each client's individual needs can be met optimally.

Another aspect that needs attention in our profession pertains to severity considerations and eligibility criteria. Currently a child may be eligible for treatment in one state or in one school district but not in an adjacent one (Apel, Hodson, Gordon-Brannan, & Shulman, 1994). Moreover, a child with mild speech deviations commonly receives the same amount of treatment time as a highly unintelligible child. As well, guidelines for dismissing a client need to be evaluated. In some instances, children stay in treatment until their next yearly Individual Education Plan meeting, even though treatment goals were achieved earlier. We need to know a great deal more about the relationships of intelligibility (also see Gordon-Brannan, 1994; Kent, Miolo, & Bloedel, 1994), severity, and treatment outcomes.

Another area needing research is disordered phonologies of children speaking other languages. We found that Spanish-speaking children with intelligibility problems had phonological deviation patterns comparable to those of their English-speaking peers (Hodson et al., 1984). In Chapter 2 of this volume, Ingram notes that "children with phonological delay show systems like normal children in their own linguistic environment rather than like phonologically delayed children from other environments." Although we found similarities in the deviation patterns that most differentiated children with disordered phonologies from their phonologically normal peers, we did find certain differences that were language specific. For example, whereas English-speaking children typically substitute /w/ for /l, r/, their highly unintelligible Spanish-speaking counterparts substituted /d/. This may be related to the nature of /l, r/ in Spanish (i.e., tap/trill). Clearly, we can learn from studying disorders, as well as normal acquisition, across languages.

Phonological awareness studies are yielding important information about enhancing emergent literacy skills of "at-risk" children (e.g., from "inner-city" homes) who have had limited exposure to literacy in their early years (e.g., Ball & Blachman, 1988). Several investigators (e.g., Bird et al., 1995; Clarke-Klein & Hodson, 1995; Webster & Plante, 1992) have provided data indicating that children with severely disordered expressive phonologies appear to also be "at risk" for not developing normal literacy skills. Data from studies enhancing metaphonological skills of children with histories of expressive phonological impairments are sparse.

Undoubtedly the area we expect the greatest gains from is technology. Currently, a number of computer analysis procedures serve as clinical/research tools (e.g., Hodson, 1992b; Long & Fey, 1988; Oller & Delgado, 1990; Shriberg, 1986). Practitioners would be delighted if computers not only analyzed deviations but also provided narrow phonetic transcriptions of the utterances. As well, interactive computer software has a great deal of potential for use in treatment sessions. Clearly, we have seen only the tip of the iceberg in technology. What will assessment and treatment for children with disordered phonologies be like in the year 2020? The possibilities seem endless!

Appreciation is expressed to Deena Helms, Jaymie Faust, and Paula Barta for assistance with various aspects of this chapter. Also, I thank Mary Louise Edwards for collaborating with me on editing this book and for her many helpful comments. A special recognition goes to Elaine Paden for her interactions and contributions to applied phonology over the years. And finally, a huge thanks to all the students and clients in our phonology clinics at the University of Illinois, San Diego State University, and Wichita State University for all they have taught me.

REFERENCES

Apel, K., Hodson, B., Gordon-Brannan, M., & Shulman, B. (1994, November). *Eligibility criteria and severity ratings: A confused state of the union.* Miniseminar presented at the annual meeting of the American Speech-Language-Hearing Association, New Orleans.

Apel, K., Shields, M., & Perrin, N. (1992, November). *Emergent literacy skills in normal and phonologically impaired children.* Paper presented at the annual meeting of the American Speech-Language-Hearing Association, San Antonio, TX.

Backus, O., & Beasley, J. (1951). *Journal of speech therapy with children.* Boston: Houghton Mifflin.

Baker, R., & Ryan, B. (1971). *Programmed conditioning for articulation.* Monterey, CA: Monterey Learning Systems.

Ball, E., & Blachman, B. (1988). Phoneme segmentation training: Effect on reading readiness. *Annals of Dyslexia, 38,* 208–225.

Bankson, N., & Bernthal, J. (1990). *Bankson-Bernthal Test of Phonology.* Chicago: Riverside.

Bernhardt, B., & Stoel-Gammon, C. (1994). Nonlinear phonology: Introduction and clinical application. *Journal of Speech and Hearing Disorders, 37,* 123–143.

Bird, J., Bishop, D., & Freeman, N. (1995). Phonological awareness and literacy development in children with expressive phonological impairments. *Journal of Speech and Hearing Research, 38,* 446–462.

Bopp, K., Bernhardt, B., & Johnson, C. (1996, May). *The effects of nonlinear phonological intervention on syntactic development.* Poster presented at the annual meeting of the Canadian Association of Speech-Language Pathologists and Audiologists, Kelowna, British Columbia.

Buteau, C., & Hodson, B. (1989). *Phonological remediation targets: Words and primary pictures for highly unintelligible children.* Austin, TX: Pro-Ed.

Cabello, A., Contreras, S., & Hodson, B. (1987). Salvadorean and Mexican-American children's phonological systems: Intelligible and unintelligible. In V. Deal (Ed.), *Minority focus: Selected abstracts from ASHA conventions 1980–1990* (p. 224). Rockville, MD: American Speech-Language-Hearing Association.

Catts, H. (1991). Facilitating phonological awareness: Role of speech-language pathologists. *Language, Speech, and Hearing Services in Schools, 22,* 196–203.

Chomsky, N., & Halle, M. (1968). *The sound pattern of English.* New York: Harper & Row.

Churchill, J., Hodson, B., Jones, B., & Novak, R. (1988). Phonological systems of speech-disordered clients with positive/negative histories of otitis media. *Language, Speech, and Hearing Services in Schools, 19,* 100–107.

Clarke-Klein, S., & Hodson, B. (1995). A phonologically based analysis of misspellings by third graders with disordered-phonology histories. *Journal of Speech and Hearing Research, 38,* 839–849.

Compton, A. (1970). Generative studies of children's phonological disorders. *Journal of Speech and Hearing Disorders, 35,* 315–339.

Compton, A., & Hutton, S. (1978). *Compton-Hutton Phonological Assessment.* San Francisco: Carousel.

Domnick, M., Hodson, B., Coffman, G., & Wynne, M. (1993, November). *Metaphonological awareness performance and training: Highly unintelligible prereaders.* Poster presented at the annual meeting of the American Speech-Language-Hearing Association, Anaheim, CA.

Dyson, A. (1988). Phonetic inventories of 2- and 3-year-old children. *Journal of Speech and Hearing Disorders, 53,* 89–93.

Dyson, A., & Paden, E. (1983). Some phonological acquisition strategies used by two-year-olds. *Journal of Childhood Communication Disorders, 7,* 6–18.

Edwards, M. (1992). In support of phonological processes. *Language, Speech, and Hearing Services in Schools, 23,* 233–240.

Edwards, M. (1994). Phonological process analysis. In E. Williams & J. Langsam (Eds.), *Children's phonology disorders: Pathways and patterns* (2nd ed., pp. 43–65). Rockville, MD: American Speech-Language-Hearing Association.

Edwards, M., & Bernhardt, B. (1973). *Phonological analyses of the speech of four children with language disorders.* Unpublished manuscript, Stanford University.

Elbert, M. (1983). A case study of phonological acquisition. *Topics in Language Disorders, 3,* 1–9.

Elbert, M. (1992). Consideration of error types: A response to Fey. *Language, Speech, and Hearing Services in Schools, 23,* 241–246.

Elbert, M., Dinnsen, D., Swartzlander, P., & Chin, S. (1990). Generalization to conversational speech. *Journal of Speech and Hearing Disorders, 55,* 694–699.

Elbert, M., & Gierut, J. (1986). *Handbook of clinical phonology.* San Diego: College Hill.

Fairbanks, G. (1954). Systematic research in experimental phonetics: A theory of the speech mechanism as a servosystem. *Journal of Speech and Hearing Disorders, 19,* 133–139.

Ferguson, C., & Farwell, C. (1975). Words and sounds in early language acquisition. *Language, 51,* 419–439.

Fey, M. (1992). Articulation and phonology: An addendum. *Language Speech, and Hearing Services in Schools, 23,* 277–282.

Fey, M., Cleave, P., Ravida, A., Long, S., Dejmal, A., & Easton, D. (1994). Effects of grammar facilitation on the phonological performance of children with speech and language impairments. *Journal of Speech and Hearing Research, 37,* 594–607.

Goldman, R., & Fristoe, M. (1969). *Goldman-Fristoe Test of Articulation.* Circle Pines, MN: American Guidance Service.

Gordon-Brannan, M. (1994). Assessing intelligibility: Children's expressive phonologies. *Topics in Language Disorders, 14,* 17–25.

Gordon-Brannan, M., Hodson, B., & Wynne, M. (1992, September). Remediating unintelligible utterances of a child with a mild hearing loss. *American Journal of Speech-Language Pathology, 1,* 28–38.

Green, M., & Edwards, M. (1992, November). *Phonological awareness skills of phonologically disordered preschoolers.* Paper presented at the annual meeting of the American Speech-Language-Hearing Association, San Antonio, TX.

Grunwell, P. (1975). The phonological analysis of articulation disorders. *British Journal of Disorders of Communication, 10,* 31–42.

Grunwell, P. (1981). The development of phonology: A descriptive profile. *First Language, 3,* 161–191.

Grunwell, P. (1985). *Phonological Assessment of Child Speech* [Test]. Windsor, UK: NFER-Nelson.

Guyette, R., & Diedrich, W. (1981). A critical review of developmental apraxia of speech. In N. Lass (Ed.), *Speech and language: Advances in basic research and practice* (pp. 1–50). New York: Academic Press.

Haelsig, P., & Madison, C. (1986). A study of phonological processes exhibited by 3-, 4-, and 5-year-old children. *Language, Speech, and Hearing Services in Schools, 17,* 107–114.

Higgs, J., & Hodson, B. (1978). Phonological perception of word-final obstruent cognates. *Journal of Phonetics, 6,* 25–35.

Hodson, B. (1978). A preliminary hierarchical model for phonological remediation. *Language, Speech, and Hearing Services in Schools, 9,* 236–240.

Hodson, B. (1980). *The Assessment of Phonological Processes* [Test]. Danville, IL: Interstate.

Hodson, B. (1982). Remediation of speech patterns associated with low levels of phonological performance. In M. Crary (Ed.), *Phonological intervention: Concepts and procedures* (pp. 97–115). San Diego: College Hill.

Hodson, B. (1986a). *The Assessment of Phonological Processes-Revised* [Test]. Austin, TX: Pro-Ed.

Hodson, B. (1986b). *The Assessment of Phonological Processes-Spanish* [Test]. San Diego: Los Amigos.

Hodson, B. (1992a). Applied phonology: Constructs, contributions, and issues. *Language, Speech, and Hearing Services in Schools, 23,* 247–253.

Hodson, B. (1992b). *Computer Analysis of Phonological Deviations.* Stonington, IL: PhonoComp.

Hodson, B. (1994a). Determining phonological intervention priorities: Expediting intelligibility gains. In E. Williams & J. Langsam (Eds.), *Children's phonology disorders: Pathways and patterns* (pp. 67–87). Rockville, MD: American Speech-Language-Hearing Association.

Hodson, B. (1994b). Helping children become intelligible and literate: The role of phonology. *Topics in Language Disorders, 14,* 1–16.

Hodson, B., Becker, M., Diamond, F., & Meza, P. (1984). Phonological analysis of unintelligible children's utterances: English and Spanish. In G. Nathan & M. Winters (Eds.), *Occasional papers in linguistics: The uses of phonology* (pp. 61–69). Carbondale: Southern Illinois University Press.

Hodson, B., Buckendorf, R., Conrad, R., & Swanson, T. (1994, November). *Enhancing metaphonological skills of highly unintelligible 6-year-olds.* Poster presented at the annual meeting of the American Speech-Language-Hearing Association, New Orleans.

Hodson, B., Chin, L., Redmond, B., & Simpson, R. (1983). Phonological evaluation and remediation of speech deviations of a child with a repaired cleft palate: A case study. *Journal of Speech and Hearing Disorders, 48,* 93–98.

Hodson, B., Nonomura, C., & Zappia, M. (1989). Phonological disorders: Impact on academic performance? *Seminars in Speech and Language, 10,* 252–259.

Hodson, B., & Paden, E. (1981). Phonological processes that characterize unintelligible and intelligible speech in early childhood. *Journal of Speech and Hearing Disorders, 46,* 369–373.

Hodson, B., & Paden, E. (1983). *Targeting intelligible speech: A phonological approach to remediation.* San Diego: College Hill.

Hodson, B., & Paden, E. (1991). *Targeting intelligible speech: A phonological approach to remediation* (2nd ed.). Austin, TX: Pro-Ed.

Hoffman, P., Norris, J., & Monjure, J. (1990). Comparison of process targeting and whole language treatments for phonologically delayed preschool children. *Language, Speech, and Hearing Services in Schools, 21,* 102–109.

Hunt, J. (1961). *Intelligence and experience.* New York: Ronald.

Ingram, D. (1974). Phonological rules in young children. *Journal of Child Language, 1*, 49–64.

Ingram, D. (1976). *Phonological disability in children*. New York: Elsevier.

Ingram, D. (1981). *Procedures for the Phonological Analysis of Children's Language* [Test]. Baltimore: University Park.

Ingram, D. (Ed.). (1983). Case studies of phonological disability. *Topics in Language Disorders, 3.*

Ingram, D. (1986). Explanation and phonological remediation. *Child Language Teaching and Therapy, 2,* 1–19.

Jakobson, R. (1968). *Child language, aphasia, and phonological universals* (A. Keiler, Trans.). The Hague: Mouton. (Original work published 1941)

Johnson, J. (1996). *Metaphonological awareness treatment: Enhancing emergent literacy skills in "at risk" first graders.* Unpublished master's thesis, Wichita State University.

Kent, R. (1982). Contextual facilitation of correct sound production. *Language, Speech, and Hearing Services in Schools, 13,* 66–76.

Kent, R., Miolo, G., & Bloedel, S. (1994). The intelligibility of children's speech: A review of evaluation procedures. *American Journal of Speech-Language Pathology, 3,* 81–95.

Khan, L., & Lewis, N. (1986). *Khan-Lewis Phonological Analysis.* Circle Pines, MN: American Guidance Service.

Long, S., & Fey, M. (1988). *Computerized profiling.* Ithaca, NY: Ithaca College, Department of Speech Pathology and Audiology.

Low, G., Crerar, M., & Lassers, L. (1959). Communication-centered speech therapy. *Journal of Speech and Hearing Disorders, 24,* 361–368.

Lowe, R. (1986). *Assessment Link between Phonology and Articulation* [Test]. East Moline, IL: LinguiSystems.

Lowe, R., Knutson, P., & Monson, M. (1985). Incidence of fronting in preschool children. *Language, Speech, and Hearing Services in Schools, 16,* 119–123.

Mann, D., & Hodson, B. (1994). Spanish-speaking children's phonologies: Assessment and remediation of disorders. *Seminars in Speech and Language, 15,* 137–148.

Marshalla, P. (1996, May). *Developmental apraxia.* Short course presented at the annual meeting of the Canadian Association of Speech-Language Pathologists and Audiologists, Kelowna, British Columbia.

McCabe, R., & Bradley, D. (1975). Systematic multiple phonemic approach to articulation therapy. *Acta Symbolica, 6,* 2–18.

McReynolds, L., & Bennett, S. (1972). Distinctive feature generalization in articulation training. *Journal of Speech and Hearing Disorders, 37,* 462–470.

McReynolds, L., & Engmann, D. (1975). *Distinctive feature analysis of misarticulations.* Baltimore: University Park.

Oller, D. (1973). Regularities in abnormal child phonology. *Journal of Speech and Hearing Disorders, 38,* 36–47.

Oller, D. (1980). The emergence of the sounds of speech in infancy. In G. Yeni-Komshian, J. Kavanagh, & C. Ferguson (Eds.), *Child phonolology: Vol. 1. Production* (pp. 93–112). New York: Academic Press.

Oller, D., & Delgado, R. (1990). *Logical International Phonetic Programs.* Miami, FL: Intelligent Hearing Systems.

Porter, J. (1989). *Phonological acquisition: Ages 3 to 7 years.* Unpublished manuscript.

Preisser, D., Hodson, B., & Paden, E. (1988). Developmental phonology: 18–29 months. *Journal of Speech and Hearing Disorders, 53,* 125–130.

Shields, M. (1996). *Enhancing metaphonological spelling skills of third graders with histories of phonological impairments.* Unpublished manuscript, Wichita State University.

Shriberg, L. (1986). *PEPPER: Programs to Examine Phonetic and Phonologic Evaluation Records* [Computer software manual]. Hillsdale, NJ: Lawrence Erlbaum.

Shriberg, L., & Kwiatkowski, J. (1980). *Natural Process Analysis* [Test]. New York: John Wiley.

Shriberg, L., & Kwiatkowski, J. (1982a). Phonological disorders II: A conceptual framework for management. *Journal of Speech and Hearing Disorders, 47,* 242–256.

Shriberg, L., & Kwiatkowski, J. (1982b). Phonological disorders III: A procedure for assessing severity of involvement. *Journal of Speech and Hearing Disorders, 47,* 256–270.

Smit, A., Hand, L., Freilinger, J., Bernthal, J., & Bird, A. (1990). The Iowa Articulation Norms Project and its Nebraska replication. *Journal of Speech and Hearing Disorders, 55,* 779–798.

Smith, N. (1973). *The acquisition of phonology.* London: Cambridge University Press.

Smith, M., Kneil, T., Hodson, B., Bernstorf, E., & Gladhart, M. (1993, November). *Rhyming abilities in children with and without impaired expressive phonologies.* Paper presented at the American Speech-Language-Hearing Association, New Orleans.

Stackhouse, J., & Snowling, M. (1992). Barriers to literacy development in two cases of developmental verbal dyspraxia. *Cognitive Neuropsychology, 9,* 273–299.

Stampe, D. (1969). The acquisition of phonetic representation. In R.T. Binnick, A. Davison, G.M. Green, & J.L. Morgan (Eds.), *Papers from the fifth regional meeting of the Chicago Linguistic Society* (pp. 443–454). Chicago: Chicago Linguistic Society.

Stoel-Gammon, J. (1987). Phonological skills of 2-year-olds. *Language, Speech, and Hearing Services in Schools, 18,* 323–329.

Stokes, D. (1992). *A comparison over time of three phonological assessment instruments with intelligibility measurements.* Unpublished master's thesis, Wichita State University.

Stone, J. (1992). *Animated literacy.* LaMesa, CA: J. Stone Creations.

Templin, M. (1957). *Certain language skills in children.* Minneapolis: University of Minnesota Press.

Tyler, A., & Watterson, K. (1991). Effects of phonological versus language intervention in preschoolers with both phonological and language impairment. *Child Language Teaching and Therapy, 7,* 141–160.

Van Riper, C. (1939). *Speech correction: Principles and methods.* Englewood Cliffs, NJ: Prentice Hall.

Webster, P., & Plante, A.S. (1992). Effects of phonological impairment on word, syllable, and phoneme segmentation and reading. *Language, Speech, and Hearing Services in Schools, 23,* 176–182.

Weiner, F. (1979). *Phonological Process Analysis* [Test]. Baltimore: University Park.

APPENDIX A

Glossary

PRIMARY DESCRIPTOR TERMS

Disordered phonology. A generic term indicating an individual's speech productions are inadequate and below expectations (without consideration of etiology).

Phonological disorder. A linguistic disorder manifested by the use of abnormal patterns in the spoken medium of language (implying no organic etiological component). **Developmental phonological disorder.** A speech disorder that occurs during the developmental period.

Phonological impairment (expressive). A generic term for speech pronunciation/phonological output difficulties in children (involving one or more levels of breakdown).

Speech delay. Speech typical of a slightly younger child (less than 1 year difference).

Speech differences. Speech and prosody/voice characteristics that differ from some demographic expectation, but are entirely consistent with one or more aspects of a person's linguistic, geographic, or cultural background. **Different development.** When a child is using patterns that do not occur normally in pronunciation development (i.e., atypical, idiosyncratic).

Speech disorders (childhood). A generic term preferred by Shriberg for all speech disorders occurring during childhood.

SPECIFIC TERMS

Alphabetic stage of literacy development. Stage at which children apply letter-sound rules to reading and spelling and can decode new words.

Anterior consonants. Consonants produced in the front part of oral/nasal cavities (e.g., labials).

Anterior/posterior contrasts. Using posterior (e.g., velars) and anterior (e.g., alveolars) consonants contrastively (e.g., *tea* vs. *key*).

Articulation. Movements of the speech mechanism to produce speech sounds.

Assembly stage of speech development. Stage that occurs around four years of age when children learn how words are joined together in connected speech (e.g., an apple/a pear).

Assimilation. Influence of one sound in a word or phrase upon another resulting in the output sounds being more alike.

Auditory stimulation/bombardment. Verbal presentation of words containing a target phoneme/pattern.

Backing. Replacing an anterior consonant with a posterior one.

Capability-focus framework. A two-factor perspective that stresses individual motivational differences as a key element in successful treatment of children with speech disorders.

Chronological mismatch. Co-occurrence of earlier phonemes/patterns with those that are characteristic of later stages of development (i.e., uneven development).

Cognitive neuropsychology. The study of cognitive processing abilities in individuals with and without brain injuries.

Conceptual process. The process of thinking and imagining, including the ability to abstract and categorize.

Consonant sequences. Two or more contiguous consonants, including those that cross syllable and word boundaries, contrasted with consonant clusters, which refer only to consonants within a syllable. Omission of one or more of these consonants is referred to as consonant sequence reduction (or cluster reduction if it is in the same syllable).

Consonant singleton. A single consonant separated from other consonants by vowels or silence.

Constraints. Restrictions on some aspect of phonology, such as restrictions on the syllable position in which a sound can occur or on the sequences of sounds that are allowable in a language or in a child's output (e.g., constraints against the occurrence of consonant clusters in a child's production).

Contrastive specification. A theory of how words are represented as features—both the plus and minus values of distinctive features are given.

Contrast training. Using minimal pairs in treatment to demonstrate differences in meaning related to sound usage.

Critical age hypothesis. The premise that children are at risk for literacy problems if speech difficulties have not resolved by the age of 5:6.

Cued articulation. Use of hand signs to teach and remind children how to pronounce and sequence sounds.

Cycles. Time periods (approximately two or three months) during which all primary deficient phonological patterns are targeted in succession.

Cycles phonological remediation approach. A treatment method that involves sequential targeting of phonemes within a phonological pattern for approximately

60 minutes each and targeting all major deficient patterns in succession for two to six hours each; patterns are recycled until they emerge in conversation.

Distinctive features. A system of attributes that differentiates one phoneme from another in a language.

Dysarthria. A difficulty in producing speech because of abnormal muscle tone.

Dyslexia. An unexpected reading and/or spelling difficulty in children (or adults) given their nonverbal cognitive abilities (i.e., specific literacy difficulties).

Dyspraxia (verbal). A difficulty in producing and/or sequencing sounds in words in the absence of obvious structural or neurological abnormalities; difficulties with motor programming.

Early developing patterns. Use of stops, nasals, and glides; syllable-initial singleton consonants; and syllableness.

Electropalatography. An instrumental technique for displaying tongue contact against the palate when producing sounds.

Feature geometry. A nonlinear approach to phonology in which features are organized hierarchically, with some being dominant over others.

Feature hierarchy. The model in which features are hierarchically arranged from the most general at the top to the most specific at the bottom.

Fronting. Replacing a posterior consonant with an anterior one.

Functional load. The phonological prominence of a particular phoneme within a language.

Generalization. Transfer of learning from one environment to another environment; includes across-sound (i.e., transfer of learning from treatment on a sound to other untreated sounds) and across-word (i.e., transfer of learning from treatment of a sound in one position to other word positions) position generalization.

Generative phonology (standard). A theory of phonology that includes formal phonological rules and abstract underlying representations to describe the sound system of a language.

Gestalt parametric stage. The unsegmented, whole-word learning that occurs during child's second year.

Gliding. The substitution of a glide for another consonant.

Graphemes. Written or printed letters, may or may not correspond to phonemes.

Homonymy. Producing the same phonetic form for two or more adult words that normally are not pronounced the same.

Indirect intervention. A treatment method that involves reinforcing children for their participation rather than for sound productions; sound errors are not corrected directly.

Infraphonology. The study of the infrastructure of speech systems, focusing on universal properties of sounds at each level of rhythmic structure.

Intelligibility. How well an individual is understood.

Inventory restraints. Restrictions on the sounds that can occur in a child's phonetic or phonemic inventory, possibly reflecting limitations on the child's phonological knowledge.

Letter knowledge. The knowledge that written letters have both a name and a sound.

Lexical items. Words.

Lexical representation. Stored knowledge about a word comprising its meaning, what it sounds like, how it is produced, how it is written, and how it can be used grammatically.

Lexicon. Containing the lexical representations.

Logographic stage of literacy development. When reading occurs by visual whole-word recognition and when spelling does not show letter-sound correspondences (see nonphonetic spelling).

Markedness. The proposal that some features (or feature values) are more basic (or less marked) than other ones.

Maximal oppositions. An unusual application of word pairs in which the sounds that differentiate the word pairs differ from each other in several parameters, such as major class (sonorant vs. obstruent), place, manner, and voicing (e.g., *see* vs. *me*).

Metaphonological skills. The ability to reflect upon the structure of an utterance as distinct from its meaning (see phonological awareness).

Metaphonological stage of speech development. The stage when children can apply their phonological processing skills, developed initially for storing and producing speech, to phonological awareness tasks.

Minimal pairs. Words that differ by only one or two features (e.g., pin/bin).

Minimal word. The hypothesis that all words have at least two moras.

Mora. A unit of timing in the prosodic structure of a word. A mora can be a vowel, the on- or off-glide of a diphthong, or a coda consonant.

Morphophonemic alternations. Alternations between two or more forms of a morpheme, with accompanying variations in the sounds that make up the morpheme (e.g., *house* vs. *houses*).

Motor planning. Individual words assembled into a single utterance ready for production.

Motor programming. Selecting phonological units and assembling these units into new combinations.

Multisyllabicity. The production of words with three or more syllables.

Naturalistic intervention. An approach to phonological remediation in which target sounds and words are presented as a natural part of the activities in which the children are engaged.

Natural phonology. A theory of phonology that focuses on phonetically motivated natural phonological processes that are said to account for sound changes that occur in dialect variation and historical language change, as well as phonological acquisition in children.

Nonlinear phonology. A phonological theory based on the principle that phonological structure consists of many tiers or levels of phonological information, and that the tiers consist of prosodic structure on the top and a feature hierarchy on the bottom.

Nonphonetic spelling. Spelling that contains no evidence of letter-sound rules (e.g., *slippery* → greid).

Normalization. The acquisition of age-appropriate speech. This occurs in young children acquiring adult-like speech, as well as in children with speech disorders who, with or without treatment, eventually acquire adult-like speech.

Normal or normalized speech acquisition/speech delay. A classification in Shriberg's Speech Disorders Classification System that is intermediate between normal or normalized speech acquisition and speech delay.

Obstruents. Voiceless consonants and their voiced cognates, including stops, fricatives, and affricates.

Onset. The part of a word that precedes a vowel, may be a single consonant or a consonant cluster.

Optimality theory. A recent nonlinear model of phonology that focuses on constraints rather than phonological rules or processes.

Orthographic experience. Exposure to the printed word through books, newspapers, magazines, alphabet friezes, plastic letters, letter games, etc.

Orthographic representations. The stored knowledge of spellings of words.

Pattern-oriented treatment. Emphasis on facilitating the development of phonological patterns (e.g., final consonants, liquids) using phonemes as a means to achieve the goal but not as the goal itself.

Persisting normal processes. Normal patterns that remain in a child's pronunciation patterns long after the age at which such patterns normally would have disappeared.

Phoneme class deficiency. The lack of a class of phonemes (e.g., stridents) because of omissions or substitutions from another phoneme class.

Phonemes. The meaningful sounds of a language.

Phonetic spelling. Spelling in which letter-sound correspondence is clear and the intended word is obvious (e.g., *cigarette* → sigaret).

Phonics. A method of teaching letter-sound correspondences to help emergent readers decode new words.

Phonological awareness. The awareness of aspects related to the sounds of one's language, including blending, segmenting, and manipulating sounds and syllables.

Phonological change. Four types of phonological change (see Grunwell, Chapter 4 of this volume) sought through phonological treatment: stabilization, destabilization, innovation, and generalization.

Phonological deficit hypothesis. An emphasis on the specific phonological processing problems found in children with dyslexia.

Phonological deviations. Broad simplifications (e.g., stopping, cluster reduction) that adversely affect intelligibility.

Phonological dyslexia. Specific reading difficulties that arise from difficulties at the alphabetic stage of literacy development, including difficulties with learning letter-sound correspondences and with phonological awareness tasks.

Phonological idiom. A more advanced production for one word than expected based on productions of other words.

Phonological input skills. Auditory processing, including auditory discrimination, memory, and sequencing, and storing lexical representations.

Phonological knowledge. What one knows about the phonology of the language.

Phonological linkage hypothesis. Literacy development and teaching dependent on making explicit links between children's phonological awareness development and their experience with the printed word.

Phonological output skills. Retrieval from the lexicon, motor programming, motor planning, and articulation.

Phonological patterns. Accepted groupings within an oral language (e.g., sound class, consonant cluster, syllable shape).

Phonological processes. Systematic sound changes that affect classes of sounds or sound sequences. A universal set of articulatory simplifications that learners apply to the words they hear.

Phonological processing. Using phonological information to process oral and written language.

Phonological processing difficulties. Problems with phonological input (auditory processing), lexical representations, and/or phonological output (speech).

Phonological processing system. A system that enables children (and adults) to deal with auditory input, storage of word knowledge, and speech output; using phonological information to process oral and written language.

Phonological representation. Stored knowledge about what a word sounds like (sufficient to recognize it when heard) and how to discriminate it from similar sounding words.

Phonological rules. More or less formal ways of capturing the sound changes of a language. These can be written formally using distinctive features and notational devices or informally using phonetic symbols or the names of sound classes.

Phonology. The signalling of meanings and the physical phonetic substance whereby meanings are transmitted; the sound system of a language.

Phonotactics. Rules defining permissible sequences of phonemes to form meaningful words.

Posterior consonant. Consonant articulated in the back of oral cavity (e.g., velars).

Postvocalic consonant. Consonant that follows a vowel in a syllable.

Prelexical stage of speech development. The first year of speech development prior to production of first words, including babble.

Prevocalic consonant. Consonant that precedes a vowel in a syllable.

Productive phonological knowledge. A speaker's competence about the sound system of a language.

Prosodic hierarchy. The theory that the prosodic structure of words is hierarchically arranged, consisting of units such as word, foot, syllable, and mora.

Prosodic structure. The ways in which individual sounds combine to form higher units of organization.

Psycholinguistic profile. A child's strengths and weaknesses in input skills, stored linguistic knowledge, and output skills.

Radical underspecification. A theory about how words are represented as features (distinctive), with only the marked value being shown; unmarked values are predicted by rule.

Redundancy rules. Rules that determine those feature values that are predictable and therefore do not need to be a part of the underlying representations of words.

Representation. The form in which the mind stores the information that underlies the phonetic form of words.

Residual errors. Speech errors that persist after nine years of age.

Rhyme knowledge. An understanding that a syllable can be divided into onset and rime (*c/at*), and that rhyming words have the rhyme in common but differ in their onsets (*c/at*, *h/at*, *m/at*).

Rime. A unit of prosodic structure that consists of an obligatory nucleus and optional coda. The part of a word that rhymes with another word (i.e., from the vowel to the end).

Segmentation. Dividing an utterance into smaller units (e.g., a sentence into words, words into syllables, syllables into onset/rime or segments, and consonant clusters into individual consonants).

Semantic categorization. Sorting words by meaning (e.g., farm animals from zoo animals).

Semiphonetic spelling. Evidence that letter-sound rules are being applied but that the intended word may not be obvious (e.g., *boat* → bot, *burglar* → bgl).

Sibilants. Consonants that can be described as "hissing"; lisps can occur on these sounds.

Sonorants. Phonemes characterized by relatively unobstructed airflow, including vowels, nasals, glides, and liquids.

Sound blending. Combining segmented sounds to form a word or nonword (e.g., *c-a-t* → cat).

Sound categorization. Sorting words by sound rather than meaning (e.g., words that have the same onsets or rimes).

Special populations. Childhood speech disorders associated with speech-hearing mechanism, cognitive-linguistic, or psychosocial involvements and needs.

Speech disorders classification system. A set of classification terms used by Shriberg to characterize each type of childhood speech disorder based on age, suspected etiology, and speech characteristics.

Spoonerism. The exchange of the beginnings of two words (e.g., *car park* → par cark).

Stability. A characteristic of mature phonological systems; a finite number of mutually exclusive terms in the system; homeostasis.

Stimulability. The degree to which a misarticulated sound can be imitated correctly.

Stopping. Substituting a stop consonant for a continuant (i.e., fricative, liquid, nasal, glide).

Stridents. Consonants characterized by forceful airflow striking back of teeth, including sibilants and also /f/ and /v/.

Structure. Syntagmatic relationships between phonological units; relationships of co-occurrence, sequence, and of structural contrast.

Supralaryngeal. The articulators above the larynx.

Syllableness. Sequencing two or three syllables.

Syllable segmentation. Dividing an utterance into syllables.

System. The paradigmatic relationships between phonological units. The relationships of replacement or substitutability and of systemic contrast.

Systematic simplification stage of speech development. A stage of speech development characterized by simplifying processes (e.g., fronting, stopping).

Systematic sound preference. One consonant used for a large range of target consonants (i.e., multiple loss of phonological contrasts).

Tetism. A phonological difficulty marked by the use of [t] for other consonants.

Underlying representations (URs). The mentally stored forms of words to which phonological processes or rules are said to apply; can be adult-like form or a unique form.

Verbal deficit hypothesis. An emphasis on verbal, rather than visual, processing deficits in children with dyslexia.

Word-finding difficulties. Problems retrieving words from the lexicon.

Word spurt. A stage of language acquisition at approximately 1:6 when children demonstrate a marked increase in their rate of word acquisition.

Index

A

Acoustic-aided auditory transcription, 121
Acoustic-aided perceptual procedures, 124
Acoustic analysis, in child phonology, 145–148, 149
Acquisition
  cross-linguistic, 26, 39
  of features, 51
  gradual, 207
  of liquids, 202
  normal *vs.* disordered phonologies, 201–202
  patterns, 22–25
  of phonological processes, chronology of, 72
  research, 38–39
  steps in, 25, 201, 202
Across sound generalization, 45
Across word position generalization, 45
Active participation, 211
Adult-onset speech disorders, 110
African American Vernacular English (AAVE), 112
Allophones, 214
Alphabetic stage of literacy development
  beginning of, 162–163
  definition of, 225
  phonological awareness and, 157, 164
Alveolars, 202, 206, 214
Amplification, low level, 53
Analogy, reading by, 159, 163
Analysis
  acoustic, 145–148
  advantage of, 69
  in childhood speech disorder assessment, 124–125
  level of, 160, 161
  methods, alternative, 125, 199–201
  phonological
    types of, 21–22
    vs. phonetic, 62–63
  process. *See* Process analysis
Anterior contrasts, 206, 208, 225
Anterior nasals, 214
Anterior/posterior contrasts, 225
Anterior stops, 214
Apraxia, speech
  delay-developmental, 116–117, 203
Arrested development, 170–176
Articulation
  characterizations of, 149

cueing, 190
definition of, 225
disorders, 48, 105
ease of, 135
errors, 105
generalization. *See* Generalization
manner of, 65
place of, 65, 169, 170, 175
precision, 170
primitive, 139
problem, 178, 188
supraglottal, 149–150
vs. phonology
in late 1960s to early 1970s, 44–46
in late 1970s thru 1980s, 46–50
for 1990s thru 2001, 50–53
Articulation tests
in complex cases, 38
pre-post, 44
standardized, problems with, 197
value of, 20–21
Articulatory/linguistic theory, 34
Assembly stage of speech development, 178–179, 184, 226
Assessment
analytical. *See* Analysis
of clinical applications, 67
contrastive, 69, 70
disordered phonological, 134, 199
distinctive features in, 54
historical aspects
in late 1970s and 1980s, 46–48
in 1990s and on to 2001, 50–51
instruments for, 190, 198, 201, 205
language, 125
methods, research and, 198, 199–201
methods for, 199–201
PACS contrastive, 96, 101, 103
PACS developmental, 99
PACS TOYS screening, 86
phonological-process-based, 5–6
procedures for, 67, 198, 199
results, 212–215
stimulability in, 54
Assimilation, 209, 214, 226
Atypical classification, 68
Auditory bombardment. *See* Auditory stimulation/bombardment
Auditory discrimination
in children with arrested speech and literacy development, 174, 175–176
longitudinal case study of, 180–181, 182, 186
tests, 166, 174, 175–176, 182
Auditory processing, 164, 166, 187
Auditory stimulation/bombardment
definition of, 226
to increase sound awareness, 53
interventions, 13
in manipulative techniques, 78
in remediation, 207, 210–211

B

Babble
canonical, 108, 142, 151, 202
infant, 138–141, 145, 177
Backing, of consonants, 124, 226
Beginning-cycle target patterns, 215–217
Behavioral disorders, 109
Behaviorism, 197–198
Binary foot structures, 32
Biolinguistic disorders, 113
Blinding, experimental, 144–145
Brain injury, 109
Brazilian Portuguese, 36

C

Canonical babble, 108, 142, 151, 202
Canonical speech, 139–140, 150
Canonical syllable, 149
Capability, 126
Capability-focus framework, 126–127, 226
Caregivers, 127
Case study
  of developmental phonological disability, 78–81
  of disordered phonology
    background information, 211–212
    beginning-cycles target patterns, 215–217
    metaphonological skills enhancement, 217–218
    phonological assessment results, 212–215
  longitudinal
    of phonological awareness development, 138, 179–188, 190–191
    of rhyme awareness, 159
Cerebral palsy, 169
Change, phonological, 73–74, 77, 230
Childhood special education classes, 204–205
Childhood speech disorders
  assessment, 119–125
  classification of, 110–119
  phonological assessment of, 61–62
  research of, 126
  residual errors in, 106–108
  special populations with, 109, 118
  speech delay in, 108–109
  treatment, 126
Child phonology
  development of, 138
  historical research in, 133–136
  historical theories in, 136–141
  methodological protections in, 141, 142–148
  theoretical growth in, 148–153
Children. *See also* Infant
  English-speaking. *See* English-speaking children
  phonological awareness
    development failure in, 164–165
  phonological impairments, 36–38
    literacy development and, 167–170
    reading problems and, 165–167
  phonologies, evaluation
    developments in, 198–202
  reading ability of, 159, 168
  reading impairment in, 165–167
  speech difficulties, literacy
    problems and, 168–169
  speech errors of, 168, 169–170
  spelling errors of, 168, 169–170
  suprasegmental characteristics of
    speech in, 121
Chinese, 145
Chronological mismatch, 74, 201, 226
Classification
  atypical, 68
  of childhood speech disorders, 110–119
  developmentally immature, 68
Cleft lip, 168
Cleft palate, 168, 211, 214, 216
Clinical applications
  assessment, 67
  case study, 77–81
  development, 70, 72–75
  procedures, 67–70, 71
  treatment, 75–78
Clinical phonology. *See* Phonology, clinical

Clinical prediction, 125
Clinical research, 125, 198, 219
Clinical treatment, 125
Closed syllable, 49, 205
Cluster realization chart, PACS, 90
Clusters
  complex, 178
  of consonants, 213, 216
  in PACS, 67
  reduction, 11, 72, 135, 178, 199, 200
  /s/, 200, 202, 206, 208, 215–216
  sequence, 175–176, 216
Coda position, 181
Cognitive-linguistic processes, 107, 108, 109
Cognitive neuropsychology, 191, 226
Collaboration, between professionals, 188
Complex cluster, 178
Computer-aided procedures, 127, 145, 219
Conceptual process, 49–50, 53, 226
Connected speech, 125, 171, 179, 188
Consonants
  backing of, 151
  clusters of, 213
  deletion of, 47–48, 72, 135, 214
  derhotacized, 107
  early-8, 115
  English language, 24, 65–66, 70
  final
    deletion, 47–48, 214
    target, 206
  fronting of, 151
  harmony, 72, 82
  late-8, 115
  middle-8, 115
  onset, 31–32
  posterior, 231
  postvocalic, 206, 209, 215
  prevocalic, 206, 214, 215, 231
  prototypical, 149
  sequence, 200, 209, 226
  singleton, 206
  target, 206
Consonant-vowel-consonant (CVC), 169, 202
Consonant-vowel (CV), 32, 135, 202, 208
Constraints, 10, 226
Contingent reinforcement, 126
Contrastive assessment
  PACS, 96, 101, 103
  performance indicators for, 69, 70
Contrastive function, 64
Contrastive phones chart, PACS TOYS, 94
Contrastive specification, 30–31, 226
Contrasts
  anterior, 202
  English consonant, 70
  errors and, 67
  minimal, 49, 182
  plosive/fricative, 78
  posterior, 202
  voiced/voiceless, 79
Contrast training, 49, 226
Conversational speech sampling, 119–120, 121, 206
Core features, 124
Covert repair hypothesis, 11–12
Craniofacial anomalies. *See* Cleft lip; Cleft palate
Critical age hypothesis, 167–168, 226
Cross-linguistic acquisition, 26, 39
Cross-linguistic research, 34–36, 82
Cued articulation, 190, 226
Cycles phonological remediation approach, 206–211
Cycle target patterns, 215–217
Cyclical model, 50

Cyclicity
definition of, 226–227
laryngeal-supralaryngeal, 79
remediation approach, 206–211

D

Dark /l/, 143, 144
Deafness, 134, 150. *See also* Hearing impairment
Deficit hypothesis, 163–164, 166, 230
Delays
children with, 36–37, 74, 163
developmental, 74, 163
of literacy development, 169, 177
phonological, 36
of speech acquisition. *See* Speech, delays
supralaryngeal developmental, 37
Dentalized lisps, 107
Dental /s/, 68, 119
Dental stop, 51
Derhotacized sounds, 107
Destabilization, 77
Development. *See also specific aspects of*
delayed, 37, 74, 163
different, 74, 225
PACS assessment, 99
patterns of, 22–25
of pronunciation, 75
uneven, 74
Developmental apraxia of speech (DAS), 116–117, 203
Developmental categories, 68
Developmentally immature classification, 68
Developmental model of phonological impairment, 21
Developmental period, 68
Developmental phonological disorders
assessment, 67, 119–125
procedures, 67–70
tools, 67–70, 219
case study, 78–81
characterization, 70, 72–75
classifications, 110–119
definition of, 225
differential diagnosis, 82
distinct, 37
gender ratio, 113, 114
residual errors in, 106–108
special populations with, 109
speech delays in, 108–109
terminology, 105
theories, 62–66, 106–119
treatment, 75–78, 126–127
Developmental phonological dyslexia. *See also* Dyslexia
phonological processing skills and, 166
Developmental profile, 71–72
Developmental reassessment, PACS, 99
Developmental speech disorders. *See specific developmental speech disorders*
Developmental verbal dyspraxia. *See* Verbal dyspraxia, developmental
Deviations
definition of, 230
in disordered phonologies, 212–215, 230
patterns, 198
Diacritic symbols, 120
Diagnostic markers, 115, 117, 121, 124, 125
Diphthongization, 143, 215
Discontinuity theory, 138
Discrimination

auditory, 166, 174, 175–176
speech-sound, 53
Disordered phonology. *See also* Impairments, phonological
assessment, 134, 199, 200
definition of, 52, 63, 225
differential diagnosis, 218
errors in, 12
identification of, 201–202
in other languages, 219
with stuttering, 11
systems, 134
Disordered speech, 81–82
Distinctive features
analysis of, 45, 64, 148, 199
definition of, 27, 227
in phonological assessment, 54
theory, 3–4, 22, 54
Distinctive feature theory, 3–4, 22
Distortions
PACS and, 67
questionable residual errors and, 118
speech-sound, 106–107, 121
Down syndrome, 150, 152, 218
/d/ target, 80
Dutch, 36
Dysarthria, 169, 227
Dyslexia
assembly stage problems and, 178
definition of, 227, 230
literacy development and, 163
phonological, 163, 171
phonological processing problems in, 165–166
Dyspraxia
definition of, 227
label of, 203
severe developmental, 211
speech errors and, 171
verbal. *See* Verbal dyspraxia
vs. phonological disorders, 218

E

Early-8 consonants, 115
Early developing patterns, 208, 227
Ear training, 53
Education of All Handicapped Children Act of 1975, 108
Electropalatography, 191, 227
English
consonant
contrasts, 70
system, 65–66
phonological acquisition of, 23–24
as second language, 112
syllables duration in, 146–147
English-speaking children
group comparisons and transcription, 142, 143
phonological development patterns in, 22–24
phonological impairments
cross-linguistic research on, 36–38
patterns of, 33–34
research on, 200, 219
vocalizations, 145
Errors
articulation, 45
in childhood speech disorders, 118–119, 168–170
contrasts and, 67
of measurement, 121
patterns of, 46–47
place/manner, 115–116
sound, 51
systematic, 135
in target words, 171
types, 53
visual, 183

Etiology, of developmental phonological disorders, 124, 127
Evaluation, 198–202
Excessive-equal stress, 117
Exclusion codes, in prosody-voice assessment, 121–122
Experimental blinding, in child phonology, 144–145
Expressive grammar, 211
Expressive phonological impairment, 181, 190
  definition of, 225
  severe, 169, 170–176

F

Familial aggregation, 113
Feature
  distinctive. *See* Distinctive features
  geometry, 8–10, 28, 227
  hierarchy of, 9, 27–29, 39, 227
Feedback, 160, 161
Final consonant
  deletion, 47–48, 214
  target, 206
Final-consonant deletion rule, 7
Final syllables, 146–147
Fluency, phonology and, 11–12
Focus, 126, 199
Foot structures, binary, 32
French, 24, 146
Fricatives, distortions of, 118, 181
Fronting
  acquisition, 72
  assessment, 31
  of consonants, 72, 124, 151
  definition of, 227
  in systematic simplification stage, 178
  of vowels, 151
/f/ target, 78–79, 205
Functional articulation disorder, 61–63, 105
Functional load, 227
Functional phonetics. *See* Phonetics

G

Gender ratio, for developmental phonological disorders, 113, 114
Generalization
  across sound, 45, 210
  across word position, 45
  definition of, 227
  patterns, 44–45, 46
  phonological treatment and, 48–49, 51, 77
Generative phonology
  applications, 134, 136
  definition of, 227
  phoneme-oriented methods and, 205
  standard approach, 4, 5, 47
  underlying representations and, 7–8
Genetic transmission, of speech delay, 113
Gestalt parametric stage, 177–178, 181, 184, 227
Glides
  acquisition, 72, 202
  clusters, 209
  definition of, 227
  in disordered phonology, 214–216
  palatal, 209
  as phonological targets, 206, 207
Glossing, 120
Glottal stops, 184
Gradual acquisition, 207
Graphemes, 157, 227
Group comparisons, in child phonology, 142–144

H

Handicaps, physical, 168–169
Hearing impairment, 207, 211–212
Hierarchy
  phonological feature, 27–29
  rhythmic, of speech, 149
Higher order rhythmic units, well-formed, 150, 153
Homeostasis, 66
Homonymy, 169, 213, 227

I

Idiom, 214, 230
Imitation tasks, 169, 170
Immature speech, 184
Impairments, phonological
  classification, 33–38
  definition of, 225
  expressive, 167, 175–176, 181, 190
  with hearing disorder, 207, 211–212
  history of, 20–26
  intervention for, 25–26
  linguistic model, 21–22
  literacy development in children with, 167–170
  medical model, 20–21
  phonological awareness and, 13–14, 125, 190
  reading, 165–167, 183, 186–188
  research on, 26–33
  sensorimotor, 203
  severe, 169, 170–176
  theories on, 34
Implicational principles, 25–26, 205
Inconsistent speech output, 184–186
Indirect intervention, 227
Individual Education Plan meeting, 219
Infant
  babble, 138–141, 145
  deafness in, 150
  Down syndrome, 150, 152
  speech, canonical stage of, 139–140
  vocalizations, 137–151, 177
Infraphonology, 149–150, 227
Initial consonant deletion, 124
Innovation, 77
Input
  definition of, 230
  skills
    absence of, 164
    phonological awareness and, 181, 185, 187, 189
    with segmentation and memory problems, 166–167
Intelligibility, 178, 187, 227
Interjudge reliability, 120, 121
Internalized representations, 47
Interventions. *See* Treatment interventions
Intrajudge reliability, 121
Inventory restraints, 228
Italian language, 24, 35

J

Junctions between words, 179, 188

K

Kinesthetic images, 207, 210
Knowledge
  definition of, 230
  least phonological, 48
  productive, 7, 48

L

Labial trills, 139–140, 151
Language
  acquisition, 25–26
  assessment, 125

characteristics of, 142
delay. *See* Delays
enhancement of, 203–205
impairment. *See specific language impairments*
longitudinal case study of, 180, 181–182
manifestations of, 63
scales, 180
sign, 205
skills, 189
therapists. *See* Speech therapist
treatment, 205
written, 166
Laryngeal node, 27, 28
Laryngeal quality, 124
Laryngeal-supralaryngeal cyclicity, 79
Late-8 consonant, 115
Lateralized lisps, 107
Late talkers, 108
Learning measurements, 126
Letter names knowledge, 157, 165, 228
Lexical decision, 172–175
Lexical disorder, 174
Lexical items, 47, 164, 184, 228
Lexical storage, 164
Lexicon
definition of, 228
inaccurate/incomplete representations of, 164
orthographic, 162
Linguistic/articulatory theory, 34
Linguistic competence, 124
Linguistic differences
in cross-linguistic research, 34–36, 39, 82
in phonological analyses, 124, 125
Linguistic model, 21–22
Linguistic research, 141
Linguistic theory, 34, 125
Linkage hypothesis, 162, 230
Liquids
acquisition, 202
beginning-cycles target patterns, 215, 216–217
deviations, 213
distortions, 118
as phonological target, 206, 207, 209
Lisps, 107, 202
Listening skills, 207
Literacy
alphabetic stage of, 164, 165, 176
beginning of, 162–163
definition of, 225
development
arrested, 170–176
delayed, 169, 177
with phonological impairment, 167–170
prognostic factors for, 167
speech and, 189
stage model of, 162–164
logographic stage of, 162, 164, 171, 176, 177, 183
phonological awareness and, 159–162
problems with, 163
developmental, 169–177
speech difficulties and, 168–169
Logographic skills, 164
Logographic stage of literacy development
alphabetic stage and, 162
definition of, 228
Gestalt parametric stage and, 177
phonological awareness and, 164
typical, 171
Longitudinal case study

of phonological awareness development, 138, 179–188, 190–191
of rhyme awareness, 159
Long-term normalization, 108, 109

M

Manipulative techniques, 78
Manner errors, 115–116
Marginal phones, 139–140
Marginal syllables, 139–140
Margins, 149–150
Markedness, 228
Maximal oppositions, 228
Mechanism processes, 107
Medical model, 20–21, 38
Memory, short-term, 163
Mentalistic view, of language, 125
Metalinguistic awareness, 52, 53
Metalinguistic techniques, 78
Metaphonology. *See also* Phonological awareness
definition of, 228
research, 200
skills, 13–14, 217–219
stage of speech development, 179, 183, 184, 189
Microcomputer-based acoustic displays, 121
Middle-8 consonant, 115
Minimal contrasts, 49, 182
Minimal pair words
definition of, 64, 228
discriminating, 166, 175
historical aspects, 49–50, 52
Minimal sets, 64
Minimal word stage, 32, 228
Molecular genetics, 127
Mora, 228
Morphophonemic alterations, 7, 178, 228
Motivational events, 126
Motoric treatment, 49–40
Motor planning, 187–188, 228
Motor programming
definition of, 228
longitudinal case study of, 186, 187–188
skills, 187
Multiple articulation errors, 105
Multisyllabicity, 207, 209, 228

N

Nasals
age for acquisition of, 202
anterior, 214
beginning-cycles target patterns and, 215–216
as phonological target, 206
Naturalistic intervention, 13, 228
Natural phonology
definition of, 228–229
history of, 4–6, 133
phonological process approach and, 1
theory of, 27, 46
vs. nonlinear phonology, 30
Natural process theory, 124, 135
Neuropsychology, cognitive, 191
Nondevelopmental childhood speech disorders, 110
Nonfinal syllables, 146–147
Nonlinear phonology
analysis procedures of, 199–200
definition of, 26–28, 229
history of, 8–10
nonsegmental descriptions and, 150–152, 153
prosodic structure in, 31–33

research on, 26–27
theory, 22, 38–39
vs. natural phonology, 30
Nonphonetic spelling, 162, 163, 229
Nonsegmental descriptions, 150–152
Nonwords
auditory discrimination, 186
spelling test, 169, 174, 175
Normalization, 107–108, 109, 127, 229
Normalized speech acquisition (NSA-X), 110
Normal speech acquisition (NSA), 110, 111, 112, 114, 116
Normal speech acquisition/speech delay (NSA/SD), 112, 114, 118, 229
Nuclei, 149–150
Nuffield Centre Dyspraxia Assessment, 168, 169, 180, 190
Nursery rhymes, 157, 159

O

Obstruents
beginning-cycles target patterns, 215–216
definition of, 229
as phonological targets, 206, 207, 208
Onset, 31–32, 165, 187, 229
Onset/rhyme segmentation, 160, 217
Open syllable, 49
Optimality theory (OT), 10, 229
Optimal match, 210
Oral-motor exercises, 203, 212
Orthographic experience, 159, 160, 165, 179, 229
Orthographic lexicon, 162
Orthographic representations, 229
Orthographic stage of literacy development, 162, 164, 179
Orthography, phonological awareness and, 159–160, 161
Otitis media, 207, 211–212
Outcomes, 76, 218
Output skills
definition of, 230
in phonological processing system, 189
problems
nature of, 165, 167, 181
in processing, 185–186, 187

P

PACS
cluster realization chart, 90
contrastive assessment, 96, 101
developmental assessment, 99
developmental reassessment, 99
phoneme realization chart, 88
screening assessment procedure, 67, 69, 70
PACS TOYS
contrastive phones chart, 94
extended realization chart, 92
screening assessment, 86
Palatal glide, 209
Palatal sibilants, 209, 217
Paradigmatic relationship, 64
Participation, 211
Pattern
definition of, 230
of deviations, 198
of error, 46–47
phonemic, 45–46, 134
in phonological analysis/assessment, 61–62, 82
symmetrical, 65, 81
targets, 206

advanced, 207
secondary, 207, 209, 217
Pattern-oriented treatment, 53, 198, 205–206, 229
Patterns, pronunciation development, 75
Percentage
of agreement, 121
of consonants correct, 115, 125
of consonants correct-revised, 112
of deviations, 198, 212–213
Perception, 121
Performance indicators, 69, 97
Persisting normal processes, 74, 229
Persisting speech difficulties, 167
Phenotype marker, 117, 125
Phoneme
class deficiencies, 200
definition of, 157, 229
distortions. *See* Distortions
in feature hierarchy, 27
realization chart, 67–68
segmentation skills, 159, 217–218
sequence, 175
Phoneme-oriented treatment, 197–198, 205, 206, 211–212
Phonemic pattern, 45–46, 134
Phonemic repertoire, 202
Phonemics. *See* Phonetics
Phonemic theory, traditional, 22
Phonetic analysis, *vs.* phonological analysis, 62–63
Phonetic feature. *See* Feature
Phonetic inventory, 31, 55, 202
Phonetic parameters, 177
Phonetic problem, 45
Phonetics, *vs.* phonology, 62, 63–64
Phonetic spelling, 163, 229
Phonetic transcription
of canonical syllables, 140
in childhood speech disorder assessment, 120–121
group comparisons and, 142–144
of word productions, 212
Phonics, 229
Phonological awareness
with arrested speech and literacy development, 170–176
assessment of, 200–201
clinical applications, 13–14
definition of, 157, 158–159, 229
development
failure in, 164–165
normal, 157
explicit, 160, 161, 178
future directions, 190–191
level of, 160, 161, 162
literacy development and, 159–162
longitudinal case study, 179–188, 190–191
metalinguistic, 52, 53
orthography effect, 159–160, 161, 179
phonological impairments and, 125, 190, 218
problems, 157–158
literacy development with, 167–170
in processing, with reading impairment, 165–167
stage model of speech development and, 176–179
tacit to explicit awareness, 160, 161
tasks, 158, 174, 187, 200
tests, 189
training program, 160–162, 191
Phonological disorders, 48, 225. *See also* Impairments, phonological; *specific phonological disorders*
Phonological dyslexia, 163, 171

Phonological knowledge, productive, 7, 47, 231
Phonological processes, 198
Phonology. *See also specific aspects of*
  clinical
    distinctive feature theory of, 3–4
    future trends, 218–219
    history of, 3–11, 197–198
    special applications of, 11–14
  definition of, 1, 230
  fluency and, 11–12
  generative, 4, 7–8, 47
  history of, 3–11
  natural. *See* Natural phonology
  nonlinear, 26–27
  vs. articulation
    late 1960s to early 1970s, 44–46
    late 1970s thru 1980s, 46–50
    1990s thru 2001, 50–53
  vs. phonetics, 62, 63–64
Phonotactics, 55, 66, 73, 77, 231
Place errors, 115–116
Place node, 27, 28
Plosive/fricative contrast, 78
Populations, with childhood speech disorders, 109
Posterior consonant, 231
Posterior contrasts, 206, 208, 225
Posterior obstruents, 208, 216
Postvocalic consonant, 206, 209, 215, 231
Praxis, 117
Prelexical stage, 177, 181
Prelexical stage of speech development, 231
Prevocalic consonant, 206, 214, 215, 231
Prevocalic obstruents, voiceless, 207, 216
Primary target patterns. *See* Target, patterns
Process analysis
  alternative, 199–201
  definition of, 22
  developmental classification and, 74
  natural phonology and, 5–6
  vs. rules, 52
Processes, phonological
  broader principles for, 136
  definition of, 198
  in sound errors, 5–6
  vs. rules, 5, 52
Processing
  auditory. *See* Auditory processing
  definition of, 230
  difficulties in, 176, 177–178, 188–189
  problems, reading impairments and, 164–167
  profiles, 190–191
  system structure, 165
Productive phonological knowledge, 7, 47, 231
Professional collaboration, 188
Prognostic factors for literacy development, 167
Pronunciation development
  with arrested speech and literacy development, 169–172
  in assembly stage, 178
  Jakobsonian thinking and, 137–138, 169–170, 171–172, 178
  patterns, 75
Prosodic hierarchy, 31, 231
Prosodic structure, 31–33, 39, 231
Prosody-voice
  in childhood speech disorder assessment, 121–124
  coding, 117

pattern, 112
profiles, 124
Psycholinguistic profile, 124, 188, 191, 231
Psychosocial processes, 107, 109

Q

Questionable residual errors (QRE), 109, 118
Questionable speech delay, 109
Quiché, 24

R

Radical underspecification, 29–30, 231
Reading. *See also* Literacy
by analogy, 159, 163
approached, 166
child's ability in, 159
experience, 160
impairments
phonological awareness and, 183, 186–187, 188
with phonological processing problems, 165–167
Realization chart
PACS, 88
PACS cluster, 90
PACS TOYS, extended, 92
Realizations, zero, 69–70
Receptive knowledge, 25
Receptive vocabulary, 180, 211
Redundancy rules, 29–30, 231
Reduplication, 72, 180
Reliability data, 121
Remediation
basic assumptions for, 207–211
description of, 48–49
phonological targets for, 206–207
steps for, 20
Representations
definition of, 230, 231
imprecise, 186
internalized, 47
lexical, 164–165
prelexical, 177
research on, 29–31
underlying. *See* Underlying representations
Research. *See specific types of*
Residual errors
in childhood disorders, 106–108, 110, 120
classification of, 118–119
definition of, 231
questionable, 109, 118
Residual errors-A (RE-A), 111, 118–119
Residual errors-B (RE-B), 111, 118–119
Reynell Developmental Language Scales, 180
Rhyme
arrested development of, 172–173
awareness, 164, 218
definition of, 231
longitudinal case study of, 159, 182–186
production, 158
in prosodic structure, 31–32
Rhythmic feet, 150
Rhythmic units, well-formed higher order, 150, 153
Rime, 217, 231
Root node, 27, 28
/r/ target, 206–207
Rules
definition of, 230
mapping, 178
vs. processes, 5, 52

S

Sampling mode, 119
Schonell Graded Word Reading Test, 183
/s/ clusters, 200, 202, 206, 208, 215–216
Screening assessment
  PACS TOYS, 86
  procedure, PACS as, 67
Segmentation
  competence, retest variability in, 117
  definition of, 231
  difficulties, 167, 171–172
  onset/rhyme, 160, 217
  of phonetic units, 149
  skills, 159, 188
    in arrested speech and literacy development, 175
    enhancement of, 217–218
    in stage model of speech development, 177–178
  sound, 141, 158, 159
  syllable, 159, 160, 217
  of targets, 169–170
  tasks, 160
Self-monitoring, 127, 210
Semantic categorization, 173, 174, 177, 182, 231
Semiphonetic spelling, 163, 231
Sensorimotor impairment, 203
Sentential stress, 117
Severity continuum, in disordered phonologies, 202
Short-term memory, 163
Short-term normalization, 107–108, 109
Sibilants, 202
  definition of, 231
  palatal, 209
Sign language, 205
Silent period, in child speech development, 138
Simplifying processes, 202
Singleton consonants, 206, 209, 215–216
Socially influenced, phonological patterns, 37
Sociolinguistic disorders, 113
Sociolinguistic distortions, 107
Sonorants, 232
Sound
  approach to reading, 166
  blending, 158, 173–174
  categorization, 161
  changes, 124
  definition of, 232
  deletion, 158
  distortions, 118
  exchange, 158
  games, 157
  manipulation, 159
  segmentation, 141, 158, 159
  sequence, 175
Sound-to-word matching, 158
Spanish-speaking clients, 142, 143, 145, 146, 200, 219
Special education classes, 204–205
Special populations, 109, 118, 121, 232
Speech. *See also* Pronunciation
  development
  connected, 125, 171, 179, 188
  definition of, 225
  delays, 107, 112
    in childhood speech disorders, 108–109, 110, 114, 178
    genetically transmitted, 113
    questionable, 109
    special populations with, 118
    subtypes, 113, 115–118, 125

vs. speech acquisition in childhood, 112, 114
development, 138, 142, 176–179. *See also specific speech development stages*
arrested, 170–171
atypical, 142, 179–188
functional, 148
stages of, 176–179
deviation continuum, 203
differences, in childhood speech disorders, 112
difficulties with, literacy problems and, 168–169
disorders. *See also* Adult-onset speech disorders; Childhood speech disorders
definition of, 225, 232
emergence, 24
errors
with spelling errors, 168, 169–170
systematic nature of, 133
immature, 184
literacy development and, 189
longitudinal case study of, 180, 181, 184
patterns, 46, 61–62, 82, 176
production, 175, 205–206
profiles, 124
rhythmic hierarchy of, 149
sampling, conversational, 119–120, 121, 206
Speech delay-developmental apraxia of speech (SD-DAS), 116–117, 203
Speech delay-developmental psychosocial involvement (SD-DPI), 117–118
Speech delay-otitis media with effusion (SD-OME), 115–116
Speech disorders classification system (SDCS), 110, 111, 113, 117, 118
Speech-hearing mechanism, 109
Speech-language pathologist, 21, 38
Speech-language therapist. *See* Speech therapists
Speech-language therapy, 180, 181
Speech segment duration, 146
Speech sounds
basic set of, 23
deletions, 121
developmental patterns, 23
discrimination, 53
distortions, 106–107, 121
errors, 46–47, 52, 106
substitutions, 121
Speech therapists, 188, 189, 190
Spelling
adolescent, 159–160
errors
in speech difficulty children, 168
with speech errors, 169–170
longitudinal case study of, 183, 187
nonphonetic, 162, 163
phonetically, 166
semiphonetic, 163
targets, 163, 183
Spoonerism, 160, 232
Stability, 66, 73, 76, 232
Stabilization, 77
Stage model
of literacy development, 162–164
of speech development, 150, 176–179
Standard error of measurement, 121, 147
Standard phonology. *See* Generative phonology
Stimulability, 54, 55, 77, 79, 232
Stops

age for acquisition of, 202
anterior, 214
definition of, 232
in disordered phonology, 214–216
glottal, 184
velar, 48
Stress, 117, 121
Stress feet stage, 32
Stridents, 202, 213, 214, 216, 232
Structural extension, 76
Structure, 65–66, 67, 232
Stuttering
with disordered phonology, 11
indirect approach to, 12–13, 218
Subgrouping, of child speech disorders, 106–109, 113–118, 179. *See also specific types of child speech disorders*
Substitution
bidirectional, 134
PACS and, 67
questionable residual errors and, 118
uncommon place and manner, 124, 135
Supraglottal articulation, 149–150
Supralaryngeal articulators, 232
Supralaryngeal cyclicity, 79
Supralaryngeal developmental delays, 37–38
Suprasegmental characteristics, 121
Swedish language, 34–35, 146–147
Syllabic symbols, 152
Syllable-final word-final (SFWF), 78, 79, 80
Syllable-initial within-word (SIWW), 78, 79, 80, 81
Syllable-initial word-initial (SIWI), 78, 80, 81
Syllableness
acquisition, 202
beginning-cycles target patterns and, 215–216
definition of, 232
as phonological target, 206, 208
Syllables. *See also* Multisyllabicity
closing, 205
deletion of, 72
duration of, 146–148
infant, 151
nonfinal *vs.* final, 146–147
prosodic structure and, 31–32
reduction of, 170
segmentation, 159, 160, 217
structure of, 49, 55, 65–66, 199
unstressed, 167
well-formed, 148–150
Symbols
diacritic, 120
syllabic, 152
Symmetry, 65, 81
Syntagma, 66
System
definition of, 232
expansion, 76
phonological
adult, 67
child, 61, 64–65
Systematic deletions, 134
Systematic errors, 135
Systematic simplification stage of speech development, 177–178, 181, 184, 232
Systematic sound preference, 74, 232
Systematic substitutions, 134

T

Target. *See also specific targets*
/d/, 80
errors in, 171
/f/, 78–79, 205

final consonant, 206
patterns, 206, 207
advanced, 207, 209
beginning-cycle, 215–217
primary, 208–209
secondary, 207, 209, 217
/r/, 206–207
reading, 183
rhyming, 172–173, 182, 184–185
/s/, 80
segmenting, 169
sound, 51, 77
spelling, 163, 183
variability and, 73
words as, 170
Tetism, 79, 232
Theories, 22, 38, 146
Tracheostomy, 109
Training material, 191
Training studies, 160–162
Transcription
assessment in childhood speech disorders, 120–121
computer-aided, 145
group comparisons and, 142–144
nonlinear approach, 151–152
Traumatic brain injury, 109
Treatment interventions
acquisition and, 25–26
approaches, 202–206
clinical applications, 12–13, 126
historical aspects, 12–13
during 1980s, 48–50
during 1990s and on to 2001, 50–53
longitudinal case study of, 187–191
motoric, 49–50
outcomes, 76, 218
pattern-oriented, 53, 198, 205–206, 229
phoneme-oriented, 197–198, 205, 206, 211–212
phonological, 75–77
planning, 76–77
research clinic, 199
techniques, 202–206
Trills, 139–140
Turkish language, cross-linguistic research, 35–36

U

Underlying representations
definition of, 232
in natural phonology, 5, 7
phonological analysis and, 125
vs. internalized representations, 47
Unusual processes, 74
Uvular trills, 139, 140

V

Variability, 73–74, 76
Variable use of processes, 74
Velar deficiency, 213–216
Velar sounds
age acquisition of, 202
in anterior/posterior contrasts, 206
in canonical babbling, 151
in posterior obstruents, 215
in primitive articulation, 139
Velar stops, 48, 51
Verbal deficit hypothesis, 165–166, 232
Verbal dyspraxia, developmental
assembly stage and, 178
auditory discrimination in, 175–176
nature of, 168, 169
prelexical stage and, 177
speech characteristics in, 170
Verbal rehearsal, 184
Visual approach to reading, 166

Visual errors, 183
Vocables, 202
Vocabulary
  development of, 23, 189
  receptive, 180
  size of, 177
Vocalizations, infant, 137–151, 177
Vocal rhythm, 150
Voiced contrasts, 79, 167, 181, 183, 187, 209
Voiceless
  contrasts, 79, 167, 181, 183, 187, 209
  prevocalic obstruents, 207, 216
  segment contrastivity and, 64–65
  stops, 208, 216
Voicing
  auditory discrimination and, 175
  context-sensitive, 72
  prevocalic, 207, 216
  segment contrastivity and, 64
Vowel-consonant (VC), 208
Vowels
  backing of, 151
  contrasts, 209
  derhotacized, 107
  fronting of, 151
  insertion of, 135
  low, 151
  prototypical, 149

W

Whole language, 162
Word
  age for recognizable, 202
  junctions, 179, 188
  real *vs.* nonword, 174, 175–176
  spelling, 169
  whole, 186–187
Word-final (WF)
  in developmental phonological disability, 79
  in disordered phonologies, 202, 205, 208, 216
  velars, 214
Word-finding difficulties, 232
Word-initial, 208–209, 214–216
Word spurt, 232
Word-to-word matching, 158

Z

Zero realizations, 69–70

About the Contributors

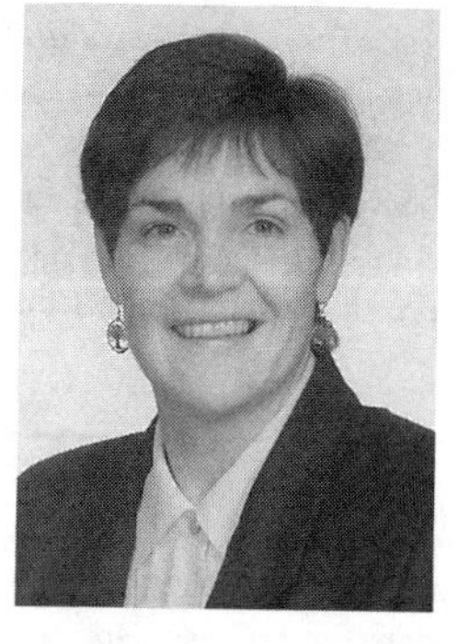

MARY LOUISE EDWARDS, PhD, is a Professor and the Chair of the Communication Sciences and Disorders Program at Syracuse University. She received her MA in Linguistics at the Ohio State University (with David Stampe) in 1970 and her doctorate in Linguistics (with Charles Ferguson) at Stanford University in 1979. Her areas of specialization include phonetics, phonology, and normal and disordered phonological development, as well as the application of phonological theories to the assessment and remediation of severe speech sound disorders in children. Edwards is the author of *Introduction to Applied Phonetics* and coauthor of *Phonology: Applications in Communicative Disorders* (with L.D. Shriberg) and *Phonogroup: A Practical Guide for Enhancing Phonological Remediation* (with M.E. Kelman). In recent years, Edwards and her colleague Edward Conture, along with several doctoral students, have been investigating the relationship between stuttering and disordered phonology in young children. Most of this research has been funded by the National Institutes of Health.

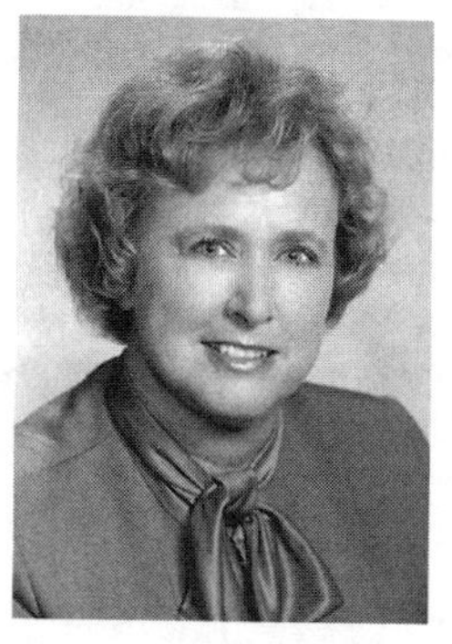

BARBARA WILLIAMS HODSON, PhD, CCC-SLP, is the author of English and Spanish versions of the *Assessment of Phonological Processes* and the developer of a computer software program, *Computer Analysis of Phonological Deviations*. In addition, she is coauthor of *Targeting Intelligible Speech: A Phonological Approach to Remediation* (with E. Paden) and *Phonological Remediation Targets* (with C. Buteau). Prior to joining the faculty at Wichita State University where she currently is a Professor, Hodson taught at San Diego State University and at the University of Illinois, the institution where she received her doctorate in 1975. She is a Fellow of the California and American Speech-Language-Hearing Associations and was the recipient of the state Clinical Achievement Award for California in 1987 and for Kansas in 1992. Hodson has been directly involved with University Phonological Remediation Clinics since 1975. Her most recent research direction has been in the area of Metaphonology.

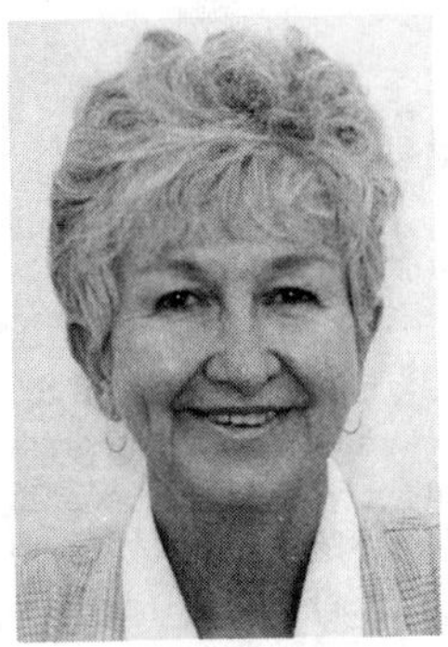

MARY ELBERT, PhD, CCC-SLP, received her doctorate from the University of Kansas in 1976, is a Professor in the Department of Speech and Hearing Sciences at Indiana University. She is coauthor of *Handbook of Clinical Phonology: Approaches to Assessment and Treatment* (with J. Gierut) and *Contrasts: The Use of Minimal Pairs in Articulation Training* (with B. Rockman and D. Saltzman). Elbert, who served a term as Associate Editor for the *Journal of Speech and Hearing Research*, is a Fellow of the American Speech-Language-Hearing Association. She has taught courses in phonological development and disorders for many years and has been the recipient of federally funded grants for the last 12 years. Her doctoral students have made major contributions to the profession.

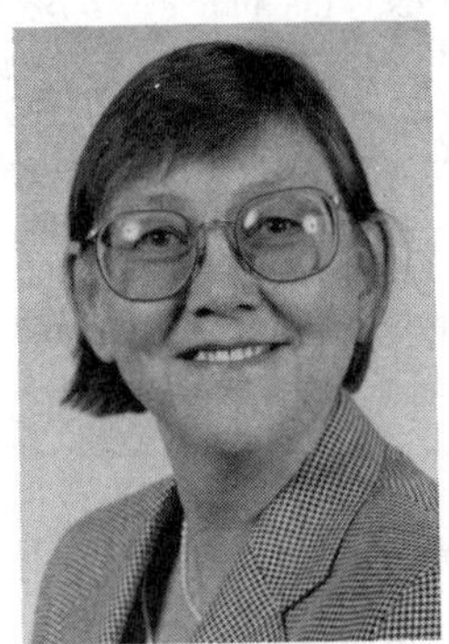

PAMELA GRUNWELL, PhD, is currently Head of the Department of Human Communication at DeMontfort University in Leicester. She received a First Class Honours Degree in Russian Studies with Czech Language and General Phonetics as subsidiary subjects, read for a Masters in Phonetics and Linguistics, and received her doctorate in 1977 (with David Crystal) at the University of Reading. She was appointed a Lecturer in Phonetics and Linguistics at the School of Speech Therapy, Birmingham Polytechnic, in 1971, where she began her collaboration with speech therapists. In 1979, Grunwell became Principal Lecturer at Leicester. She was appointed to a personal Chair in Clinical Linguistics in 1986 and became an Honorary Fellow of the Royal College of Speech and Language Therapists in 1987. Grunwell is the author of *The Nature of Phonological Disability in Children, Clinical Phonology, Phonological Assessment of Child Speech*, and *Analysing Cleft Palate Speech*, and she is the editor of *Developmental Speech Disorders*.

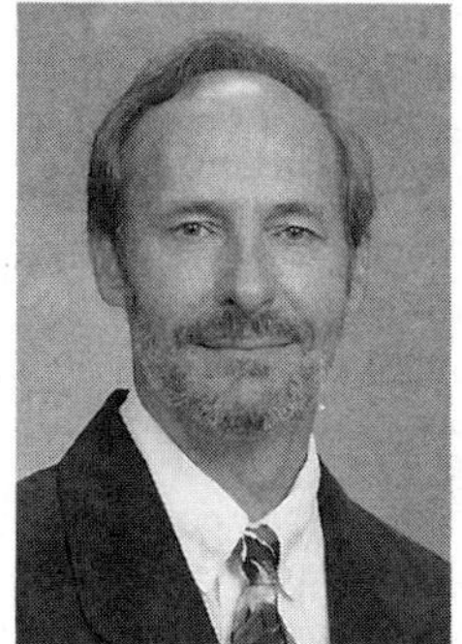

DAVID INGRAM, PhD, who is a Professor in the Department of Linguistics at the University of British Columbia, received his BS in French and Linguistics from Georgetown University and his doctorate in Linguistics from Stanford University in 1970. The first two years following his doctorate were spent as a Research Associate and Associate Director of Research at the Institute of Childhood Aphasia at Stanford University. During this period, he published his first articles on specific language impairment in children. Ingram's publications deal with language disorders as well as normal language acquisition. His 1976 book, *Phonological Disability in Children*, was a major impetus for viewing speech-sound deviations from a phonological perspective. Ingram also is the author of *Procedures for the Phonological Analysis of Children's Language* and *First Language Acquisition: Methods, Description, and Explanation.*

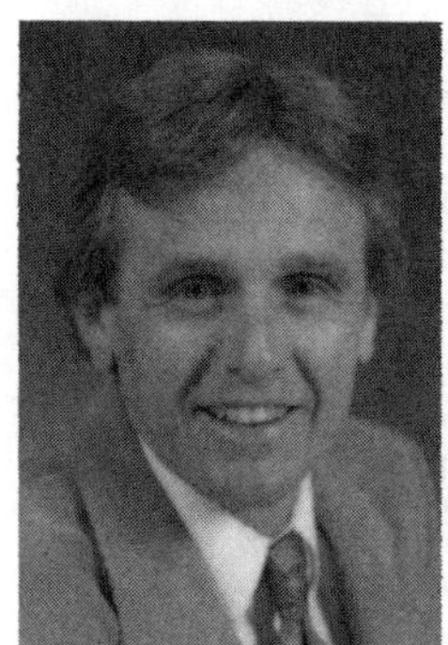

D. KIMBROUGH OLLER, PhD, completed his doctorate in Psycholinguistics at the University of Texas in 1971. Since that time he has been a faculty member at the University of Washington and the University of Miami, where he currently is a Professor of Psychology and Pediatrics. For the past 20 years, Oller has been Codirector of the Language and Hearing Program, a multidisciplinary research and graduate education effort at the University of Miami. Oller's research has focused on the development of both theory and empirical evidence regarding the human capacity for speech, with special emphasis on the development of vocalizations in infancy. Much of this work has involved infants and children with disorders of communication, especially those with profound hearing impairment and Down syndrome. Oller is the codeveloper of a comprehensive computer software program, *Logical International Phonetic Programs* (with R. Delgado). Other areas of his research include artificial hearing and bilingualism in infants and children.

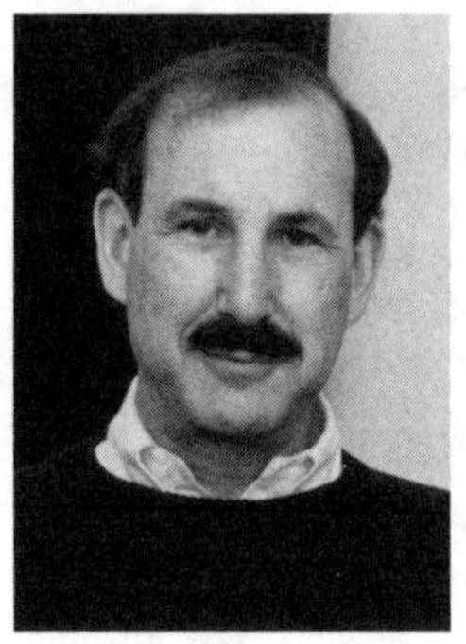

LAWRENCE D. SHRIBERG, PhD, CCC-SLP, is a Professor of Communicative Disorders in the Department of Communicative Disorders, University of Wisconsin—Madison. Shriberg, who is a Fellow of the American Speech-Language-Hearing Association, received his doctorate from the University of Kansas in 1970. He is Codirector of the Phonology Clinic, a service and research facility associated with the Phonology Project at the Waisman Center on Mental Retardation and Human Development. Shriberg's principal research interests focus on the etiologies and maintaining causes of childhood speech disorders. With long-term collaborator Joan Kwiatkowski, Shriberg's treatment research focuses on a two-factor framework that places primary emphasis on children's motivation for speech change. Shriberg is the coauthor of *Natural Process Analysis* (with J. Kwiatkowski) and *Clinical Phonetics* (with R. Kent) and is author/developer of *PEPPER: Programs to Examine Phonetic and Phonologic Evaluation Records*.

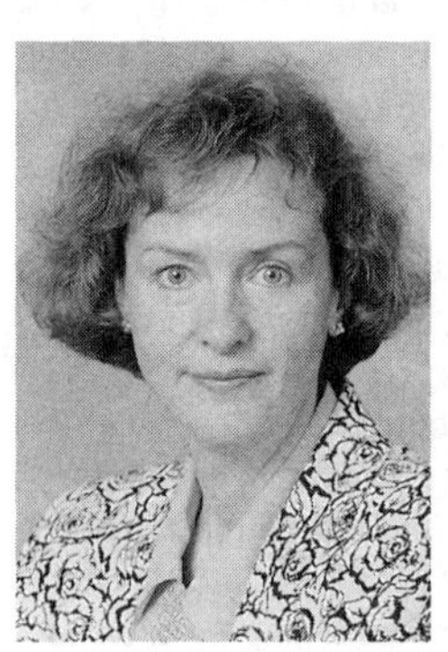

JOY STACKHOUSE, PhD, is a Senior Lecturer in the Department of Human Communication Science at University College London. She has worked as a Speech Therapist in North Wales and at the Birmingham Children's Hospital, has been a Lecturer at the National Hospital College of Speech Sciences, London, and is Head of the Speech Therapy School at Birmingham Polytechnic. Stackhouse, who received a First Class Honours Degree in psychology at Birkbeck College, London, completed her doctorate in 1989 (with Margaret Snowling) at University College London in the area of phonological dyslexia. She and Snowling are coeditors of *Dyslexia, Speech, and Language: A Practitioner's Handbook*. Stackhouse and her colleague Bill Wells have developed a psycholinguistic framework and processing model for investigating children with speech and literacy problems. They currently are working on a series of texts and assessment materials to use with children with spoken and written language difficulties.